# Group Therapy With Children and Adolescents

# Group Therapy With Children and Adolescents

*Edited by*
Paul Kymissis, M.D., and
David A. Halperin, M.D.

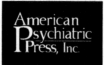

American Psychiatric Press, Inc.

Washington, DC
London, England

**Note:** The authors have worked to ensure that all information in this book concerning drug dosages, schedules, and routes of administration is accurate as of the time of publication and consistent with standards set by the U.S. Food and Drug Administration and the general medical community. As medical research and practice advance, however, therapeutic standards may change. For this reason and because human and mechanical errors some-times occur, we recommend that readers follow the advice of a physician who is directly involved in their care or the care of a member of their family.

Copyright © 1996 American Psychiatric Press, Inc.
ALL RIGHTS RESERVED
Manufactured in the United States of America on acid-free paper
99  98  97  96     4  3  2  1
First Edition

American Psychiatric Press, Inc.
1400 K Street, N.W., Washington, DC   20005

**Library of Congress Cataloging-in-Publication Data**
Group therapy with children and adolescents / edited by Paul Kymissis
   and David A. Halperin. — 1st ed.
      p.     cm.
   ISBN 0-88048-654-6 (alk. paper)
   1. Group psychotherapy for teenagers.     2. Group psychotherapy for
   children.     I.   Kymissis, Paul, 1944-          .    II.   Halperin, David A.
      [DNLM:   1. Psychotherapy, Group—in infancy & childhood.
   2. Psychotherapy, Group—in adolescence.  3. Psychotherapy, Group—
   methods.     WS 350.2.G8824 1996]
RJ505.G7G768      1996
   616.89′152′083—dc20
   DNLM/DLC
   for Library of Congress                                                    95-19715
                                                                                  CIP


British Library Cataloguing in Publication Data
A CIP record is available from the British Library.

# Contents

## SECTION III
## Groups in Specialized Settings and Special Populations

### SECTION IV
### Groups in Broader Societal Context

### SECTION V
### Research

# Contributors

**Fern J. Cramer Azima, Ph.D.**
Associate Professor of Psychiatry, McGill University, Montreal, Canada

**David W. Brook, M.D.**
Professor of Community Medicine, Mount Sinai School of Medicine, Adjunct Professor of Clinical Psychiatry, New York Medical College, and Board of Directors, American Group Psychotherapy Association, New York, New York

**Velleda C. Ceccoli, Ph.D.**
Clinical Assistant Professor of Psychiatry, New York University Medical School, New York, New York

**Yechezkel Cohen, Ph.D.**
Executive Director, B'nai B'rith Women—Residential Treatment Center, Supervising and Training Analyst, Israel Psychoanalytic Institute, and Faculty, Department of Psychology, Hebrew University, Jerusalem, Israel

**Kathryn R. Dies, Ph.D.**
Adjunct Assistant Professor, Department of Psychology, University of Maryland, College Park, Maryland, and Associate Administrator for Clinical Services, Dominion Hospital, Falls Church, Virginia

**Penelope Buschman Gemma, M.S., R.N., C.S.**
Research Nurse Clinician, The Presbyterian Hospital in the City of New York, and Assistant Professor of Clinical Nursing, Columbia University School of Nursing, New York, New York

**Harvey Roy Greenberg, M.D.**
Clinical Professor of Psychiatry, Albert Einstein College of Medicine, and Supervisor/Lecturer in Adolescent Psychiatry, Bronx Children's Psychiatric Center, Bronx, New York

**Mala R. Gupta, M.D.**
Clinical Instructor in Psychiatry, Albert Einstein College of Medicine, Bronx, New York, and Medical Director, Acute Adolescent Clinic, Four Winds Hospital, Katonah, New York

**David A. Halperin, M.D.**
Associate Clinical Professor of Psychiatry, Mt. Sinai School of Medicine, and Adjunct Associate Professor of Psychology, John Jay College, City University of New York, New York, New York; and Associate Director of Group Therapy and Training Analyst, Contemporary Center for Advanced Psychoanalytic Studies, Livingston, New Jersey

**Jo Rosenberg Hariton, Ph.D.**
Lecturer in Social Work in Psychiatry, Cornell University Medical College, New York, New York

**Don R. Heacock, M.D.**
Associate Professor of Clinical Psychiatry, New York Medical College, Valhalla, New York, and Director, Child and Adolescent Psychiatry, Lincoln Medical and Mental Health Center, Bronx, New York

**Susan Hou, M.D.**
Postgraduate Year 4 Resident, Department of Psychiatry, University of Pennsylvania School of Medicine, Philadelphia, Pennsylvania

**Michael G. Kalogerakis, M.D.**
Clinical Professor of Psychiatry, New York University, New York, New York

**Paulina F. Kernberg, M.D.**
Associate Professor of Psychiatry, Cornell University Medical College, New York, New York, and Director, Child and Adolescent Psychiatry, The New York Hospital, Westchester Division, White Plains, New York

**Irvin A. Kraft, M.D.**
Emeritus Professor, University of Texas School of Public Health, and Clinical Professor of Psychiatry, Baylor Medical School, Houston, Texas, University of Texas Medical School—Houston, and University of Texas Medical School—Galveston

**Paul Kymissis, M.D.**
Professor of Clinical Psychiatry and Pediatrics, New York Medical College, and Director, Division of Child and Adolescent Psychiatry, New York Medical College/Westchester County Medical Center, Valhalla, New York

**Elaine Leader, Ph.D.**
Private consultation practice; and Cofounder and Executive Director, Teen Line, Cedars-Sinai Medical Center, and Former Coordinator, Adolescent Group Psychotherapy Training Program, Cedars-Sinai Medical Center, Los Angeles, California

**Erica M. Loutsch, M.D.**
Associate Professor of Clinical Psychiatry, New York Medical College, Valhalla, New York

**Brendan McCormack, M.B.B.S.**
Consultant Psychiatrist, St Ann's Hospital and Harperbury Hospital, London, England; and Clinical Director and Consultant Psychiatrist, Cheevertown House, Templeogue, Dublin, Republic of Ireland

**Emily Nash**
Program Director, Creative Alternatives of New York, New York, New York

**Sheila A. Orbanic, R.N., M.S.**
Clinical Coordinator, Eating Disorders Day Hospital, and Director of Program Development, Silver Hill Hospital, New Canaan, Connecticut

**Arnold Wm. Rachman, Ph.D.**
Clinical Associate Professor of Psychiatry, New York University School of Medicine, and Training and Supervising Analyst, Psychoanalytic Institute, Postgraduate Center for Mental Health, New York, New York

**Stanley Schneider, Ph.D.**
Executive Director, Summit Institute, Professor of Psychology, Michlalah Jerusalem Women's College, and Training Coordinator, Israel Institute for Group Analysis, Jerusalem, Israel; Adjunct Professor of Social Work, Wurzweiler School of Social Work, Yeshiva University, New York, New York; and Professor of Guidance/Counseling, Bar Ilan University, Ramat Gan, Israel

**Alberto Serrano, M.D.**
Professor of Psychiatry and Pediatrics and Vice Chair, Department of Psychiatry, University of Pennsylvania School of Medicine, and Medical Director, Philadelphia Child Guidance Center, Philadelphia, Pennsylvania

**P. Wells Shambaugh, M.D.**
Clinical Instructor in Psychiatry, Harvard Medical School at The Cambridge Hospital, Boston, Massachusetts

**Ellyn Shander, M.D.**
Director, Eating Disorders and Dissociative Disorders Program, and Consultant, Journey to Healing Program for Survivors of Sexual Abuse, Silver Hill Hospital, New Canaan, Connecticut

**Valerie Sinason, B.A. Hons, P.G.T.C., M.A.C.P.**
Consultant Child Psychotherapist, Tavistock Clinic, London, England

**Edward S. Soo, M.S.**
Editor, *Journal of Child and Adolescent Group Therapy*

**Henry I. Spitz, M.D.**
Clinical Professor of Psychiatry, College of Physicians and Surgeons, Columbia University, and Director, Group Psychotherapy Program, New York State Psychiatric Institute, New York, New York

**Susan T. Spitz, A.C.S.W.**
Clinical Instructor of Psychiatry, Department of Psychiatry, College of Physicians and Surgeons, Columbia University, New York, New York

**Sandra Swirsky Strome, C.S.W., B.C.D.**
Private practice, New Rochelle, New York

**Arthur J. Swanson, Ph.D.**
Chief Psychologist, St. Barnabas Hospital, Bronx, New York

# Foreword

Long established as a major treatment modality, group therapy has focused generally on the adult population, with scant attention being paid to its use with children and adolescents. The reasons for this focus are not clear, because the method is ideally suited for use with adolescents, often as the treatment of choice; properly adapted, it also works well with younger children.

Social interaction is a key aspect of the developmental process. Quite naturally, social interaction is very likely to be afflicted if there is any disturbance of normal development. When psychopathology supervenes, peer relations are almost invariably affected. Therapeutic intervention that directly addresses the interrelationships of childhood society tackles a vital aspect of a child's life and is likely to benefit the child more broadly than interventions that do not deal with these interrelationships. For example, self-esteem may be closely related to the success or failure of attempts at socialization.

From another perspective, both the normal needs of children and adolescents and the specific forms that emotional disturbance is likely to take during the growing years make a group therapy approach particularly appropriate. The need to be liked, to find validation of one's ideas, to develop social skills, and to become a respected member of a group is universal among children. Similarly, alienation during the chumship period, feelings of inadequacy vis-à-vis one's peers in the academic setting, gang membership, and teenage pregnancy all partially represent failures to negotiate age-appropriate social adjustment in a healthy manner. The impact on a youth's life is often devastating.

The use of group therapy with young people has not, of course, been limited to the various forms of social pathology. Individual psychopathology, from the psychoses through personality disorders and psychoneuroses, frequently includes a group therapy experience as part of the comprehensive treatment plan. In these cases, group therapy is commonly neither the only nor the major modality that is used, yet its contribution is frequently unique and critically important.

As the technique has evolved over the past several decades, many varieties of group therapy have been developed and have found application in child and adolescent psychiatry. The present book provides an in-depth discussion not only of the theory and practice of group psychotherapy as used with children and adolescents, but also of the many varieties that have evolved as clinicians have sought new ways of tackling old problems. Thus, there are chapters on groups formed of adolescents with eating disorders, those who are suicidal, and others who abuse drugs. Inpatient and outpatient groups are both considered. Education-oriented groups are discussed, along with the more traditional psychoanalytic approaches. We offer a discussion of diagnostic groups, as well as groups that make use of theater. Other, more general expositions of group formation and development round out a generous potpourri that is both stimulating and complete.

The editors have wisely included a chapter on supervision. Training to work with children and adolescents in group therapy is an essential part of every quality fellowship in child and adolescent psychiatry and should be available as an option to the general psychiatry resident. Despite the logistical difficulties in establishing and maintaining groups, especially on an outpatient basis, clinicians in private practice, especially those who work with adolescents, frequently refer patients for group therapy. It is discouraging when such efforts come up empty and the teenager must do without the benefits of an added modality of treatment that offers so much.

In earlier days, zealots among the proponents of the new technique maintained that it effectively superseded individual psychotherapy. Such pointless internecine squabbling about the best way of helping those in need has fortunately long since been discarded, at least where individual and group therapy are concerned. (Sadly, we are living in a time when a broader and even more nefarious battle is being waged, that between biological and psychodynamic psychiatry.) Sensible clinicians are prepared to avail themselves of all the help they can get from the full spectrum of treatment modalities currently available.

It should be noted that, at the time of this writing, the tidal wave sweeping the United States of cutting costs in health care can be expected to lead, among other things, to even greater use of group therapy. Though this trend may have obvious benefits, thoughtful clinicians everywhere will be vigilant to ensure that such choices are driven not by financial but by appropriate clinical considerations. This important book provides the clinician with solid preparation to make just such judgments.

*Michael G. Kalogerakis, M.D.*

# Introduction

The transition from childhood to adolescence is a trajectory marked by the change from isolation to socialization and peer affiliation. In a remarkable, rapid process, children change from helpless infants who cling in fear to their parents to persons exploring their external environment, taking the first timid, and then the increasingly confident, steps to group play and then education in a group setting. Finally, adolescents complete their socialization in that most characteristic institution: the gang, group, or fraternity, with its positive and negative potential for the final transition into adulthood.

Yet despite the importance of group processes as a central aspect of the individual's transitions, psychotherapy for children and adolescents is seen in primarily individual terms. The therapist attempts to replicate a parenting situation that might have been or should have been, without recognizing that after the child's entry into schooling, the group plays an increasing role in maturation. One has only to compare and contrast the intense and time-consuming telephone calls that play so preeminent a role in adolescent culture to the strained conversations between adolescent and parent or adolescent and therapist to appreciate that as children begin to enter the nonfamilial world their contacts with their crowd assume a significance and importance that far surpass individual involvements.

The editors have a profound commitment to the importance of group modalities in the treatment of children and adolescents. Although there is extensive literature on the use of group modalities in working with adults, the literature on the use of group approaches in working with children is surprisingly sparse, particularly when the importance of groups to children and adolescents is considered. *Group Therapy With Children and Adolescents* represents the individual theoretical and practical vantage points of the individual authors. However, this book is designed to deal with a wide variety of topics and is organized so that the later chapters build on the preceding ones.

Initially, the history of group psychotherapy with children and adolescents is discussed by an eminent participant in that history, Irvin Kraft. The next three chapters by Paul Kymissis, Kathryn Dies, and P. Wells Shambaugh consider in depth the theoretical issues that arise in working with children and adolescents in group psychotherapy. Particular attention is paid to the evolution that occurs in working with groups and the importance of a theoretical background in framing interventions within the group psychotherapeutic process.

The authors of three of the chapters in the next section (Mala Gupta, Jo Rosenberg Hariton, Paulina Kernberg, Arthur Swanson, Harvey Roy Greenberg, Arnold Rachman, and Velleda Ceccoli) consider the use of group psychotherapy in treating children and adolescents. They discuss the use of this therapy for diagnostic purposes, as well as more technical issues of actual group intervention. All of the authors are eminent practitioners who share with the reader their approach(es) to working with groups. Because this type of psychotherapy does not exist in a vacuum, Edward Soo discusses supervision in child and adolescent group psychotherapy.

Chapters 9–17 represent an extension of group psychotherapy into specialized settings and populations. Sandra Swirsky Strome and Erica Loutsch discuss the use of other creative modalities in a group setting. Emily Nash describes the therapeutic use of the theater with adolescents.

Penelope Buschman Gemma, Brendan McCormack, and Valerie Sinason consider group psychotherapy in the context of working with severely limited patients. Substance use and abuse are the focus of much of the work with children and adolescents. The theoretical and practical aspects of this work are discussed in detail within the chapters contributed by David Brook and Henry and Susan Spitz. Their work emphasizes the interfacing of theoretical and practical issues that necessarily forms the underpinning for any meaningful work with adolescents who use or abuse substances. Ellyn Shander and Sheila Orbanic discuss groups of patients with eating disorders. Finally, Don Heacock contributes a sensitive chapter on work with suicidal adolescents in group therapy.

The final chapters of the book reflect the editors' desire to examine groups and group psychotherapy within a broader societal context. Elaine Leader's chapter on the Teen Line represents a model of utilizing group dynamics in peer support among adolescents. Alberto Serrano and Susan Hou's chapter focuses on the importance of culture and ethnicity in group processes and therapy. Similarly, in their chapter, Stanley Schneider and Yechezkel Cohen, in their scholarly interweaving of world events and individual experience, discuss the impact of world events on children and adolescents. David Halperin deals with the issue of how cults can affect children and adolescents in a most destructive manner.

The final chapter, by Fern Cramer Azima, deals with research in the entire field. No individual book can cover every aspect of group processes and group psychotherapy with children and adolescents. However, we think that this book is comprehensive and encourages the reader to examine this vast arena.

We would like to thank our families for their patience and understanding during the preparation of this book. Also, we would like to thank the chairmen of our respective departments, Dr. K. Davis of Mt. Sinai School of Medicine and Dr. E. Brownstein of New York Medical College, for their encouragement and support. We would like to thank Iris Laufman, executive secretary at the Division of Child Psychiatry of New York Medical College, for her valuable assistance. Finally, we would like to thank Claire Reinburg of American Psychiatric Press for her patient support and assistance.

*Paul Kymissis, M.D.*
*David A. Halperin, M.D.*

# SECTION I

# General Issues

# CHAPTER 1

# History

*Irvin A. Kraft, M.D.*

The history of group psychotherapy with children and adolescents encompasses many themes, some of which I describe in this chapter. These themes differ from those involved in the history of adult group psychotherapy because strong elements of nascent and physiological development significantly influence all of them—for example, group composition.

Historically, the overreaching conceptualizations of western societies accepted a basic framework of development. As Aries (1962) summarized, "It is as if, to every period of history, there corresponded a privileged age and a particular division of human life: 'youth' is the privileged age of the seventeenth century, childhood of the nineteenth, adolescence of the twentieth." (p. 32)

One might suggest that socioeconomic factors, such as parental financial status, allow time for leisure, for further education, and for delay in entering the workplace. In this century, childhood began to lose its special social characteristics in favor of adolescence.

As children and adolescents became more differentiated and acquired discriminating characteristics, deviations from those distinguishing traits could be seen as behavior susceptible to discipline.

My appreciation to Patricia Reed for her help with this manuscript.

3

With the popularization of Freud and other work such as Gesell's delineation of normal problems of development, deviancy could be seen more as a treatable condition than a cause for discipline.

Historically, the treatment of deviant behavior in children and adolescents was itself based on a dyadic relationship with the psychiatrist, and later the psychoanalyst and the psychotherapist, conceptualized as healers. In that general thematic context, Pratt's seminal discovery of a group format paved the way for others to experiment. Kessler (1966) pointed out that Moreno worked in 1909 with group productions of children who acted out written plays—soon to play out their problems without a script. Moreno followed in 1911 with "a children's theatre for spontaneity." Bender and Woltman (1936) also pioneered in using puppet shows for children with behavior problems. The comprehensive bibliography of group psychotherapy by Corsini and Putzey (1957) cited 54 references before 1936, none of which applied directly to children and adolescents.

## ◆ Definitions

At this point, we need to define group psychotherapy per se and more specifically its use with children and adolescents. Group psychotherapy is a form of therapy in which two or more patients meet with one or more therapists to alter behavioral and cognitive patterns. The therapist has a psychodynamic concept of change and uses that in the therapeutic process. This process assumes that change occurs via external and internal forces at work within the patient that are derived from the unique interactions occurring in a group setting. The same psychodynamic processes, including transference and other phenomena ordinarily described in dyadic therapy, occur with children and adolescents, except that a wider, more extensive set of techniques must be used to take advantage of the unique qualities and development in these patients.

Pervading these therapeutic endeavors are the themes we discuss here as historically relevant to children and adolescent group psychotherapy.

# ◆ Locations

To do group psychotherapy, one needs first of all a place in which to work. Among the first places described in the literature were hospitals as primary sites (e.g., Bender and Woltman 1936), social agencies, and children's agencies. Group therapy existed in 1934 at the Jewish Board of Guardians as "recreational therapy" in the Big Sister Department (Slavson 1944). Burlingham (1938) reported on the therapeutic effects of a play group for preschool children. Another pioneer, Durkin (1939), described her extemporaneous application of Dr. John Levy's relationship therapy to a summer play group. Also, Gabriel (1939) described her experiment in group treatment at a neighborhood center for boys and girls in a discussion-oriented play group.

The mid-1940s witnessed an increased number of articles. For observation and treatment in a social agency, Gula (1944) used a group of adolescents mostly under 17 years of age who had extreme isolation problems. Hewitt and Gildea (1945) successfully used a homogeneous group within a larger aggregation of summer campers. They mentioned similar group therapy by Redl (1944) for diagnostic purposes. Bollinger (1945) also used group therapy at a children's center, and Margolis (1946) spoke of her work with selected children in activity group therapy in a similar setting.

In 1947, the most used primary sites continued to be clinics and nonhospital settings (Bettelheim and Sylvester 1947; Fleming and Snyder 1947; Fraiberg 1947; Hamilton 1947; Holland 1947; Slavson 1947). The literature expands at a high rate thereafter, with numerous articles dealing with multiple modalities of group psychotherapy in varied nonhospital settings (Alpert 1957; Barnes et al. 1957; Becker 1948; Dana and Dana 1959; Davids 1955; Fabian 1954; Freeman and King 1957; and others in the decades following).

Bender and Woltman (1936, 1937) published some of the earliest reports of group psychotherapy in hospitals, describing the use of puppet shows and plastic materials as therapeutic devices with groups of children in hospitals. From 1937 on, the frequency of articles about group therapy with children in hospitals was less than one per year. The articles covered its use in a pediatric service (Dubo 1951), where the emphasis was on specific disease entities such as tuberculosis. Few articles before 1960 described a planned group therapy program on pediatric wards. Clinicians used group therapy for teaching psychological aspects of pediatric illnesses to nursing and medical students who participated in their own groups. Chronic disorders, such as asthma, lent themselves to group psychotherapy (Ghory 1965–1966).

The emphasis in the literature shifted to reports of group psychotherapy in psychiatric hospitals (Adams 1976; Anderson 1968; Stewart and Axelrod 1947). Socioeconomic factors plus advances in medical technology altered the average stay of children in pediatric settings (e.g., in Texas Children's Hospital, with over 300 beds, an average stay is less than 7 days). Psychiatric hospitals in the late 1980s and onward realized the impact of managed care, health maintenance organizations, and other insurance programs. The training and education of personnel doing group psychotherapy of children in these hospitals varied greatly, often suggesting ethical questions about quality and standards for this and other treatment modalities.

In 1995, group therapy occupied a settled role in psychiatric hospitals. Some controversy still swirls around frequency, the qualifications of the therapists, financial issues, and the efficacy of group therapy. The last topic, however, seems to go unresearched.

Other socioeconomic factors played behind-the-scenes roles in influencing settings (as well as techniques). For example, in an urban setting with quite adequate public transportation, adolescent groups of various ages could maintain attendance without needing their parents to transport them. In other settings, parents or surrogates brought the children or adolescents by car, which created scheduling problems—especially after the mid-1970s in the United States, when inflation and other economic vectors drove perhaps 50% of mothers into the work force, as is still the case today. Currently, managed care and other insurance factors significantly affect psychotherapists. It is not possible to do more than hint at these other considerations influencing outpatient group therapy. Little comment about these factors exists in the literature.

## ◆ Approaches and Models

One can posit that the work done in child and adolescent group psychotherapy, like all clinical efforts in this field, follows one or more of the following four approaches to human behavior: the biological, the psychodynamic, the sociocultural, or the behavioral model (Lazure 1979). Group psychotherapy of children and adolescents had a psychodynamic model, predominantly a classical psychoanalytic one, into the 1960s. Sociocultural vectors gained recognition with the growth of general systems theory and its offshoots, especially with the bursting forth in the late 1960s and early 1970s of transactional analysis, gestalt, encounter therapy, and other techniques. Behavioral approaches (Rose 1972) commingled with others but did not live up to their promise. The biological model interwove itself with little recognition beyond the developmental physiology of the body and the nervous system inherent in childhood and adolescence. Now in the 1990s, with the advances of neuroscience, new tools—for example, single photon emission computed tomography (SPECT) and positron-emission tomography (PET)—seem to demonstrate the biological underpinnings of depression, manic-depressive manifestations, obsessive-compulsive disorders, and panic states.

## ◆ Group Therapists and Leaders

The qualifications and characteristics of the group leaders remain ill defined to this day. With the immense increase in the number of freestanding psychiatric hospitals in the 1980s (England and Coler 1993; Patrick et al. 1993), thousands of adolescents and children underwent hospitalization. These hospitals offered group therapy as a standard therapeutic modality; most, if not all, patients underwent it, frequently with therapists of questionable or uncertain qualifications and training. In a way, the message came through that anyone could perform in the role of the therapist.

Slavson (1943) stated that the therapist's personality and attitude was highly important for enabling the children to feel accepted and loved. This ideal existed for activity group therapy. Early on, the psychoanalytic view of transference emphasized the ability of the therapist to handle a deluge of various unconscious manifestations of hostility from eight or so group members. Therapists leading adolescent groups confronted material that inevitably recalled their own (perhaps troubled) adolescent experiences.

With the high interest felt in the 1960s in therapeutic communities, the role of the social sciences in the training of the therapist received strong emphasis, especially for those working with children and adolescents. Early pioneers recognized that leadership required traits additional to those generally considered necessary for adult group psychotherapy. Flexibility, perceptiveness, activity, warmth, creativity, understanding, empathy, self-awareness, and responsiveness were needed to meet the quickly shifting productions of these patients. One can suggest that no single portrayal of the leadership role suffices; rather, active roles emerge during the sweep of the sessions. The group therapy literature showed a lack of studies on the effects of the therapist's personal characteristics and behavior, both verbal and nonverbal, on the group process.

Moreno (1966) in the early 1940s began training nonprofessionals because he believed training for group therapy was quite different from that for individual therapy and, of course, that for psychoanalysis.

MacLennan (1975) emphasized the multifaceted requirements for group therapists, including a life stage and developmental level of the therapist compatible with those of the group members. It is important to recognize that a leader might have great understanding and empathy for one age group and not for another. She pointed out that the acceptability of the leader might vary according to class, race, sex, and age. For example, if the children in a group come from low-income families, should the therapist have a similar background? Would group members of one racial group be unwilling to work with a leader who belongs to another racial group (Lolhstein 1985)? MacLennan pointed out that the pursuit of academic degrees and professional training may not have much in common with the real requirements of group leadership, especially with children and adolescents.

Another feature of leadership is cotherapy (usually involving two therapists) and the nature of the relationships between the therapists. The literature has little to say about gauging their abilities to work together. I found few references about when cotherapy began and developed. Schiffer (1947a) wrote of group therapy involving children from families with an absent father or with other parental changes or losses; these children benefited from having two group therapists, preferably of different sexes. Schiffer (1984) commented that dual transference could be more effective than single and could help create a surrogate psychological family. In Slavson's text (1947) none of the authors mentions the use of cotherapists.

# ◆ Types of Clients and Patients

## Delinquent Adolescents

The treatment of delinquent adolescents played a major role in the development of adolescent group therapy. Until the early 1960s, the theory and techniques in group therapy of adolescents frequently focused on delinquent adolescents (Raubolt 1989). The settings in which group therapy occurred varied greatly; treatment of delinquent adolescents usually happened wherever they were confined (Kraft 1983). The community often wanted delinquents segregated from the rest of society. As a result, delinquent adolescents often went to institutions to be rehabilitated.

## Hospital Inpatients and Institution Residents

Early treatment of children and adolescents on an inpatient basis was reported by Cameron (1953). The development of inpatient units for the psychiatric treatment of adolescents at the Maudsley Hospital in England in 1947 quickly produced problems with their adolescent patients, because the hospital routinely admitted adolescents over the age of 12 to its adult wards. The adolescents' high activity level and intolerance of adults led to recognition of the fact that the adolescents needed to be separated from the older patients. On the other hand, the gap existing between adolescents and children and the difference in their needs made combining these two groups impractical. Two years later, in 1949, a separate adolescent unit was opened (Cameron 1953).

The problems of institutionalized adolescents become particularly severe because of the degree of deprivation and assault the adolescents often experienced before being confined (Phelan 1960). Group and individual psychotherapy proved to be an effective technique; indeed, therapists agreed that adolescent delinquent boys in residential treatment responded with enthusiasm both to the fact of belonging to a group and to the therapeutic influence provided by both types of therapy (Slavson 1950). Slavson further stated that an important facet of residential and inpatient treatment was maintenance of a favorable environment, created through positive, caring interpersonal relationships among the staff of the institution.

Historically, the gains made by adolescents from group psychotherapy were typically based on long-term treatment. In an institutional setting, though, group therapy must be adapted to the problems of the adolescents because of their ongoing and constant struggle against authority, the intensification of that struggle with incarceration, and the uncertainty of length of stay.

## Outpatients

Predominantly, both child and adolescent group psychotherapy tended to be in an outpatient setting, which often presented a physical environment that strongly influenced the type of care offered. The square footage required for a traditional activity group program represented a significant financial commitment. Perhaps this fact encouraged the development of interview, or interview-activity, group therapy for latency-age and adolescent patients—modifications of the original activity group model invented by Slavson. Interview-activity group therapy involved the verbal interaction of therapist and children, with comments on transference and group actions.

Slavson, Moreno, Durkin, and other pioneers wrote of work done in outpatient settings. Clinics, teaching units, camps, and other sites were used for groups. Therapy-induced changes in behavior constituted the goals of most of these efforts. The patients came from varied sources: private referrals, the courts, community mental health centers, and child guidance center populations.

## Schoolchildren

Early on, schools were sites for this type of therapy. Moreno's work in 1932 involved schools (Moreno 1966), and he also wrote of using group therapy in elementary schools. Another early work, by Davis

(1948), which appeared in a school journal, described group therapy to help children gain social acceptance in the first grade. Buchmueller and Gildea (1949) focused attention on parents in relation to their school-age children with behavior problems. Group therapy was applied to remedial reading (Berl 1959) and other academic problems early on. Schiffer's work (1984) over a 20-year period began in the mid-1950s with therapeutic play groups.

By the 1970s, a number of investigators, including Schiffer and Slavson (1975), had published accounts of interesting and creative attempts to help in schools. Chigier (1963) worked with troubled children, meeting 1 hour a week, with normal pupils acting as auxiliary therapists. Davidson (1965) used small groups as adjuncts to counseling by school counselors. Over a 12-year period, Pasnau et al. (1971, 1976) worked successfully in an urban school district, using a structured activity group program to develop preventive mental health activities. Rhodes (1973) reported on short-term work (six or eight sessions) stressing behavioral modification. Berman (1953) reported on a combined seminar and group psychotherapy for teachers in a public school setting. Kraft (unpublished data, January 1960) replicated this work in 1957–1959 and found this combination extremely valuable in a public junior high school. Interestingly, few reports deal with group therapy of adolescents in schools.

## ◆ Selection and Number of Group Members

The selection of patients posed difficulties from the beginnings of group therapy. Durkin (1939) worked with children under 4 years of age. Ginott (1961) and others treated preschool-age children. Gradually, a consensus grew that patients should be divided into about six groups that roughly coincide with developmental epochs: preschool and early school age (4–8 years old), late latency (9–11 years old), puberty (12–13 years old), early adolescence (13–14 years old), middle adolescence (15–16 years old), and late adolescence (17–18 years old) (Duffy and Kraft 1966–1967; Kraft 1971; Quin and Egan 1969).

As work with children and adolescents continued, other developmental considerations assumed more significance. Schamess (1986) described selection of patients based on their phase-specific developmental needs. As early as 1947, Slavson realized that activity group therapy missed out with youngsters who could not control their exuberance and aggressiveness in the unrestrained, free-acting nature of activity groups. Slavson (1947) suggested that no one pattern of group therapy fitted all types of patients. He also stated that a clinical judgment of the child's ego strength and superego construction was basic to including the child in a group.

Certain exclusion factors exist in child and adolescent groups. For example, battered patients who have been prostitutes or who have been deeply involved with the drug scene do not fare well in these groups. Rachman and Heller (1976) and others developed group techniques specifically for drug-using adolescents. Sadly, the modern world for these youngsters includes activities not really known or discovered in decades past: drug abuse by latency-age children; tens of thousands of runaways exposed to prostitution, exploitation, and now AIDS.

In effect, many different subsets of children have been involved in the evolution of group therapy. These subsets include learning-disabled children (Barcai 1973; Berl 1951; Hinds and Roehke 1970; Ledebur 1977), mildly retarded children (Mehlman 1953; Schiffer 1964), handicapped children (Colman et al. 1976), exceptional children (Slavson 1955), schizophrenic children (Speers and Lansing 1965), pregnant adolescents (Kaufman 1967), and children in foster care (Lee and Park 1978).

The number of patients in a group varied vastly and still does, depending on the circumstances of the therapists and the community. Interestingly, Joseph Pratt began groups for undernourished children in 1908, a time when many children obviously fell into that category. Clinics, inpatient services, residential units, and day hospitals have a ready supply of patients.) Usually, the preferable group size is 8–10 for adolescents and a smaller number for children. In private settings, circumstances dictated the number of patients involved, at least in inaugurating an open-ended group. In some circumstances, an open-ended adolescent group survives for many years (Richmond 1971). Therapists of adolescent groups that start from scratch often have to screen 20 or so applicants to get 10 ongoing patients.

## ◆ Families

A basic question is how the therapy group relates to the child or adolescent's family of origin, because that biosocial edifice remains a powerful influence on the child's performance and productivity within his or her therapy group. Multiple impact therapy, developed in the mid-1950s by MacGregor (1964), was reported to have favorable results for 75% of the families in an 18-month follow-up. That format directly involved parents and offspring with several therapists for 2 or more days; it breached the family's defenses and gave them opportunities to regroup and redo their intrafamilial patterns of behaving and relating with one another. This and other forms of family therapy aimed at altering the functioning of the family, as well as that of the putative patient. These methods had applicability to various settings. As a variant of group psychotherapy for children and adolescents, family therapy evolved from the 1940s to the present time.

Some therapists excluded young children from family therapy. Mendell (1975) described a unique approach to counseling families and using group therapy for problems of adolescents. He used family sessions to observe and study the family system as a whole and its individual subsystems. Each parent and the adolescent obtained treatment in separate groups, along with individual sessions when indicated. Psychoanalytic psychodynamics usually dominated the theoretical underpinnings of these endeavors. Ackerman (1958) described family and individual therapy sessions with an 8-year-old child.

In treating youngsters, therapists recognized early on the role of parents, primarily mothers. Literature surveys (Corsini and Putzey 1957; Lubin and Lubin 1987; Slavson 1950) showed four articles before 1947 and six articles from 1950 through 1953 dealing with mothers and seven articles from 1948 through 1953 that were concerned with parents. Little emerges regarding specific goals and connections with the group experiences of the children and adolescents. The mothers tended to focus initially on their children's problems, then shifted the focus to their husbands and finally to themselves and their own psychodynamic interplay with their children and their spouses.

Various techniques for group therapy of mothers included having them observe their preschool children in a therapy group via a one-way mirror. Kartha and Ertel (1976) reported on short-term group therapy for mothers of children with leukemia. Bice (1949), Durkin et al. (1944), Glatzer (1947), and others described various modifications of mothers' groups, all oriented to the child patient's areas of difficulty. In 1993, the use of mothers' groups remains a valid and helpful technique that perhaps is not exploited as fully as it could be.

## ◆ Sex of Group Members

The sex of the child or adolescent patient influences the kind of group psychotherapy used and sometimes the choice of male or female therapist(s). Usually, clinics have a 3:1 ratio of boys to girls, which impedes forming coed groups. Generally, the literature throughout its evolution emphasized single-sex groups. When coed groups were tried, the group process itself reflected the presence of both sexes and generally worked satisfactorily. Some believed that this combination presented hazards, as shown in the literature of the 1940s and early 1950s. Others found that sexual acting out tended not to occur.

## ◆ Rules and Structure of Meetings

Rules and regulations governing the groups varied with the situations and the therapists. Generally, most therapists set limits and boundaries concerning injury to self or others, room damage, and most other destructive patterns of behavior (Kessler 1966; Schiffer 1984).

Most groups met once a week and occasionally twice a week—except those in hospital settings. The length of time per session tended to be 1 hour for the early age groups, extending to 1½ hours or longer for late-latency and adolescent groups.

# ◆ Closed and Open Groups

Schiffer (1947b) strongly urged that activity groups, and probably interview-activity groups, be closed groups; in other words, that patient composition should be unchanged from start to finish. Open groups tend to be better accepted with adolescents (Richmond 1971). Early childhood groups, on the other hand, tend to be closed. Few authors specify with precision the duration of a group's life, although school times, vacations, and other features tend to circumscribe somewhat the duration and uninterruptedness of such groups.

# ◆ Summary

Where is child and adolescent group psychotherapy today? What has it achieved? Abramowitz (1976) complained that "available evidence regarding group therapy outcome with children is inconclusive, but nonetheless discouraging (p. 325)." It is to be hoped that, as Dies and Riester (1986) expressed it, "We will cling more tenaciously to our optimism that there is some substance to the claims that group psychotherapy with children can be highly beneficial (p. 191)." This very immature state of research on efficacy and therapeutic outcome applies to group therapy with adolescents as well as children (Azima and Dies 1989). Group therapy works (Riester and Kraft 1986), but how it works, and what treatment conditions are most effective, remain undetermined.

Group psychotherapy of children and adolescents has woven a rich and varied tapestry in its evolution over 60–70 years. This chapter only briefly hints at the complexity of its themes. Yet despite its apparent efficacy and usefulness, this mode of therapy still struggles to achieve a rightful place in the spectrum of child and adolescent care. Its practitioners believe in it; will managed care, the government, and others accept our clinical impressions? Dies and Riester (1986) suggested that research on group psychotherapy of children and adolescents should become significantly sophisticated and that it is time for the field to grow up.

# ◆ References

Abramowitz CV: The effectiveness of group psychotherapy with children. Arch Gen Psychiatry 33:320–326, 1976

Ackerman NW: Group psychotherapy with a mixed group of adolescents. Int J Group Psychother 5:249–260, 1955

Ackerman NW: The Psychodynamics of Family Life: Diagnosis and Treatment of Family Relationships. New York, Basic Books, 1958

Adams MA: A hospital play program: helping children with serious illness. Am J Orthopsychiatry 46:16–24, 1976

Alpert A: A special therapeutic technique for certain disorders in prelatency children. Am J Orthopsychiatry 27:256–70, 1957

Anderson JE: Group therapy with brain damaged children. Hosp Community Psychiatry 19:175–176, 1968

Aries P: Centuries of Childhood. New York, Knopf, 1962, p 32

Azima FJ Cramer, Dies KR: Clinical research in adolescent group psychotherapy: status, guidelines, and directions, in Adolescent Group Psychotherapy. Edited by Azima FJ Cramer, Richmond LH. Madison, CT, International Universities Press, 1989

Barcai A: A comparison of three group approaches to underachieving children. Am J Orthopsychiatry 43:133–141, 1973

Barnes M, Schiff E, Albee C: The collaboration of child psychiatry, case work, and group work in dealing with the mechanism of acting out. Am J Orthopsychiatry 27:377–386, 1957

Becker M: The effects of activity group therapy on sibling rivalry. Journal of Social Casework, June 1948

Bender L, Woltman AG: The use of puppet shows as a psychotherapeutic measure for behavior problem children. Am J Orthopsychiatry 6:341–354, 1936

Bender L, Woltman AG: The use of plastic material as a psychiatric approach to emotional problems in children. Am J Orthopsychiatry 7:283–300, 1937

Berl ME: The relationship of group psychotherapy to remedial reading group. Group Psychology 4:60, 1951

Berman L: Mental hygiene for educators: report on an experiment using a combined seminar and group psychotherapy approach. Psychoanal Rev 40:319–332, 1953

Bettleheim B, Sylvester E: Therapeutic influence of the group on the individual. Am J Orthopsychiatry 17:684–692, 1947

Bice HV: Psychological services for cerebral palsied. Nervous Child 8:183–192, 1949

Bollinger DM: Group therapy at the children's center. Nervous Child 4:221–227, 1945

Buchmueller AD, Gildea MC-L: Group therapy project with parents of behavior problem children in public schools. Am J Psychiatry 106:46–52, 1949

Burlingham S: Therapeutic effects of play group for pre-school children. Am J Orthopsychiatry 8:627–638, 1938

Cameron K: Group approach to inpatient adolescents. Am J Psychiatry 109:657–661, 1953

Chigier E: Group therapy in a school by the school physician in Israel. Journal of School Health 33:471, 1963

Colman MD, Dougher CA, Tanner MR: Group therapy for physically handicapped toddlers with delayed speech and language development. J Am Acad Child Psychiatry 15:395–413, 1976

Corsini RJ, Putzey LJ: Bibliography of Group Psychotherapy, 1906–1956. New York, Beacon House, 1957

Dana RH, Dana JM: Systematic observation of children's behavior in group therapy. Psychol Rep 24:134, 1959

Davids M: Integration of activity group therapy for a ten year old boy with case work services to the family. Int J Group Psychother 5:31–44, 1955

Davidson PW: Comment on the small activity group project of the Montbello Unified School District. Journal of School Health 35:423, 1965

Davis RG: Group therapy and social acceptance in a first-second grade. Elementary School Journal, December 1948

Dies RR, Riester AE: Research in child group therapy: present status and future directions, in Child Group Psychotherapy: Future Tense. Edited by Riester AE, Kraft IA. Madison, CT, International Universities Press, 1986, p 191

Dubo S: Opportunities for group therapy in a pediatric service. Int J Group Psychother 1:235–242, 1951

Duffy JH, Kraft IA: Beginning and middle phase characteristics of group psychotherapy of early adolescent boys and girls. Journal of Psychoanalysis in Groups 2:23–29, 1966–1967

Durkin HE: Dr. John Levy's relationship therapy as applied to a play group. Am J Orthopsychiatry 9:583–598, 1939

Durkin HE, Glatzer HT, Hirsch A: Therapy of mothers in groups. Am J Orthopsychiatry 14:68–75, 1944

England MJ, Coler F: Discussion of "Use of inpatient service by a national population: do benefits make a difference?" J Am Acad Child Adolesc Psychiatry 32:153–154, 1993

Fabian A: Group treatment of chronic patients in a child guidance clinic. Int J Group Psychother 4:243–252, 1954

Fleming L, Snyder W: Social and personal changes following nondirective play therapy. Am J Orthopsychiatry 17:101–116, 1947

Fraiberg S: Studies in group symptom formation. Am J Psychiatry 17:273–289, 1947

Freeman H, King C: The role of visitors in activity group therapy. Intern J Group Psychother 7:289–301, 1957

Gabriel B: An experiment in group treatment. Am J Orthopsychiatry 9:1946–1969, 1939

Ghory JE: The short-term patient in a convalescent hospital asthma program. J Asthma Res 3:243–247, 1965–1966

Ginott H: Group Psychotherapy with Children. New York, McGraw Hill, 1961

Glatzer HT: Selection of mothers for group therapy. Am J Orthopsychiatry 17:477–483, 1947

Gula M: Boy's House: the use of a group for observation and treatment. Mental Hygiene 28:430–437, 1944

Hamilton G: Psychotherapy in Child Guidance. New York, Columbia University Press, 1947

Hewitt H, Gildea MC-L: An experiment in group psychotherapy. Am J Orthopsychiatry 15:112–127, 1945

Hinds WC, Roehke HJ: A learning theory approach to group counselling with elementary school children. Journal of Counseling Psychology 17:49–55, 1970

Holland G: Treatment of a case of behavior disorder through activity group therapy, in The Practice of Group Therapy. New York, International Universities Press, 1947

Kartha M, Ertel IJ: Short-term group therapy for mothers of leukemic children: what professional staff can do to help parents cope with chronic illness. Clin Pediatr (Phila) 15:803–806, 1976

Kessler J: Psychopathology of Childhood. Englewood Cliffs, NJ, Prentice-Hall, 1966

Kraft IA: Child and adolescent group psychotherapy, in Comprehensive Group Psychotherapy. Edited by Kaplan HI, Sandock BJ. Baltimore, MD, Williams & Wilkins, 1983, pp 223–234

Lazure A (ed): Outpatient Psychiatry Diagnoses and Treatment. Baltimore, MD, Williams & Wilkins, 1979, pp 3–12

Ledebur GW: The elementary learning disability process group and the school psychologist. Psychology in the Schools 14:62–66, 1977

Lolhstein L: Group therapy for latency age black males: unplanned interventions, setting, and racial transferences as catalysts for change. Int J Group Psychother 35:603–623, 1985

Lubin B, Lubin AW: Comprehensive Index of Group Psychotherapy Writings. Madison, CT, International Universities Press, 1987

MacGregor R, Ritchie AM, Serrano A, et al: Multiple Impact Therapy With Families. New York, Grune and Statton, 1964

MacLennan BN: The personalities of group leaders: implications for selection and training. Int J Group Psychother 29:177–183, 1975

Margolis L: Critera for selection of children for activity group therapy. Smith College Studies in Social Work, September 1946

Mehlman N: Group play therapy with mentally retarded children. J Abnormal Social Psychology 48:53–54, 1953

Mendell D: Combined family and group therapy for problems of adolescence: a synergistic approach, in Adolescent Group Therapy. Edited by Sugar M. New York, Bruenner Mazel, 1975

Moreno JL (ed): The International Handbook of Group Psychotherapy. New York, Philosophical Library, 1966

Pasnau RD, Williams L, Tallman FF: Small activity groups in the school: Report of a twelve year research project in community psychiatry. Community Mental Health 7:303–311, 1971

Pasnau RD, Meyer M, Davis LJ, et al: Coordinated group psychotherapy of children and parents. Int J Group Psychother 26:59–103, 1976

Patrick C, Padgett DK, Burns BJ et al: Use of inpatient srvices by a national population: Do benefits make a difference? J Am Acad Child Adolesc Psychiatry 32:144–152, 1993

Phelan JF: Recent observations in group psychotherapy with adolescent delinquent boys in residential treatment. Int J Group Psychother 10:174–175, 1960

Quin DC, Egan MH: preadolescent girls in "transitional" group therapy. Am J Orthopsychiatry 39:263–264, 1969

Rachman AW, Heller ME: Peer group psychotherapy with adolescent drug-abusers. Int J Group Psychother 26:373–383, 1976

Raubolt RR: The clinical practice of group psychotherapy with delinquents, in Adolescent Group Psychotherapy. Edited by Azima FJ Cramer, Richmond LH. Madison, CT, International Universities Press, 1989, pp 143–162

Redl F: Diagnostic group work. Am J Orthopsychiatry 14:53–67, 1944

Rhodes SL: Short term groups of latency age children in a school setting. Int J Group Psychother 23:204–216, 1973

Richmond LH: Some further observations on private practice and community clinic adolescent psychotherapy groups. Group Process 6:57–65, 1971

Riester AE, Kraft IA (eds): Child Group Psychotherapy: Future Tense. Madison, CT, International Universities Press, 1986

Rose SD: Treating Children in Groups. San Francisco, Jossey-Bass, 1972

Schamess G: Differential diagnosis and group structure in the outpatient treatment of latency age children, in Child Group Psychotherapy: Future Tense. Edited by Riester AE, Kraft IA. Madison, CT, International Universities Press, 29–71, 1986

Schiffer M: Activity group therapy with exceptional children, in The Practice of Group Therapy. Edited by Slavson SR. New York, International Universities Press, 1947a, pp 59–72

Schiffer M: Children's group therapy: Methods and case therapy and residential treatment. Am J Orthopsychiatry 17:312–325, 1947b

Schiffer M, Slavson S: Group Psychotherapies for Children: A Textbook. New York, International Universities Press, 1975

Schiffer M (ed): Children's Group Therapy, Methods and Case Histories. New York, Free Press, 1984

Slavson SR: Introduction to Group Therapy. New York, Commonwealth Fund and Harvard University Press, 1943

Slavson SR: Group therapy at Jewish Board of Guardians. Mental Hygiene 278:414–422, 1944

Slavson SR: The Practice of Group Therapy. New York, International Universities Press, 1947

Slavson SR: Bibliography on Group Psychotherapy. Group Therapy Brochure No. 32. New York, American Group Therapy Association, 1950

Speers RW, Lansing C: Group Therapy in Childhood Psychoses. Chapel Hill, NC, University of North Carolina Press, 1965

Stewart KK, Axelrod PL: Group therapy on children's psychiatric ward: experiment combining group therapy with individual therapy and resident treatment. Am J Orthopsychiatry 17:312–325, 1947

# CHAPTER 2

# Developmental Approach to Socialization and Group Formation

*Paul Kymissis, M.D.*

An understanding of normal child development is essential for the accurate diagnosis and effective treatment of children and adolescents. It is a prerequisite for an appreciation of both normal and pathological behavior in children, because what may be characterized as appropriate within one age group may be seen as inappropriate and pathological in another.

Group psychotherapy is no exception to this rule. The peer group plays an important role in the growth and development of all children. In terms of the growth and development of children, the peer group is perhaps as significant as their genetic endowment and the individual parent-child relationship. Each stage of development has its own characteristic mode of relating. Knowledge of the normative mode is essential if the therapist is to be an effective group therapist.

In the nonverbal animal world, it has been suggested that the process of development contains critical periods; only during these periods does learning of certain skills occur. Lorenz (1952) claimed that imprinting of specific behavior occurs only at specific times during the animal's development. The applicability of the concept of critical periods to human beings has been challenged (Bemporad 1980). Clearly, human development is in many ways different than animal development. Although there are no clearly defined critical periods in human development, there may be *optimal periods* when under appropriate environmental circumstances particular tasks are more easily mastered and learning takes place more rapidly. Other authors have referred to these periods as *sensitive periods* (Wolff and Feinbloom 1969). Moreover, in addition to the developmental processes that are genetically programmed, the environment plays an important and often decisive role in human development.

Kohut (1977) suggested that empathic mirroring is essential to promoting the optimal growth of the self. According to Kohut, children need continuous validating experiences from others (parents, friends, peers) to thrive. Children are attached to the mother in a symbiotic bond after birth. In normal children, this phase is followed by the process of separation-individuation (Mahler et al. 1975). Children subsequently begin to move away from the mother and simultaneously develop body differentiation from her. Children start to explore those inanimate objects (blankets, bottles, toys, etc.) provided by the mother, which will later become their *transitional objects*. Fear of separation from the mother is a constant source of anxiety for 2-year-olds (Kestenbaum 1980). The availability of transitional objects and the presence of other figures help children deal with the anxiety of separation. As children begin improving their motor skills and organize language and speech, they are able to move away from the mother and start relating to peers.

As children grow, they move through various developmental stages that are characterized by specific tasks. These tasks need to be mastered adequately for the process of maturation and growth to continue successfully.

The process of development does not take place in a vacuum. Rather, it unfolds in a context. Bronfenbrenner (1989) wrote about human growth from an ecological perspective. He saw "development as a progressive, mutual accommodation between the growing human being and his environment" (p. 188). He noted that there is a reciprocal interactive process in which the developing individual affects his or her environment and the environment simultaneously influences the individual. From this perspective, the significant others, life events, and experiences can delay, speed, or change the developmental process. From an ecological point of view, traumatic experiences and abusive environments can be obstacles to normal development.

Likewise, positive events (such as peer group experiences) can foster and facilitate further development. Harlow (1971) called the phenomenon of a child trying to learn by relating to peers *social exploration.* Bandura (1989) suggested that most social learning takes place by observing others and the results of their actions. These others are persons in the child's immediate social environment (e.g., parents, siblings, teachers, and peers).

In addition, children learn from models and heroes, not simply by imitating their behavior but by developing new judgmental standards, learning new rules of behavior, and incorporating the ideals they symbolize.

## ◆ Developmental Theories and Group Formation

Piaget's contributions have improved our understanding of how children move beyond egocentricity toward viewing objects and events from the other's perspective (Ginsburg and Opper 1979). Children refine, redefine, and validate their opinions through their interactions with others. In the process of learning, children need to act and socially interact. At every stage of cognitive development, children acquire new skills and abilities. Four-year-olds start classifying things, and between the ages of 7 and 11 years, they are able to do concrete operations. They become able to focus on several aspects of a situation simultaneously. After the age of 6, children start using words as the primary medium for the codification of various experiences (Sarnoff 1980). Children start to develop a sense of independence, which is accompanied by the fear of being small and vulnerable. Children start to defy their parents and, paradoxically, develop the fantasy of taking over the parental role.

According to Piaget, after the age of 11, children move to the stage of formal operations. They are able to reason, connect phenomena, and see alternate choices to given situations. Along parallel lines, Erikson (1963) described the psychosocial development of the child within the context of a social environment. In Erikson's developmental theory, each stage is characterized by the certain way children relate to others. The child's early sense of identity is developed according to the principle *I am what I get*. Later on, the child moves toward the stage of *autonomy versus shame and doubt*. The sense of the self is not related to the child being a passive recipient but rather an active doer. Therefore, the identity is related to the principle *I am what I will be*.

During the latency age (industry versus inferiority), the child defines his or her identity as *I am what I learn*. Children begin to learn social skills, collect items, and participate in cooperative efforts. Children also begin to produce, get recognition, share their belongings, relate to others, and develop the concept of finality and completion.

Finally, adolescence is characterized by the ending of childhood and the beginning of youth. Adolescents struggle to establish their identity and defend themselves against role confusion. This struggle in adolescence takes place in the no-man's-land between childhood and adulthood. Adolescents need heroes, peers, and their own in-group to move successfully toward adulthood. They test the self and others in going to extremes. They mourn the loss of childhood, are often preoccupied with death, and deal with anxiety in trying to find the meaning of life. Blos (1962) suggested that some adolescents so fear the end of their childhood that they try to remain adolescents indefinitely. Adolescents struggle to move beyond dependent relationships and toward the ability to give and love. Blos (1962) described this struggle as a movement from object-dependency to object-love.

## ◆ A Developmental View of Children's Groups

Most developmental theories recognize the importance of peer relationships, friendships, and play as major factors in human development. The peer group is a powerful system that, in conjunction with the child's genetic endowment and ecological context, greatly affects the child's emotional and intellectual growth.

Thus, a prerequisite for the group leader is to be aware of the developmental needs of the various members of the group. The effective group leader should know what to expect from every child within the group and what constitutes age-appropriate peer-to-peer interaction.

Above all, the group leader must have a conviction that group psychotherapy with children of various ages can be used to unlock developmental arrests and facilitate the movement toward the next developmental phase. Thus, one of the roles of the therapeutic group experience is to foster healthy development and become a catalyst for growth.

In the past, most dynamically oriented psychotherapists emphasized the parent-child relationship. However, there is an increasing recognition that although it is true that the child originally relates only to the parents, peers become more and more influential and important as development progresses. They become the major system for socialization, play, friendships, acquiring life skills, learning social values, and developing moral judgment (Grunebaum and Solomon 1980). The group therapist builds on this recognition.

## ◆ Friendships and Play

In the process of group formation, play and friendships have a prominent role. Play is one of the characteristics of humankind and is present in persons of all ages. Erikson (1963) stated that play permits the individual to step outside the social reality and assume new dimensions of body awareness through jumping, climbing, running, and so forth. In the process of play, the ego feels superior to the environment and moves beyond the confines of space and time, with a sense of control and mastery. In the context of play, relationships and friendships are very important. Friends are loyal to each other, satisfy each other's emotional needs, and validate each other's identity (Brain 1975). There are various stages in the development of friendships (Grunebaum and Solomon 1980, 1982). Each of these stages has its own characteristics.

During the first year of life, infants see their peers in an enjoyable way. Initially their play is parallel, but later on they play in an interactive way by sharing toys and exchanging items. Around the age of 3 years, children can start to socialize. They learn to take turns and wait for the others to finish their task. Around the age of 4 years, some children develop an imaginary friend. This is seen more frequently among firstborn and only children. By the age of 6 years, children start focusing on the other person and start learning that there are different ways to look at the same issue. They start to realize that their acts have certain consequences. By the age of 7 years, they insist that they need to be understood, and between 8 and 10 years of age, children begin to see the other person's perspective. During this stage, they start forming their own groups and exchanging presents, and peer pressure becomes a major force in their lives. At this age, they begin to have exclusive friends, write in each other's autograph books, and have long conversations on the telephone. Sex becomes a source of anxiety and curiosity in preadolescents. In adolescence, it becomes a central theme for discussion and exploration.

As they develop, adolescents begin to rely even more on their peer group in their effort to achieve independence from their parents (Lewis 1976). Indeed, adolescents often participate in school clubs, sport teams, religious groups, or even join street gangs and cults to get a new sense of self and freedom.

## ◆ Clinical Implications

In organizing children's therapy groups, it is important to keep in mind the children's developmental characteristics, needs, and abilities. The criteria for selecting the members of the group include age, diagnosis, level of intelligence, and stage of development. One must always remember that what is normal and appropriate for a certain age group may be abnormal and pathological for another.

Because children begin socializing with peers around the age of 3 years, the youngest group of children would be a *nursery* group that would include children aged 3–5 years. Within this group, play would be the major instrument to foster interaction and achieve group cohesion. Some of the toys for this group could be a dollhouse, dolls, cars, trucks, animals, blocks, and airplanes.

Five- and six-year-olds could be included in a *kindergarten* group. At this age, children have improved their motor and verbal skills. They are able to draw pictures and be engaged in verbal interaction. Foulkes and Anthony (1971) described the "small table technique" for the kindergarten group: five children sit around a round table, divided in five sections by lines and color. Each child has his or her own territory with sets of toys and animals. In the beginning of the group session, the play is parallel and the territories are respected. Later on, the boundaries get crossed, personal themes emerge, and the group process begins. Subsequently, common themes emerge (e.g., the aggressive brother, the absent father), which Foulkes and Anthony refer to as "the collective fantasy" of the group. This group could meet twice weekly for 30–40 minutes.

The following stage is latency. For practical reasons, the latency-age groups are divided into *early-latency–age groups* (7- to 9-year-olds) and *late-latency–age groups* (10- to 12-year-olds). During this stage, children can understand the other's point of view and therefore can use puppets and role playing.

Slavson and Schiffer (1975), who pioneered activity groups for children, divided the group session in half. In the beginning, the children are involved in an activity, and the second part is a talking period. Foulkes and Anthony (1971) used the "small room technique" for children of this age group, who cannot be expected to stay in a chair for 60 minutes. This group chooses its activity. Most children in this age group have many questions. They deal with rivalry, dreams, scapegoats, and many heroes.

Adolescent groups can also be divided into *early-adolescence* groups (12- to 15-year-olds), and *late-adolescence* groups (16- to 18-year-olds). The adolescent group is a major challenge for the group therapist. Foulkes and Anthony (1971) wrote about the use of the "small circle" technique with adolescents. In a bare room, without distraction, the members sit in a small circle in comfortable chairs. Silence creates anxiety. Adolescents either don't talk at all or talk too much. Frequently, they use hyperbolic language. When they become anxious, they start being silly and disruptive. They want guidance, and, at the same time, they want the freedom to make their own choices. Some therapists keep the sexes separate in the early-adolescence group because these groups can become overanxious over heterosexual themes. However, coed groups are used for late-adolescence groups.

In an effort to foster cohesion, the therapist searches for common themes, treats the group as a whole, and assists the group to look for the latent theme behind the manifest content. Rachman (1975) developed a theoretical model in which he focused on the resolution of the major adolescent conflict of identity consolidation versus identity confusion. He used Erikson's developmental views on adolescence in the context of group therapy. These groups enabled adolescents to move from infantile dependency on parental figures toward separation and individuation. In the group, the peer affiliation became the major developmental force. Rachman calls groups focusing on identity formation a "lifesaving device." The adolescents in the group can find out who they are, where they belong, and where they want to go.

Zabusky and Kymissis (1983), who worked with hospitalized adolescents on an inpatient unit, used the focus of identity formation for patients awaiting placement. The adolescent's anxiety about the unknown and the feeling of not being wanted were major stressors, creating more identity confusion. The therapeutic group experience, which focused on the adolescents' struggle to establish their identity, was found to be particularly helpful. Group approaches with hospitalized adolescents included all types of modalities starting with analytic groups, focused behavioral techniques, and treatment of specific target symptoms (Stein and Kymissis 1989).

Kymissis (1989), in a multiple group therapy experience on an adolescent unit, organized various groups according to the developmental, clinical, and therapy needs of the patients. These included the morning group, the doctor's group, the social worker's group, the psychologist's group, and the vocational counselor's group. In addition to the verbal channel of communication and use of discussions, the *synallactic group image therapy* technique was used. Originally developed by Vassiliou (1968), this technique uses verbal communication as well as nonverbal communication (drawings by the patients) to catalyze the group process and regulate the level of anxiety.

When adolescents become anxious, they become resistant and sometimes it is impossible for them to continue participating in the group. Many therapists refuse to work with adolescent groups because of the turbulence these groups experience. Therefore, techniques that provide structure for the session and regulate anxiety while allowing for freedom of expression are developmentally appropriate for adolescent groups. Some of the goals of adolescent groups are to enable adolescents to develop skills for coping with anxiety and to find security in themselves. Also, the adolescents need to find new and acceptable ways to gratify aggressive and sexual drives and to resolve issues relating to sexual identity (Scheidlinger 1982).

# ◆ Phases of Group Development

In addition to the developmental stages each individual goes through, therapy groups have been observed to move through developmental phases (MacKenzie and Livesley 1984). The group moves through a sequence of transformations toward more interactional complexity. MacKenzie and Livesley described the following stages of group development: engagement, differentiation, individuation, intimacy, mutuality, and termination. This frame of thinking is useful for evaluating and understanding specific group events.

Although most authors have described adult groups, child and adolescent groups undergo similar transformations and development. The life span of children's groups is usually shorter than that of adult groups. Because children grow and their developmental needs constantly change, the group should be readjusted accordingly. As the members of the group develop and acquire new skills, the group also becomes a different forum in terms of its complexity, power, and effectiveness.

# ◆ Discussion

Although individual development is often presented as a rigid system of monolithic rules, it is also a very important and useful concept in group psychotherapy for children. Development is not a static, mechanical construct. It is a dynamic and transactional process. Children do not simply follow a predestined path with various developmental stages, but are active agents and can greatly influence the course of their growth.

Most children are referred for treatment because of problems they have in their relationships with others (parents, teachers, peers, etc.). It has been suggested that the most important factor in the prediction of the future outcome and prognosis of children with psychological problems is their ability to have successful peer relationships (Sundby and Keyberg 1969). The understanding of development should be a basic element in training group therapists for children. Children are not simply smaller adults, and their basic problems are not that they are just incomplete adults. The child should rather be considered the parent of the adult. Therefore, children need to be understood as separate individuals with their own characteristics, vulnerabilities, and abilities.

Human development has different aspects: physical, emotional, cognitive, and social. The adequate understanding of all these aspects is a sine qua non for the child and adolescent group therapist. The criteria for selecting children for group therapy should include their developmental stage. Age should not be the only criterion for placing a child in a particular group. What a child knows, how much he or she understands, and what his or her potentials are should all be included in the evaluation process to assign a child to a particular group.

Groups of children and adolescents who are appropriately matched with respect to development form cohesion early and become therapy groups faster than other groups organized only on the basis of biological age. Also, children of similar developmental ages share common goals and tasks, and these can become important factors in fostering early cohesion. The technical aspects of working with children's groups should also be viewed within the developmental frame. What is therapeutic and appropriate for one age could be nontherapeutic and inappropriate for another age. For example, action in adult groups is considered as a manifestation of resistance, whereas with young children action is encouraged and is integrated in their therapeutic experience.

Communicating with children is a special art. It should be always kept in mind that it is a two-way process. The grammatical structure, vocabulary, and phraseology should be adjusted according to the developmental level of the child. For example, the language of childhood is simple, brief, direct, and concrete. Children say what they mean. Many times, it is not necessary to search for the latent meaning of a child's communication because it is clear and identical with the manifest expression.

Group therapists who work with children may be much more active than those who work with adults. They may confront, support, set rules and limits, interpret, and give information. At the same time, they must respect the group process and provide an opportunity for the group to mobilize its own resources.

Especially for younger children, play has an important role and should be used with caution and skill. Children can become overstimulated by certain activities (e.g., punching a bag). If that happens, the group could end up in disruption and chaos. Also, activities that are not appropriately structured could have a nontherapeutic group experience as an end result. Quite frequently, the boundaries between a therapy group and a social, educational, or recreational group may seem blurred. Therapy is derived from the Greek word *therapeuein,* which means "to serve the healing process." The role of the therapist is to create the right atmosphere and facilitate and catalyze the therapeutic process so that the group will not become simply a social gathering. In addition to play, any other technique used should be adjusted to meet the developmental needs and capabilities of the group members.

Group therapy for children and adolescents can be helpful as a diagnostic tool to better understand the patients in their natural peer environment, can alleviate their symptoms, and can assist them in their growth. It is a powerful force that could enable children to navigate successfully their tumultuous developmental channels and move toward growth and maturity.

## ◆ References

Bandura A: Social cognitive theory, in Annals of Child Development. Edited by Vasta R. Greenwich, CT, Jai Press, 1989, pp 1–60

Bemporad J: Theories of development, in Normality and Psychopathology. Edited by Bemporad J. New York, Brunner/Mazel, 1980, pp 3–42

Blos P: On Adolescence: A Psychoanalytic Interpretation. New York, Free Press, 1962

Brain R: Friends and Lovers. New York, Basic Books, 1975

Bronfenbrenner U: Ecological systems theory, in Annals of Child Development. Edited by Vasta R. Greenwich, CT, Jai Press, 1989, pp 187–249

Erikson EH: Childhood and Society. New York, WW Norton, 1963

Foulkes SH, Anthony EJ (eds): Group Psychotherapy: The Psychoanalytic Approach. London, Penguin Books, 1971

Ginsburg H, Opper S: Piaget's Theory of Intellectual Development. Englewood Cliffs, NJ, Prentice-Hall, 1979

Grunebaum H, Solomon L: Toward a peer theory of group psychotherapy, I: on the developmental significance of peers and play. Int J Group Psychother 30:23–49, 1980

Grunebaum H, Solomon L: Towards a theory of peer relationships, II: on the stages of social development and their relationship to group psychotherapy. Int J Group Psychother 32:283–307, 1982

Harlow HF: Learning to Love. San Francisco, CA, Albion, 1971

Kestenbaum JC: Early childhood: the toddler years in child development, in Normality and Psychopathology. Edited by Bemporad J. New York, Brunner/Mazel, 1980, pp 99–120

Kohut H: The Restoration of the Self. New York, International Universities Press, 1977

Kymissis P: Multiple group therapy with hospitalized adolescents, in Group Psychodynamics: New Paradigms and New Perspectives. Edited by Halperin D. Chicago, IL, Year Book Medical Publishers, 1989, pp 270–279

Lewis M: Clinical Aspects of Child Development. Philadelphia, PA, Lea & Febiger, 1976

Lorenz K: King Solomon's Ring. London, England, Methuen, 1952

MacKenzie RK, Livesley JW: Developmental stages: an integrating theory of group psychotherapy. Can J Psychiatry 29:247–251, 1984

Mahler M, Pine F, Bergman A: The Psychological Birth of the Human Infant. New York, Basic Books, 1975

Rachman AW: Identity Group Psychotherapy With Adolescents. Springfield, IL, Charles C Thomas, 1975

Sarnoff AC: Normal and pathological psychological development during the latency age period in child development, in Normality and Psychopathology. Edited by Bemporad J. New York, Brunner/Mazel, 1980, pp 146–173

Scheidlinger S: Focus on Group Psychotherapy. New York, International Universities Press, 1982

Slavson SR, Schiffer M: Group Psychotherapies for Children: A Textbook. New York, International Universities Press, 1975

Stein M, Kymissis P: Adolescent inpatient group psychotherapy, in Adolescent Group Psychotherapy. Edited by Azima FJ Cramer, Richmond LH. Madison, CT, International Universities Press, 1989, pp 69–84

Sundby H, Keyberg P: Prognosis in Child Psychiatry. Baltimore, MD, Williams & Wilkins, 1969

Vassiliou G: An introduction to transactional group image therapy, in New Directions in Mental Health. Edited by Riess B. New York, Grune & Stratton, 1968, pp 133–172

Wolff PH, Feinbloom RI: Critical periods and cognitive development in the first two years. Pediatrics 44:999–1006, 1969

Zabusky G, Kymissis P: Identity group therapy: a transitional group for hospitalized adolescents. Int J Group Psychother 33:99–109, 1983

# CHAPTER 3

# The Unfolding of Adolescent Groups: A Five-Phase Model of Development

*Kathryn R. Dies, Ph.D.*

A child is born, and with that event begins a relationship that will unfold in a fairly predictable manner. Initially, there is a connectedness between parent and child that is a basic ingredient in the development of trust, as well as an as yet uncomprehended interpersonal bond. From this first stage of development, the child moves into a stage that comprises processes that begin to test both the viability of the bond and the sense of self as a separate being. These life goals continue throughout the ensuing years as the youngster progresses through the stage of separation and individuation to establish an independent mode of functioning while remaining in the protected environment of the parent-child relationship.

Once the child has resolved these issues of connectedness with accompanying independence, there is a lengthy period of exploration of the intricacies of relationships and skill development that defines the child's developing personality and strengthens the relationships within which this process occurs. The final stage in the child's growth is a second separation and individuation progress (Winnicott 1953) that is marked by the solidification of acquired skills and the hopeful expectation that these skills will be a sufficient foundation from which an adult life can emerge.

In many ways, the developmental phases of an adolescent psychotherapy group parallel these stages of human development (K. R. Dies 1991, 1992; MacLennan and K. R. Dies 1992). The group therapy process has been described as providing a "transitional object" that facilitates the adolescent's establishment of a self perspective that is separate from the family of origin, but one that continues in a sense of connectedness with others (Levin 1982; Zabusky and Kymissis 1983).

## ◆ Setting the Stage for Developmental Theory History

The concept of recognizable phases of development in therapy groups is not new. For more than four decades, writers have described this unfolding process (e.g., Bales and Strodbeck 1951; Beck 1974; Bennis and Shepard 1956; Bion 1959; Brabender 1985; Garland et al. 1965; Lacoursiere 1980; MacKenzie and Livesley 1983; Schutz 1966; and Tuckman 1965), and their characterizations of the process have reflected their theoretical orientations.

Until recently, the emphasis has been on explicating the developmental stages of adult groups, mirroring the more general emphasis in the field of group psychotherapy literature. Thus, the adult literature is first reviewed as an anchoring point for understanding the developmental process of psychotherapy groups conducted with adolescents. This review provides meaningful frames of reference given the proposition that virtually all groups—regardless of the members' ages, the setting, or the theoretical orientation of the leaders—progress through very similar phases of growth.

Several dynamics of group work warrant examination: short term versus long term, structured versus unstructured, and open versus closed. These realities of the group's life may affect the developmental phases.

A phenomenon of today's mental health field is an emphasis on psychotherapy that is briefer, less costly, and provided in an outpatient rather than inpatient setting. Thus, short-term group psychotherapy for adolescents has gained in popularity in recent years, seeking to maximize the therapeutic gain for each group member while containing treatment costs. As this practice has been instituted in many settings (e.g., outpatient clinics, schools, private practice, hospitals), adolescent groups with a duration of 10–12 sessions have become the norm. What is the impact of this abbreviated time frame on the unfolding process of the group?

A study of mine (K. R. Dies 1986) charted the developmental progress of short-term inpatient groups that comprised eight sessions held within a 2-week period, that is, Monday through Thursday for 2 consecutive weeks. These groups, with the exception of one, each evidenced discernible phases of group development. In general, these phases consisted of initial attempts to form connections among the members; a period of struggle, discontent, and negotiation; a working phase; and termination. It is speculated that groups of a shorter duration, such as the "agenda" group (Yalom 1983), are less likely to experience discrete phases of development.

The second dynamic relevant to the developmental progress of groups is the level of structure provided by the leaders and how this structure is influenced by the requirements for time-limited group work. Because most developmental theories of the past were predicated on long-term groups, frequently with little active leadership intervention, the challenge to therapists of the brief therapy groups is to maximize the benefits derived from the treatment. This requirement has become associated with a more active, directive leadership style (K. R. Dies 1992; K. R. Dies and R. R. Dies 1993; R. R. Dies 1985; R. R. Dies and K. R. Dies 1993a; Vinogradov and Yalom 1989). As such, the more directive leaders are able to structure the group in such a way as to move the members toward increased interactions, thereby facilitating the establishment of an environment within which treatment can occur. In the sections that follow, phase-specific leadership is discussed to highlight this fostering of the group's evolution.

The effect of open versus closed groups on the developmental process is quite significant, not in terms of disrupting that process, but in how it is manifested. In time-limited groups with a closed membership, the developmental stages discussed herein are generally quite predictable, assuming that the members are capable of interacting in such a way that each group session builds on the previous ones. There is a stability across time, and the members become increasingly familiar with one another's strengths and weaknesses. Most important, trust is established among them.

An open therapy group (one in which the individual short-term membership changes over time) follows a slightly different, albeit predictable, pattern. In these groups, each time a new member is added, the members are likely to regress to an early stage of development during the integration process. Similarly, each time a member leaves the group, thereby altering the former dynamics, the entire group experiences the termination. These events are in distinct parallel to the developmental processes of the family in that when an infant is born, older siblings may briefly regress to prior levels of functioning; for example, they may again wish to nurse or need to be toilet trained. However, the older siblings do not remain at that regressed level for a significant period of time, and with parental tolerance and support, they quickly resume their age-appropriate behaviors. Later-born children frequently develop at a faster rate than their older siblings. This can be attributed to the fact that their teachers extend beyond the parental dyad to include older brothers and sisters, who assist them in learning the ropes. In groups, the addition of a new member may return the membership to a previous level of interaction while the new member is integrated. However, the membership has numerous resources for demonstrating the norms of the group to this new member; thus, the integration process is enhanced, and the members are able to return to their earlier mode of interaction.

Having briefly considered the roles of short-term versus long-term groups, the impact of active, directive leadership that seeks to provide structure, and the dynamics of closed versus open-ended groups, let us review some of the earlier descriptions of group development.

## ◆ Selected Highlights of Early Developmental Models

Among the earliest writers to posit a theory of group development were Bennis and Shepard (1956). In their outline, groups were portrayed as moving through six preliminary stages of organization before beginning the basic work phase. These substages were presented under two general headings: "Authority Issues" and "Interdependence–Personal Relationships." The authors emphasized the importance of the group's overcoming these obstacles as a way of achieving the consensual validation among the members that allows for therapeutic work.

In phase 1 (Authority Issues) Bennis and Shepard stressed the group members' struggles with dependency and power relationships. The authors divide this phase into three substages: 1) dependence/submission, 2) counterdependence, and 3) revolt and resolution. The progression through these substages culminates in the group members' confrontation with the group leader as preparation for movement into the second phase (Interdependence–Personal Relationships). The subphases associated with this portion of the group's process are 4) enchantment and solidarity, 5) disenchantment, and 6) consensual validation. As these subphases unfold, the group members bond and experience a expectation of benefit, followed by concern and a distrust for the capacity of the group to meet individual needs, culminating in the integration of their expectations and fears in the acceptance of the group process.

Bion (1959) described the pattern of group development consisting of the members' increased capacity to engage in constructive therapeutic work. The first area of focus is issues of dependency, during which the concern centers on the desire for direct guidance from the group leaders. Recognition of the dependency needs during this initial period provides an entrée into the second stage of development, wherein the members confront issues of authority and control and choose one of two ways of dealing with the emotions generated: fight (challenging the leaders) or flight (avoiding). Resolution of these conflicts leads to pairing as group members defensively form supportive alliances to cope with ambiguity inherent in the group's development. As these three developmental issues (dependency, fight or flight, and pairing) are resolved, the members eventually form what Bion postulates is the work group.

A concise and meaningful theory of group development was presented by Tuckman (1965), who synthesized prior research findings and then current theoretical models into the sequence familiar to many group leaders: "forming," "storming," "norming," and "performing." These descriptive labels convey the developmental task that is considered most salient for each stage of the group. As members convene for the first time at the beginning to the group's life cycle, forming represents their exploration of superficial socioeconomic and educational background information as members seek a means of initially connecting with one another. However, the perceived pressure to become more involved, coupled with an ambiguity about the group's structure, creates an environment of concern. This unsettling dynamic leads members to pursue a definition of the parameters that will guide their subsequent interactions. This storming process is manifested by increased competition among the members, followed by a press to resolve the competitiveness and establish a more cooperative mode of interaction that will provide the foundation for defining group norms. As norms are clarified, boundaries and individual limits are solidified, and the members join together to create a safe environment within which they can embark on the intense exploration of the inter- and intrapersonal issues.

Tuckman described this final stage of the model of development as continuing over sustained periods of time, during which the focus is on the group as a supportive structure for individual growth. This part of the group's life cycle involves the integration of individual members' complex issues, which are dealt with in a more open manner. The members are increasingly self-disclosing, relying on the trust established in earlier phases. Tuckman did not define an ending phase, but many contemporary writers, in accounting for the reality of termination, have added the phase of *adjourning* to his model (Beck 1974; Brabender 1985; MacKenzie and Livesley 1983).

The stage theory of Lacoursiere (1980) follows the general outlines of his predecessors and adds a stage of *transition,* bridging the group's movement from the earlier to the later phases of growth. Lacoursiere began by defining the initial or *orientation* stage of the group's life cycle, positing that during this phase, members generally have positive expectations, evidence a tempered eagerness to begin the process, and, at the same time, experience a certain amount of anxiety as they begin an uncharted progress. In these times of uncertainty, members display a significant amount of dependency on the leaders to define the group's purpose and, in so doing, seek to contain their anxieties in fantasies of the leaders taking full responsibility for the group's work.

After a brief period of evolution, feelings of *dissatisfaction* arise. These feelings appear when the group members' expectations about the leaders are not realized. The transitional phase included by Lacoursiere represents the group members' attempts to resolve their discontent and to use this resolution to propel them forward to greater productivity. A rapprochement occurs between reality and the group members' fantasies, with the evolution of a more realistic set of assumptions and thereby a reduction in the animosity among members and between members and leaders.

These events provide the first evidence of cohesiveness and enable the group to proceed to the stage of *production*. Positive feelings again emerge, as does the members' anticipation of the potential of their interactions. However, at this time in the group's life, these optimistic outlooks are founded more concretely in reality and thus form a solid foundation from which members can engage in higher levels of interaction. In so doing, members further refine their interpersonal skills. The *termination* stage marks the end of the group's work, as members acknowledge their accomplishments while accepting a sense of loss that accompanies their final interactions. Lacoursiere stated that the stage of termination is most often signaled by external time boundaries, such as the ending of the contract for short-term groups or the departure of a member in ongoing, or open-ended, group.

## ◆ A Developmental Model for Adolescent Groups

The following model posits five phases of development that adolescent groups traverse in the course of their life cycle. The stages are, in many ways, parallels of adult psychotherapy groups; however, the developmental issues to be discussed in conjunction with each phase deal with those stages particularly salient to the youthful population. The stages are *initial relatedness, testing the limits, resolving authority issues, working on self,* and *moving on.*

## Stage 1: Initial Relatedness

The goals of the beginning stage of a group's life cycle center on clarifying expectations, educating members regarding group processes, and addressing issues of engagement. These dynamics begin to surface with the earliest considerations of group composition. As leaders evaluate the potential group members, they search for goodness of fit among members, in other words, balancing commonalities with complementary qualities. Questions of homogeneity or heterogeneity of ages, gender, and symptoms are among the considerations of leaders assembling psychotherapy groups. (For a complete discussion of these composition issues, see MacLennan and Dies 1992).

The decisions made by the group leaders regarding who will be selected for membership form the foundation from which subsequent group development will emerge. How leaders address the prospective members' expectations about the group experience and educate them about individual roles in group directly influences not only the members' initial capacity to relate to one another, but also their subsequent interactions.

Member expectations about group therapy can be quite misleading. For example, many adolescents enter into group treatment with the idea that they will attend the sessions and talk about the problems that they are having with people in their lives such as parents, siblings, teachers, and significant others. They believe that their reports will be personal and historical (i.e., involving events that occur outside the boundaries of the group sessions), and they will most likely direct their stories to the group leader, looking to these figures of authority to correct or "heal" their problems. Prospective members may anticipate that there will be a process of questions and answers during which the group leaders will offer advice and "psychologize." Through these words of wisdom, the adolescent will experience some significant insight (an Aha! phenomenon). This enlightenment will be followed by a cathartic release, and with that emotional outpouring will come the "cure." This scenario is quite different from that of most leaders.

From the perspective of group leaders, it is not the outside, historical material that is important, but rather the manner in which the adolescents manifest their behaviors within the context of the group.

Thus, the interpersonal and the here and now are central in the treatment process. The group, not the therapist, is the agent of change. Through a process of mutual exploration, in which the adolescents engage in self-disclosure and feedback, the youthful group members gain in self-understanding that can lead to greater self-acceptance and feelings of self-worth and acquire strategies for dealing with life's difficulties.

During the initial phase of the group's involvement, then, leaders are focused on building appropriate expectations for what is to be accomplished during their time of working together. This process of clarification is one in which the leaders do a significant amount of education. These educational procedures include the definition of member roles, temporal guidelines for attendance and punctuality, confidentiality, and such extragroup concerns as outside socializing (R. R. Dies and K. R. Dies 1993a, b). These procedural guidelines form the structure within which the group will unfold, and, as such, are an integral part of the first stage of development.

As the adolescents meet for the first time, the task of forming connections among the members begins. The leaders seek to instill a positive climate within which the work of the group can take place. From the onset, the group leaders present themselves in such a way as to be models for the behaviors they hope to see develop in their group members. They demonstrate an appropriate level of openness and self-disclosure: in other words, a level sufficient to create an atmosphere of honest sharing but not of such potency as to threaten their cautious charges (R. R. Dies and Teleska 1985). For example, a leader may acknowledge that regardless of the number of groups conducted, the leader continues to experience a certain amount of nervousness at the beginning of a new group. This acknowledgment serves to model the type of sharing that is appropriate for this early stage of development as well as establish a norm for the group members' interactions. At the same time, the leader is seeking to normalize the as yet unspoken concerns of the youthful members. Through this type of openness in the leaders' responses to the group process, members learn to interact with one another in a similarly open fashion. By exploring their shared reactions to being in a psychotherapy group, members become familiar with one another and build a foundation for future exchanges.

Similarly, the leaders create a safe, secure environment within which adolescents can explore new dimensions of their behaviors by seeking to convert any negative exchanges or behaviors into more positive, productive forms of interaction. For example, the group may be confronted with the controlling, disruptive style of a monopolizer. This is an individual who may be attempting to deal with his or her own feelings of vulnerability, anxiety, or passive-aggressive tendencies through taking control of the interaction of the group members. At the same time, this talkative member may be providing a service to the remainder of the group by alleviating their press to participate in the group process. A frequent intervention in this situation is for the leader to ask the rhetorical question, "I wonder why the group is allowing Harry to do this?" Although this strategy may be useful in adult groups, it has the potential to generate in youthful members feelings of being punished or reprimanded for their actions, or lack thereof. Thus, the group has done something wrong by allowing Harry to do "this," and the "this" is talking.

It is unlikely that any leader would consciously seek to criticize a group member's initiative to share with other members. Yet there is the dilemma of how the leaders can encourage the participation of all group members rather than have one member monopolize the group time. While the leaders are working to establish an inviting climate within which interpersonal sharing can take place and members can form connections with one another, they may choose to simply intervene: "Harry, can we stop you a minute? You're saying a great deal, and when someone says so much, it is often difficult to take it all in. Let's stop and all take a look at some of these issues." The leaders can then restate or recast some of what Harry has been saying in a way as to invite the involvement of other group members. In so doing, the maladaptive behavior of monopolizing has been curtailed, and the preferred norm of turn taking and involvement of all members has been reinforced. All this has been done in a way that maintains a supportive, safe group climate conducive to exploration and learning. By choosing to delay confronting the group members' underlying dynamics until a more trusting climate has evolved, leaders are enhancing the retention of members and minimizing the potential for premature terminations. There will be ample time for confrontations once the security of the environment has been established.

As the engagement process of stage 1 unfolds, leaders help members identify commonalities among themselves. For many youthful members, the knowledge that other teens experience similar struggles and feelings can be quite therapeutic and can serve to reduce their sense of isolation and separateness. For example, adolescents who have grown up in alcoholic families frequently are unaware of the similarity between their personal struggles with intense negative feelings and those experienced by peers in analogous conditions. As the adolescents become aware that group members have comparable feelings, the framework is set for the exploration of additional therapeutic factors that are an integral part of the group therapy experience (Vinogradov and Yalom 1989). In the early process, the occurrence of altruism among the members is unique to the therapy group. In other words, members come to recognize their capacity to put aside their own concerns for a period of time and to focus on the issues of their peers. This altruism can be very gratifying and may generate within these adolescents a sense of power and self-control that heretofore had been missing from their perceptions of themselves. To the extent that the teenagers can set aside their own struggles and attend to the concerns of others, they come to recognize their capacity to make choices, even in the face of emotional pain.

Thus, the earliest stage of the group life cycle involves a supportive, directive leadership that works to facilitate the development of initial trust among group members and to establish some of the ground rules for meaningful interactions. Regardless of the leaders' skill and well-intended interventions, this period of cautious acceptance will give way to a time of questioning and discontent on the part of the members as they struggle to confirm the viability of the treatment process, thereby shifting the focus to the group's second stage of development.

## Stage 2: Testing the Limits

During adolescence, the challenges of separation and individuation are confronted, and youths seek to establish an identity that is an outgrowth of, but separate from, that of their family of origin. In light of these developmental tasks, the work that is accomplished during the second phase of the group's life cycle is critical in facilitating the adolescents' efforts to master the challenges they face. During this process, the central pursuit of the group's leaders is to create an atmosphere conducive to the exploration of the members' options, selecting aspects of their identity that are complementary to their self-views and integrating those parts of self that continue to generate feelings of discomfort. Throughout this process, the teens look to leaders, and to one another, for acceptance and validation.

The developmental task of the second stage of the group's life cycle, then, is one in which the adolescents strive to determine whether the group leaders will be appropriately available to them as they struggle for identity, or whether these adults will fall into negative patterns similar to those exhibited by other authority figures in their lives. Thus, the adolescents, by testing the limits, are exploring the leaders' commitment to the group members and the group process. This phase of group also closely approximates the developmental issues that teens face in their daily lives. In challenging the leaders, the youths may be seeking to determine both the leaders' level of tolerance and to understand their own capacity to function as part of a group while maintaining their separate identities.

Others (Levin 1982; Zabusky and Kymissis 1983) discussed the group process as a transitional object for adolescents as they move from their attachment to the family of origin to seek identities that are separate and apart from this nucleus. The safe, accepting environment of the group allows adolescents to begin to define new parameters of self by first asserting themselves and challenging the leadership. As this process unfolds, leaders with the stamina to serve as a container of the adolescents' negative expressions, seeking to explore rather than to challenge, serve the group's developmental need for tolerance and enable the members to move toward the phase of working together.

## Stage 3: Resolving Authority Issues

Hand in hand with limit testing and the accompanying desire to find that leaders tolerate their expressions of anger, frustration, and concern, the group members benefit significantly from the collaborative work between themselves and the leaders to negotiate and resolve their interpersonal struggles. Once the leaders have demonstrated their capacity to withstand the challenges of individual members and the group as a whole, the developmental task that follows is one of negotiation and resolution.

For example, in the pregroup contracting period (K. R. Dies 1991, 1992), the group members may have been advised of a no smoking guideline. During the limit-testing stage, the members may express their frustration with the policy and the authority behind such a policy. They may ask, "Whose group is this anyway?" Leaders who are willing to entertain the adolescents' displeasure and seek to clarify what is behind their feelings of frustration are likely to be quite instrumental in helping these youngsters experience an openness from adults that is not generally an aspect of their daily existence. In other words, rather than rebuking the teens and avowing that there is no realistic basis for their feelings, leaders attempt to validate these experiences and to convey a concern for the discomfort of the members. This does not, however, translate into a negotiated change in the guideline. Here, the group environment becomes a microcosm for reality. The fact that a situation evokes displeasure and that a resolution is sought does not automatically result in an alteration of the boundaries. In the third stage of the group's life, leaders share with members the leaders' concern for the members' feelings and explore other aspects of the group climate that may also create frustration, searching for those areas where negotiations can legitimately lead to change in the group policies.

Through the processes of the third stage of the group's life, leaders and members work together to define those elements of group guidelines that represent firm boundaries. Distinguishing between those guidelines that remain intact, despite the discomfort they may evoke, and those guidelines that may represent areas of negotiation is an integral part of this phase. As a variety of issues cycle through the group, the adolescent members have the opportunity to examine themselves vis-à-vis their limits and their developing skills for self-assertion. The leadership goal during this stage is to encourage increasing trust between the members and leadership and among the members themselves. The establishment of trust is critical in affording the members the necessary frame within which to continue their interpersonal work and intrapersonal learning in the next phase of the group.

## Stage 4: Working on Self

Adolescence is a time when teens appear to experience more comfort in learning from one another than they do from adult figures. With this in mind, the fourth stage of the group is a time during which leaders reduce their level of activity, thereby creating the opportunity for the members to assume greater responsibility for their treatment. The central events at this time include increased member-to-member activity, opportunities for behavioral practice so that members may acquire more productive interpersonal skills, and concerted efforts to enhance self-understanding and to have members generalize from the treatment setting to their lives outside the group.

To encourage greater member responsibility, leaders approach this phase of group development with the goal of reducing their level of activity so that they create an environment within which the teens may engage in more self-initiated behaviors. One strategy that may facilitate this shift in focus from leader direction to member direction is for the leaders to alter the pacing of their interactions to offer members frequent but brief interventions. In so doing, leaders continue to maintain clear boundaries, but by limiting their verbal expressions, they effectively promote the transition of responsibility to the adolescents. With reduced leader involvement, the exchanges among the members will likely increase, a strategy that further enhances the treatment outcome in that member interaction is directly related to increased cohesion and trust in the group process.

To set the stage for this shift in their activity level, leaders may openly apprise the members of their intentions. At the same time, leaders can enhance the process by sharing with the adolescents the reasoning behind their decreased involvement. For example, leaders may announce their perception of the members' growing skills and their confidence in the adolescents' capacity to be more self-directing. This intervention encourages the type of work that is inherently a part of the working-on-self phase of the group while concomitantly limiting the opportunity for the teens to misread the leaders' change in behavior.

A second task of the fourth stage of the group's life cycle is the inclusion of behavioral practice to continue to develop and solidify the members' interpersonal skills and self-understanding. These skills are the outgrowths of increased member-to-member interaction, the products of structured exercises, and the benefits reaped as the adolescents recognize intrapersonal weaknesses as reflected in the intergroup process of self-disclosure and feedback. The opportunity to practice new behaviors may also emerge from role-playing, role reversals, or *fishbowl techniques*—in which a subgroup of members act out an alternate behavior and then receive feedback from the other members serving as observers. Each of these strategies provides an arena within which the youthful group members can work to incorporate behaviors into their repertoire that complement their growing sense of identity and that most succinctly demonstrate to others and to themselves the intrapersonal characteristics that are most compatible with their perceived identities.

At other times, leaders may comment on the group's process to highlight for the members behaviors that have been identified as problematic outside the group and that have subsequently been demonstrated within the microcosm of the group. Thus, using the here-and-now examples of problematic behaviors, leaders and members can work together in seeking to establish patterns of interactions that are more adaptive and that will serve to generate a more positive sense of self as the adolescents both view themselves in their new behavioral patterns and receive feedback from their peers.

The success of the working-on-self phase of the group is measured directly by the members' ability to generalize their learning from the group climate to their lives outside the safety of the treatment setting. Thus, the third task of the working stage of the group emphasizes the need for members to translate their actions from the current treatment setting to their world outside the group. This process is frequently an extension of the within-group practice of new skills. Because members are encouraged to work on refining their behaviors between group sessions through homework assignments, they can discover the aspects of the new behaviors over which they have control and also identify those areas that would benefit from continued work. In keeping with the less active role of the leaders during this phase of development, these extragroup assignments are often initiated by the members themselves, either as self-suggestions or peer suggestions for how members may practice their newly acquired ways of conduct.

The cycle of self-disclosure, feedback, acknowledgment, practice, and generalization composes the adolescents' fourth stage of group development. Generally, this stage is recognized as where the major portion of the treatment occurs. As this process approaches an end, either by way of the temporal signal of the group's ending or whenever a member has accomplished pregroup goals, the final stage of the group's life cycle is signaled.

## Stage 5: Moving On

The developmental tasks of the termination phase of the group encompass the consolidation of acquired learning and the integration of feelings of loss that accompany the ending of the members' time together. In a society that is fraught with losses, it is inherently beneficial for teenagers to develop a capacity to experience loss and integrate those difficult feelings into their overall sense of well-being. As such, the work of the group continues throughout this process of ending.

Given the discomfort people of all ages tend to experience when confronted with loss, a primary goal of leaders during this final stage is to keep the members focused on their emotional reactions to bringing closure to the group process. It is not unusual to find members resorting to denial in their press to avoid any painful encounters with one another or with the leaders. A frequent strategy to circumvent dealing with ending is for one or more members to suggest that the group get together for a party, a reunion, or some other type of event that is offered as a reason not to have to say good-bye.

Leaders may begin with recognition of the positive feelings that are expressed in the members' desire to continue their relationships; however, in reality, the group will end, and there is work yet to be done as members share their feelings with one another. Members are asked whether they experience any personal or group issues as unresolved, and leaders assume a more active role in assisting the adolescents in working through these issues.

Leaders guide the teenage members on their journey through this unfamiliar territory, conveying their support and encouraging the expression of a full range of emotions: sadness, regret, happiness, and peace. The leaders can model yet another type of behavior by sharing their own sense of regret that the group is coming to an end. Just as the leaders may model openness by describing their own experience of anxiety as a group begins, the leaders may say at the termination, "No matter how many groups I have ended with, I still feel a sense of sadness when each one comes to an end." In so doing, it is possible for leaders to set an example for how one seeks to integrate and tolerate, rather than avoid or withdraw, in the face of difficult emotions.

As the members work on termination issues, it becomes clear that in adolescent groups there is a particular reason for the choice of moving on as the descriptive phrase for the final phase of the group's life cycle. Adolescents' completion of the group treatment process often parallels and facilitates their second separation and individuation process. The ending marks the beginning of the next phase of their lives.

## ◆ Conclusion

The five-stage developmental model closely parallels the phases of human development and seeks to address the distinctive developmental needs of the adolescent population. The active, directive leadership style accompanying each of the five stages is seen to complement those characteristics reported to be valued by the youthful consumers of this treatment modality: in other words, group members value clinicians who "manage that charmed balance between supportive care and objective discernment, between a willingness to interact emotionally with a young person and a respect for his need for separateness and autonomy" (Meyer and Zegans 1975, p. 22).

## ◆ References

Bales RF, Stordbeck FL: Phases in group problem solving. Journal of Abnormal Social Psychology 46:485–495, 1951

Beck AP: Phases in the development of structure in therapy and encounter groups, in Innovations in Client-Centered Therapy. Edited by Wexler DA, Rice LN. New York, Wiley, 1974, pp 421–463

Bennis WG, Shepard HA: A theory of group development. Human Resources 9:415–437, 1956

Bion WR: Experiences in Groups. New York, Basic Books, 1959

Brabender VM: Time-limited inpatient group therapy: a developmental model. Int J Group Psychother 35:373–390, 1985

Dies KR: Members' perception of therapists' behavior in short-term psychotherapy groups (unpublished doctoral dissertation). College Park, MD, University of Maryland, 1986

Dies KR: A model for adolescent group psychotherapy. Journal of Child and Adolescent Group Therapy 1:59–70, 1991

Dies KR: Leadership in adolescent psychotherapy groups: strategies for effectiveness. Journal of Child and Adolescent Group Therapy 2:149–159, 1992

Dies KR, Dies RR: Directive facilitation: a model for short-term group treatment, II. The Independent Practitioner 13:177–184, 1993

Dies RR: Leadership in short-term group therapy: manipulation or facilitation. Int J Group Psychother 35:435–455, 1985

Dies RR, Dies KR: Directive facilitation: a model for short-term group treatment, I. Independent Practitioner 13:103–109, 1993a

Dies RR, Dies KR: The role of evaluation in clinical practice: overview and group treatment illustration. Int J Group Psychother 43:77–105, 1993b

Dies RR, Teleska PA: Negative outcome in group psychotherapy, in Negative Outcome in Psychotherapy and What to Do About It. Edited by Mays DT, Franks CM. New York, Springer, 1985, pp 118–141

Garland J, Jones H, Kolodney R: A model for stages of development in social work groups, in Exploration in Group Work: Essays in Theory and Practice. Edited by Bernstein S. Boston, MA, Boston University School of Social Work, 1965, pp 17–71

Lacoursiere R: The Life Cycle of Groups: Group Developmental Stage Theory. New York, Human Sciences Press, 1980

Levin S: The adolescent group as transitional object. Int J Group Psychother 32:217–232, 1982

MacKenzie KR, Livesley WJ: A developmental model for brief group therapy, in Advances in Group Psychotherapy: Integrating Research and Practice. Edited by Dies RR, MacKenzie KR. New York, International Universities Press, 1983, pp 101–116

MacLennan BW, Dies KR: Group Counseling and Psychotherapy With Adolescents. New York, Columbia University Press, 1992

Meyer JH, Zegans LW: Adolescents perceive their psychotherapy. Psychiatry 38:11–22, 1975

Schutz WC: The Interpersonal World. Palo Alto, CA, Science and Behavior Books, 1966

Tuckman BW: Developmental sequence in small groups. Psychol Bull 63:384–399, 1965

Vinogradov S, Yalom ID: Group Psychotherapy. Washington, DC, American Psychiatric Press, 1989

Winnicott DW: Transitional objects and transitional phenomena: a study of the first not-me possession. Int J Psychoanal 34:89–97, 1953

Yalom ID: Inpatient Group Psychotherapy. New York, Basic Books, 1983

Zabusky GS, Kymissis P: Identity group therapy: A transitional group for hospitalized adolescents. Int J Group Psychother 33:99–109, 1983

# CHAPTER 4

# Developmental Models of Adolescent Groups

*P. Wells Shambaugh, M.D.*

M any investigations over the past 40 years have showed that small groups move through phases as they develop from collections of individuals to cohesive social entities. Although they shade into one another, phases are readily discernible. They are few in number and are arranged in a few sequences or patterns. Word pictures of phases in sequence are called developmental models. Some models also include word pictures of the performance of the leader.

Developmental models are symbolic constructions; they are ideal images not found in the real world (Hill and Gruner 1973). They are both descriptive and prescriptive. They are synoptic maps that help therapists apprehend the group interaction; at the same time, they urge therapists to emulate the leader's ideal performance and create the ideal group. Because models apply to all small groups, leaders of therapy groups can readily transpose their models to other settings.

Models help theorists, also. They open up possibilities in the theorists' search for an integrative, comprehensive model of group psychotherapy (Salvendy 1991). Models inspire them to purvey intricate, appealing, and usually untestable theories.

I wish to thank K. R. Dies, Ph.D., I. A. Kraft, M.D., R. B. Lacoursiere, M.D., S. Scheidlinger, Ph.D., and M. Sugar, M.D., for their generous assistance.

# ◆ Overview of Developmental Models

Despite their utility, there are only two major developmental models of adolescent therapy groups and a very small body of literature. In contrast, there are many adult models and a vast body of literature. Around 1959, Hill and a colleague found that they had collected over 100 distinct theories of group development (Hill and Gruner 1973). By 1994, I had collected approximately 180 models and 120 descriptions of development in a library of adult group development that included about 340 articles, six books, and two doctoral dissertations.

Recent trends promise to reduce the imbalance. The literature on group therapy of adolescents is no longer sparse (Scheidlinger 1985); rather, it is flourishing (Scheidlinger and Aronson 1991). Therapists of adolescent groups have moved beyond justifying the modality to pursuing other interests, such as comparing their theories with those of group therapists who work with other ages (Kraft 1989). Researchers on adult groups have changed their focus. They have heeded the call of Cissna (1984) to stop proving that groups develop and start investigating the development of a variety of groups (Verdi and Wheelan 1992).

## Adolescent Models

There are two established developmental models of adolescent therapy groups. The *classical model,* which is better known, restates the early discovery that adolescents resist involvement in therapy groups. The classical model has three stages: the beginning, the phase of resistance; the middle, the phase of work; and the end, the phase of termination. Garland et al. (1965) contributed the other developmental model (the *Garland et al. model)*. It has five stages: *pre-affiliation, power and control, intimacy, differentiation,* and *separation* (described in the section on the Garland et al. model). Many adolescent group therapists eschew both models. A few invoke adult models, but most apprehend group development in their own terms.

Both developmental models are flawed. Investigators have not correlated the sequence of the classical model with the sequences of adult models. They have used adolescent psychology to justify it, neglecting theories of adult group development. They have described age-specific modifications of the leader's performance (Scheidlinger 1985), but not the theoretical justification (Rachman 1989). The Garland et al. model has been overshadowed by similar adult models. Outside the fields of social work and the group therapy of children, its following has been very limited.

Recently, investigators have proposed two adolescent models that have ties to other models. Scheidlinger and Aronson (1991) offered a hybrid model that joins the Garland et al. model to the classical model. After adducing a number of adult models as well as the Garland et al. model, Dies (1991, 1992) asserted that the stages of adolescent group therapy development followed a pattern similar to those of adult groups. She proposed a five-stage model, described below in the section "Regular Sequence."

## Adult Models

Several prominent models of adult therapy groups illuminate the development of adolescent therapy groups.

Bennis and Shepard (1956) proposed a complicated sequence of phases. Based on their experience with training groups (experiential groups originated by Kurt Lewin), they stated that groups develop from a phase of "preoccupation with authority relations" to one of "preoccupation with personal relations" (p. 417). In each phase, there were three subphases.

Two major reviews of the literature clarified the sequence of phases. Tuckman's review (1965) was the first to appear. After reviewing 55 articles dealing with small group development, he proposed a model with four stages: *forming, storming, norming,* and *performing*. Later, Tuckman and Jensen (1977) appended a fifth stage: *adjourning* (the *Tuckman model*).

In a review of approximately 100 developmental studies, Lacoursiere (1980) refined the Tuckman model. Based on the affective tone and degree of resistance, he divided the first stage into *orientation* (or *positive orientation*) and *negative orientation*. Most groups begin with positive orientation and follow the regular sequence of the Tuckman model. Others, mostly therapy groups of involuntary participants, begin with negative orientation and follow modified "resistive se-quences" (p. 173).

Many investigators assume that development is intrinsic to small groups; however, a few maintain that the leader's vision and perfor-mance are critical (e.g., Bion 1961, Kernberg 1984, Shambaugh 1989).

## Investigative Methods

In sum, despite promising trends and two new models, development of adolescent therapy groups is a very limited field. There are only two established models, and both have serious flaws. To investigate, I used the method of Tuckman (1965) and Lacoursiere (1980): a comprehen-sive review of the literature.

By manual and computerized search, I collected 33 studies dealing with the development of adolescent therapy groups and 7 dealing with the performance of the classical therapist. Based on these studies and on the pertinent adult models, I describe the classical model and the Garland et al. model. Then, I review the studies that invoke neither model. Finally, I discuss the results and propose a new model.

## ◆ Classical Model

The classical model is simple and close to the group interaction. It appears in nine studies (27%).

## Early Reports

Five pioneering studies introduced the model. Two included separa-tion (termination).

All five described a difficult first stage. The early meetings of a mixed group of early adolescents were disorderly and disorganized; the therapists functioned as distant authority figures (Duffy and Kraft 1966–1967). In the *initial phase* of a group of fatherless, pubescent boys (Sugar 1967), the members were defiant and hostile; firm limits were required. In the *pre-engagement period* of a group of hospitalized, acting-out, female early adolescents (Moadel 1970), the girls manifested various forms of group and individual resistance; the therapist was firm, but flexible. In the *initial phase* (Kimsey 1969), the poor attendance of a group of outpatient, delinquent boys required external control; their aggressivity and hypermobility required internal control. At the start of groups of outpatient male delinquents (Didato 1970), the boys were suspicious, hostile, and defiant; their erratic attendance prompted the therapist to reach out, endeavoring to strengthen a positive transference.

In all cases, the middle phase was cohesive and productive. Duffy and Kraft's group (1966–1967) was cohesive and discussed a wide range of adolescent problems; the therapists were guides and translators of behavior. In the middle phase, Sugar's boys (1967) verbalized more, mourned for their lost fathers, and related positively to the therapist as a father figure. Moadel's group (1970) was a unified, stable medium for the members to test out and validate new attitudes and solutions; some depended on and identified with the therapist and the staff. The *second phase* in Kimsey's group of delinquents (1969) approximated psychoanalytic group psychotherapy; in addition to aggression, it dealt with love and tenderness. The delinquents in Didato's group (1970) developed new reactions, erected their own subculture, and identified with the therapist's social values.

Two studies included a last phase. Sugar (1967) reported that the boys studied reacted to the *termination* phase with mixed feelings of gladness and sadness and some reactivation of feelings of loss and rejection. In the *period of separation* (Moadel 1970), the attitudes of the girls in Moadel's group studied varied from deep feelings of loss to assertive self-reliance.

## Confirmatory Studies

Three reports confirmed and embellished the classical model. Two included separation (termination).

Two reports were anecdotal. The "borderline and character-disordered" boys in Levin's group (1982) initially were unmotivated, resentful poor attenders; later, they used the group as a good transitional object. A group of sexually abused girls evolved through different stages (Lubell and Soong 1982). In the beginning, the girls spoke of the isolation they felt; in the *middle or work* stage, they revealed feelings of loss and anger; and during the *termination* stage, they spoke of their hope for the future.

Scheidlinger (1985) codified the classical model. In the *beginning* of treatment, the members struggle with issues of trust regarding the adult therapist and each other. In the *middle phase,* they become deeply involved and work intensively. They perceive the therapist and peers as new objects, while the old familial objects are reactivated in the parent and sibling transference. The group becomes a "kind of substitute family, a protective transitional object encountered before venturing forth into the world" (p. 108). At the *end* of treatment, deep feelings of mourning and loss emerge, sometimes coupled with behavioral relapses.

Averill et al. (1973) applied the classical pattern to the course of group therapy of institutionalized delinquent boys. However, resistive sequence (c) gives a better fit; see the section below on this sequence.

## Later Study

Scheidlinger and Aronson's presentation of their hybrid model (1991) was the only later study. It included separation (termination).

Adopting the terms of the Garland et al. model, the authors called the early stages *pre-affiliation* and *power and control;* the therapist was "an accepting, caring yet firm person" (p. 111). Next, came two classical stages: the *middle phase* of intensive work and the *final phase* of termination.

## Performance of Therapist

The classical therapist's performance has both strategic and tactical components.

The strategic component does not change as the group develops. Occasionally, the therapist functions as a parent, often as a teacher, and always as an analyst (Phelan 1974). He or she does not interpret too deeply (Kraft 1961). The therapist is active and often directive, expresses caring and concern, and shares personal thoughts and information (Hurst and Gladieux 1980). He or she understands the normal developmental phases and tasks of adolescence (Corder et al. 1980) and maintains an intermediate position on the chronological and maturational ladders (Azima 1972). The therapist is guided by a vision or model of a cohesive, openly interacting group (Dreiss 1986) and has a genuine wish to create such a group and sufficient skill to do so (Meeks 1973).

The tactical component varies. The therapist trusts the members and, as the group matures, allows them more responsibility for its conduct (Hurst and Gladieux 1980). In the beginning phase, he or she provides structure, firm limits, and an exemplar of self-disclosure (Hurst and Gladieux 1980); in the middle phase, more confrontation and interpretation (Scheidlinger 1985); and in the last phase, effective work with separation anxiety (Phelan 1974).

# ◆ Garland et al. Model

The same year that Tuckman's model (1965) appeared, Garland et al. proposed another model that is very similar (Garland et al. 1965). It was based on these researchers' experience with social work groups of children and adolescents.

In all, three studies (9%) used the Garland et al. model, plus the article by Scheidlinger and Aronson (1991) on their hybrid model (see the section "Later Study," above).

## Five Stages of the Model

There are five stages, each involving a major task. The therapist's role is facilitating task completion.

The first stage, *pre-affiliation,* is characterized by approach and avoidance behaviors that express the members' ambivalence about involvement. The therapist provides structure and allows gradual engagement. In the stage called *power and control,* the members rebelliously strive to attain some autonomy while retaining the therapist's protection and support. The therapist clarifies the issues and encourages a balance between full-blown catharsis and repressive conformity. In *intimacy,* the third stage, the members form personal, family-like relationships. Sometimes, they call the therapist the "Club Mama" or "Pop" and compare their peers to siblings. The therapist decides how much personal material to encourage and how to deal with it.

The fourth stage is *differentiation*. The members see one another and the therapist as distinct individuals and the group experience as unique. Leadership is shared; roles are functional. The therapist lets the group run itself and becomes more of a resource person. The fifth stage, *separation,* involves termination. The members evaluate the experience and find new resources; they may recapitulate former group relationships and experiences. The therapist facilitates evaluation, supports outside interests, and helps the members come to terms with their ambivalence.

## Confirmatory Studies

Four studies invoked the model, but only three were confirmatory. They included separation (termination).

Two studies featured groups that followed the full, unmodified sequence. During the first three stages of a mixed group of late adolescents and young adults, new members fulfilled the stage-specific function the group most needed; the last two stages were satisfactory, without newcomers to represent them (Sinason and Kirtchuk 1985). Downes (1987) explored the development of a group of adolescent females from a feminist psychological orientation; the major findings correlated with the five stages.

The third study is Scheidlinger and Aronson's presentation of their hybrid model (1991). As discussed previously, it joins the Garland et al. model to the classical model.

One report involves a misapplication. Wayne and Weeks (1984) applied the Garland et al. model to their group of abused girls. However, the first period was so brief and superficial that development did not start until the second period (Lacoursiere 1980, p. 135). With this emendation, resistive sequence (a) fits this group (see below).

## ◆ Other Studies

Twenty-one studies (64%) did not invoke either model of adolescent group therapy. They featured two types of groups. A few began with some eagerness and positive expectations (positive orientation) and followed the regular sequence of the Garland et al. and the Tuckman models. Most began with hostility and resistance (negative orientation) and followed one of Lacoursiere's three resistive sequences (1980, p. 173).

To avoid confusion, I use the terms of the Garland et al. model for the phases after orientation.

## Regular Sequence

I found three studies (9%) that followed the regular sequence. All three described groups that moved into differentiation; however, only one study discussed separation. All three therapists were initially controlling and supportive.

Two groups followed the unmodified pattern. Supported by the therapists' structures, a group of sexually abused girls were relieved to talk about the trauma; subsequently, the group members tested the therapists, were involved and forthcoming, and discussed normal adolescent issues (Furniss et al. 1988). According to Dies's model (1991, 1992), in stage 1, *initial relatedness,* the members share superficial personal facts while the therapist provides structure and a positive climate; subsequent phases are *testing the limits, resolving authority issues, working on self,* and *moving on.*

One group traversed an extra phase. The hospitalized anorectic girls described by Piazza et al. (1983) initially focused on externals and fondly dubbed the group "Sweet 'N Low"; the therapists recounted personal experiences and prevented destructive interaction. In later stages, the girls discussed intragroup trust and competition; shared experiences and praised each other's progress; talked about sibling rivalry, loss, and fears of improving (an extra stage); and brought up appropriate adolescent problems.

## Resistive Sequence (a)

Resistive sequence (a) is negative orientation, intimacy, differentiation, and separation. The stage of power and control is lacking. I located eight studies (24%) that depicted resistive sequence (a). All eight featured groups that moved into differentiation, but none discussed separation.

In six studies, the groups strictly followed the pattern outlined above.

Five studies were qualitative. Aichhorn's "aggressive group" of institutionalized delinquent boys (Aichhorn 1935; Rachman and Raubolt 1984) traversed three phases: intense outbursts of aggression, diminished aggression and bonding to the workers, and preparations for outside life. Groups of institutionalized male offenders (Thorpe and Smith 1952) passed through a *therapist-centered testing operation,* a *group-centered testing operation,* a *therapist-centered acceptance operation,* and a *group-centered acceptance operation.* Combined, the two testing operations correspond to negative orientation; the two acceptance operations correspond to intimacy and differentiation. Groups of inner-city Hispanic acting-out males progressed through an *initial stage* of feeling powerless and frustrated, a *second stage* of empathetically sharing experiences and feelings, and a *third stage* of choosing between the old patterns of behavior and the new, group-generated patterns of behavior (Millán and Chan 1991). A group of unwed adolescent mothers evolved through *phase I: testing and denial, phase II: awareness and group identity,* and *phase III: self-examination* (Haagen et al. 1976).

Wayne and Weeks's group of abused girls (1984) fits into resistive sequence (a). After a brief honeymoon of best behavior, it moved through stages of scapegoating, rivalry, and therapist-directed anger; personal revelations and positive feelings for the therapists; and increasing openness and self-awareness.

The quantitative study was by Hill and Gruner (1973). Following the Hill Interaction Matrix category system, they analyzed tape-recorded sessions of two groups of institutionalized, delinquent boys (cf. Lacoursiere 1980, pp. 116–121). Both groups followed the hypothesized course of *orientation, exploration,* and *production.*

Two articles featured groups that moved through an extra stage. A mixed group of hospitalized, severely disturbed adolescents evolved through *phase I: formation, phase II: structure established, phase III: maturation* (an extra phase marked by preoccupation with immature heterosexuality), and *phase IV: peak maturity* (Powles 1959). Groups of pregnant adolescents gradually expressed personal feelings, interacted with one another and assumed polarized emotional roles, challenged the leaders' authority (an extra phase), discussed issues related to self-image and self-determination, and initiated termination (Adams et al. 1976).

## Resistive Sequence (b)

Resistive sequence (b) is negative orientation, power and control, intimacy, differentiation, and separation. I found nine studies (27%) fitting this pattern. Four described groups that moved into differentiation, but none discussed separation.

Eight studies discussed groups that strictly followed the pattern. Seven of these studies were qualitative.

Five of the qualitative studies featured groups that stopped at the stage of intimacy.

Three of the five were anecdotal. A group of institutionalized male delinquents (Schulman 1952) went through three phases in relating to the therapist: antagonism toward authority figures, distrust and hostility toward the therapist, and growing acceptance of his honesty and benign trustworthiness. Groups of institutionalized, delinquent girls (Gadpaille 1959) advanced through three phases: *open defiance, testing,* and early *self-awareness.* Less frequently, a phase of group *silence* followed that of testing; it was related to feeling rejected by the therapist. In the *initial stage* the severely traumatized and disturbed hospitalized boys in Ramos and Richmond's group (1991) were negativistic, mistrustful, and resistant. In later stages, they challenged the therapist's authority and shared their traumas.

Two of the five highlighted developmental mechanisms. Skynner (1971) described an outpatient clinic group of young adolescent boys that progressed through phases of guardedness and resentment of authorities, testing and provoking the therapist, and speaking more openly and relating positively to the therapist. Then Skynner presented the theory, reminiscent of Slater's theory (1966), that members dependently view the therapist as an omnipotent, autocratic parent figure, revolt and depose him, and finally accept him back in a more equal relationship. Drawing on both psychoanalytic and modern ethnographic theory, Spinner and Pfeifer (1986) discussed the progress of a group of ego-impaired boys through an *initial phase* of chaos, rebellion, and intense scapegoating; a *therapeutic peer group culture* based on ritualized theft; and a *more complex peer group culture* with norms of acceptable behavior.

Two qualitative studies indicated progress into differentiation. Groups of institutionalized delinquent boys passed through a series of phases: resisting relating to the therapist, testing the therapist, feeling positively toward the therapist, and intermittently working through personal problems (Shellow et al. 1958). Based on four reports summarized here (Gadpaille 1959; Schulman 1952; Shellow et al. 1958; Thorpe and Smith 1952), MacLennan (1968) offered this pattern: resistance to any treatment, banding together and testing the therapist, ambivalence about the therapist and testing each other, and gradual self-revelation and self-examination.

Bernfeld et al.'s quantitative study (1984) featured a mixed group of institutionalized adolescents that moved into differentiation. Using Dimock's coding system (1970), the authors scored the members' role behaviors. As hypothesized, development followed Dimock's three-stage model, the *middle phase* of which spans the stages of power and control and of intimacy. The sequence corresponds to resistive sequence (b), through differentiation.

One article featured a group that passed through two extra phases en route into differentiation. A mixed group of adolescents with muscular dystrophy (Bayrakal 1975) negotiated the phases of *dependence-flight, independence, regression* (an extra stage marked by destructive, violent fantasies, covert fear of death, and minimal cohesion), *interdependence, disenchantment* (a second extra stage characterized by heterosexual preoccupations, hopelessness about the future, and dissipation of harmony and illusory cohesion), and *resolution*.

## Resistive Sequence (c)

Resistive sequence (c) is the uncommon arrangement of negative orientation, positive orientation, power and control, intimacy, differentiation, and separation. I found one study (3%) that followed this pattern. The group strictly adhered to the full sequence of development, including separation.

This pattern fits Averill et al.'s description (1973) of the process of group therapy of institutionalized delinquent boys. In turn, the members are negative and suspicious, dependently want to please the therapist and receive a magical cure, are enraged when this cure is not forthcoming, share their inner lives and value the relationship with the therapist, evaluate and understand themselves, and dissolve the dependency relationship and prepare to terminate.

# ◆ Discussion

## Criticism of Literature

The literature I reviewed can be criticized for a number of reasons.

Some classes of patients are overrepresented. Ten studies (30%) are older reports about therapy groups of delinquents. When pregnant, acting-out, and abused adolescents are added, 18 studies (54%) are accounted for. I. A. Kraft (personal communication, December 1992) and M. Sugar (personal communication, December 1992) pointed out that this composition does not accurately reflect present-day caseloads. However, developmental models are mythic images that have a universality and validity that transcend the membership and the moment (Shambaugh 1989; Slater 1966). How closely a model fits the development of a particular group is always indeterminate (Hill and Gruner 1973). What needs to be done is similar to Cissna's advice (1984) to researchers of adult groups—to investigate and compare the development of a wide variety of adolescent groups. Garland et al. (1965) reached the same conclusion (p. 27).

Most of the studies lacked rigor. Almost all were anecdotal. Nineteen (58%) featured a single group. Many were submitted by the therapist, and only two were quantitative. Developmental studies of adult therapy groups have similar flaws. Nearly all are anecdotal; very few are quantitative. Nonetheless, it is impressive that all the adolescent studies can be fitted into a few models and sequences, just as Tuckman (1965), Tuckman and Jensen (1977), and Lacoursiere (1980) fitted all the adult studies into their models. However, the fit is not ideal.

A number of groups moved through extra phases. Four (21%) of the 19 studies of groups that moved into the differentiation phase described an extra phase between intimacy and differentiation. Its many forms express the group members' increasing individuation and self-esteem (Saravay 1978). Although the Garland et al. and Tuckman models do not include this stage, many adult models do (e.g., Bennis and Shepard 1956; Saravay 1978; Shambaugh 1989). Perhaps it would be better to call it an optional, rather than an extra, phase.

Two studies described an extra phase following power and control. It sporadically appeared in groups of delinquent girls (Gadpaille 1959). Feelings of having been rejected or let down by the therapist sometimes precipitated a period of group silence. The group of adolescents with muscular dystrophy traversed this extra stage as well as the later optional stage (Bayrakal 1975). Destructive, violent fantasies and covert fear of death appeared. Group cohesion was minimal. This constellation resonates with the pain of adolescent separation-individuation (Blos 1966, p. 12). It is occasionally noted at this point in the development of adult groups. Slater (1966, p. 134) associated it with fears of group death, Farrell (1976) with possible group disintegration. Understandably, it was accentuated in a group of adolescents with a progressive, crippling, and ultimately fatal disease.

A major problem is incomplete development. Twenty-four studies (73%) did not include the final phase: separation. Five of these studies featured groups that followed resistive sequence (b), but stopped at the phase of intimacy. The other studies discussed groups that followed complete patterns, but only through differentiation. Sixteen studies included an explanation. Most frequently, the issue was programmatic. To illustrate: some reports covered only a circumscribed time or a limited number of phases, several referred to defections or discharges of patients or to the therapist's leaving, and the two quantitative studies did not consider termination. A few gave miscellaneous explanations, such as a therapist's not accepting the efficacy of long-term group therapy for delinquents. In three instances, the group was still meeting when the report was submitted. The eight studies that gave no explanation are reminiscent of early adult reports, which routinely ignored termination.

Despite these issues and problems, termination is a sensitive, critical phase of the group treatment of adolescents (e.g., Dies 1991; Phelan 1974; Scheidlinger 1985). I urge investigators to give the stage the attention it deserves.

A final criticism refers to this literature as literature. The articles suggest that the classical model has fallen into disuse. M. Sugar (personal communication, December 1992) disagreed. He believes that the classical model continues to have a large following.

## The Adolescent Models and Resistive Sequences

A paramount issue is the apparent incommensurability of the two established adolescent models and the resistive sequences.

The Garland et al. model begins and ends problematically. Should the first phase be considered positive or negative orientation? Lacoursiere (1980) gave it a positive rating (p. 124). However, he pointed out that although the literature supported the dichotomy between positive and negative orientation, the varying orientations of the group members probably dictated a continuum of beginnings (pp. 141, 171). Garland et al. (1965) wrote that the members showed their mixed feeling about involvement in the group by behaving in conflicted ways (p. 35); the authors called the first phase "ambivalent" (p. 30).

The last stage of the Garland et al. model is unusually complicated. It includes a number of reactions to termination, which emerge in flashes and clusters and may not be in sequence (pp. 57–62).

The sequence of the classical model and resistive sequence (a) are not congruent. According to Lacoursiere (1980), a group beginning with negative orientation must pass through the stage of intimacy if it is to attain the stage of differentiation (p. 171). If the middle stage of the classical model corresponds to differentiation, where is the stage of intimacy?

It appears that the middle stage of the classical model corresponds to the phase of intimacy rather than to that of differentiation. According to adult developmental theory, the stage of intimacy is characterized by cohesion, harmony, increasing openness and involvement, identifications, a family transference, and a network of norms and roles, with the leader cast as a benevolent protector (Bennis and Shepard 1956; Saravay 1978; Shambaugh 1989; Slater 1966; Tuckman 1965). The members fantasy that the group is a miniature utopia (Gibbard and Hartman 1973). For adolescent groups—if sense of identity is substituted for role definition, transitional object is substituted for utopia, and allowance is made for the greater salience of the adolescent therapist—I submit that the middle stage just described is an acceptable description of the middle stage of the classical model.

The equivalency of the classical middle stage and the stage of intimacy reduces the classical sequence to a shortened version of resistive sequence (a). It corresponds to the common variant of resistive sequence (b) that also stops before reaching differentiation.

Why these groups do not develop further is not entirely clear. One reason must be that therapists who espouse short models, such as the classical model, mold their groups accordingly. M. Sugar (1967; personal communication, January 1993) offered other possibilities: restrictive therapeutic contracts with the youngsters and their parents, the limitations of depth psychotherapy with adolescents, and the group members' own expectations and wishes.

The adult literature is not very helpful. Occasionally investigators have discussed developmental arrest resulting from errors in therapist technique or from faulty group composition (e.g., Kuypers et al. 1986). A few theorists have related distorted and shortened development to the therapist's ideology or treatment philosophy (e.g., Shambaugh 1989).

Clearly, this important issue requires careful study.

## ◆ Conclusions

My investigation clarifies the sequence and the model of adolescent group development.

The three resistive sequences pattern development. Resistive sequence (a) occurs nearly twice as often as resistive sequence (b). Resistive sequence (c) is rarely encountered. Groups that begin with positive orientation and follow the regular sequence are unusual.

Variations of the resistive sequences often occur. The most significant are the absence of a phase of separation, arrest at intimacy, and the presence of an extra phase between intimacy and differentiation.

To summarize the developmental model that emerges from these studies: it begins with the stage of negative orientation. The members react to the new situation with hostility, distrust, and resistance; the therapist provides structure, sets limits, and encourages gradual involvement. Some groups then negotiate the stage of power and control, in which issues of status and rebellion are thrashed out; the therapist maintains a task orientation while allowing appropriate autonomy. Other groups proceed directly to the stage of intimacy, in which the group is a supportive place where personal issues are discussed. It is an idealized family, with the therapist as a good parent. In the next phase, differentiation, the members relate to the therapist and to one another as distinct individuals while gaining more self-understanding. The discussions cover a wide range of adolescent issues. The therapist is more of a resource person than a parent. Separation is painful and met with resistance. If the therapist persists, the members deal with deep feelings of loss as they review and at times relive the group experience.

# ◆ References

Adams BN, Brownstein CA, Rennalls IM, et al: The pregnant adolescent—a group approach. Adolescence 11:467–485, 1976

Aichhorn A: Wayward Youth. New York, Viking Press, 1935

Averill SC, Cadman WH, Craig LP, et al: Group psychotherapy with young delinquents: report from a residential treatment center. Bull Menninger Clin 37:1–70, 1973

Azima FJ Cramer: Transference-countertransference issues in group psychotherapy for adolescents. International Journal of Child Psychotherapy 1:51–70, 1972

Bayrakal S: A group experience with chronically disabled adolescents. Am J Psychiatry 132:1291–1294, 1975

Bennis WG, Shepard HA: A theory of group development. Human Relations 9:415–437, 1956

Bernfeld G, Clark L, Parker G: The process of adolescent group psychotherapy. Int J Group Psychother 34:111–126, 1984

Bion WR: Experiences in Groups and Other Papers. New York, Basic Books, 1961

Blos P: On Adolescence: A Psychoanalytic Interpretation. New York, The Free Press, 1966

Cissna KN: Phases in group development: the negative evidence. Small Group Behavior 15:3–32, 1984

Corder BF, Haizlip TM, Walker PA: Critical areas of therapists' functioning in adolescent group psychotherapy: a comparison with self-perception of functioning in adult groups of experienced and inexperienced therapists. Adolescence 15:435–442, 1980

Didato SV: Delinquents in group therapy: some new techniques. Adolescence 5:207–222, 1970

Dies KR: A model for adolescent group psychotherapy. Journal of Child and Adolescent Group Therapy 1:59–70, 1991

Dies KR: Leadership in adolescent psychotherapy groups: strategies for effectiveness. Journal of Child and Adolescent Group Therapy 2:149–159, 1992

Dimock HG: How to Observe Your Group (Leadership and Group Development Series, Part II). Montreal, Canada, Concordia University, 1970

Downes MA: The development of an adolescent females' psychotherapy group: a feminist psychological orientation (Order No DA 8716080). Dissertation Abstracts International 48:1149-A, 1987

Dreiss JE: Building cohesiveness in an adolescent therapy group. Journal of Child and Adolescent Psychotherapy 3:22–28, 1986

Duffy JH, Kraft IA: Beginning and middle phase characteristics of group psychotherapy of early adolescent boys and girls. Journal of Psychoanalysis in Groups 2:23–29, 1966–1967

Farrell MP: Patterns in the development of self-analytic groups. J Appl Behav Sci 12:523–542, 1976

Furniss T, Bingley-Miller L, van Elburg A: Goal-oriented group treatment for sexually abused adolescent girls. Br J Psychiatry 152:97–106, 1988

Gadpaille WJ: Observations on the sequence of resistances in groups of adolescent delinquents. Int J Group Psychother 9:275–286, 1959

Garland JA, Jones HE, Kolodny RL: A model for stages of development in social work groups, in Explorations in Group Work: Essays in Theory and Practice. Edited by Bernstein S. Boston, MA, Milford House, 1965, pp 19–49

Geertz C: Religion as a cultural system, in The Interpretation of Cultures. Edited by Geertz C. New York, Basic Books, 1973, pp 87–125

Gibbard GS, Hartman JJ: The significance of utopian fantasies in small groups. Int J Group Psychother 23:125–147, 1973

Haagen EK, Rosenberg J, Richmond A: A group therapy experience with unwed adolescent mothers: repairing the mother-child bond. Transnational Mental Health Research Newsletter 18:11–15, 1976

Hill WF, Gruner L: A study of development in open and closed groups. Small Group Behavior 4:355–381, 1973

Hurst AG, Gladieux JD: Guidelines for leading an adolescent therapy group, in Group and Family Therapy 1980. Edited by Wolberg LR, Aronson ML. New York, Brunner/Mazel, 1980, pp 151–164

Kernberg OF: The couch at sea: psychoanalytic studies of group and organizational leadership. Int J Group Psychother 34:5– 23, 1984

Kimsey LR: Out-patient group psychotherapy with juvenile delinquents. Diseases of the Nervous System 30:472–477, 1969

Kraft IA: Some special considerations in adolescent group psychotherapy. Int J Group Psychother 11:196–203, 1961

Kraft IA: A selective overview, in Adolescent Group Psychotherapy. Edited by Azima FJ Cramer, Richmond LH. Madison, CT, International Universities Press, 1989, pp 55–68

Kuypers BC, Davies D, Glaser KH: Developmental arrestations in self-analytic groups. Small Group Behavior 17:269–302, 1986

Lacoursiere RB: The Life Cycle of Groups: Group Developmental Stage Theory. New York, Human Sciences Press, 1980

Levin S: The adolescent group as transitional object. Int J Group Psychother 32:217–232, 1982

Lubell D, Soong WT: Group therapy with sexually abused adolescents. Can J Psychiatry 27:311–315, 1982

MacLennan BW: Group approaches to the problems of socially deprived youth: the classical psychotherapeutic model. Int J Group Psychother 18:481–494, 1968

Meeks JE: Structuring the early phase of group psychotherapy with adolescents. International Journal of Child Psychotherapy 2:391–405, 1973

Millán F, Chan J: Group therapy with inner city Hispanic acting-out adolescent males: some theoretical observations. Group 15:109–115, 1991

Moadel Y: Adolescent group psychotherapy in a hospital setting. Am J Psychoanal 30:68–72, 1970

Phelan JRM: Parent, teacher, or analyst: the adolescent-group therapist's trilemma. Int J Group Psychother 24:238–244, 1974

Piazza E, Carni JD, Kelly J, et al: Group psychotherapy for anorexia nervosa. Journal of the American Academy of Child Psychiatry 22:276–278, 1983

Powles WE: Psychosexual maturity in a therapy group of disturbed adolescents. Int J Group Psychother 9:429–441, 1959

Rachman AW: Identity group psychotherapy with adolescents: a reformulation, in Adolescent Group Psychotherapy. Edited by Azima FJ Cramer, Richmond LH. Madison, CT, International Universities Press, 1989, pp 21–41

Rachman AW, Raubolt RR: The pioneers of adolescent group psychotherapy. Int J Group Psychother 34:387–413, 1984

Ramos N, Richmond AH: Adolescent group therapy in an inpatient facility. Group 15:81–88, 1991

Salvendy JT: Group psychotherapy in the late twentieth century: an international perspective. Group 15:3–13, 1991

Saravay SM: A psychoanalytic theory of group development. Int J Group Psychother 28:481–507, 1978

Scheidlinger S: Group treatment of adolescents: an overview. Am J Orthopsychiatry 55:102–111, 1985

Scheidlinger S, Aronson S: Group psychotherapy of adolescents, in Adolescent Psychotherapy. Edited by Slomowitz M. Washington, DC, American Psychiatric Press, 1991, pp 101–119

Schulman I: The dynamics of certain reactions of delinquents to group psychotherapy. Int J Group Psychother 2:334–343, 1952

Shambaugh PW: The cultural theory of small group development, in Group Psychodynamics: New Paradigms and New Perspectives. Edited by Halperin DA. Chicago, IL, Year Book Medical Publishers, 1989, pp 29–46

Shellow RS, Ward JL, Rubenfeld S: Group therapy and the institutionalized delinquent. Int J Group Psychother 8:265–275, 1958

Sinason V, Kirtchuk G: The function of the new member in an adolescent group. Psychoanalytic Psychotherapy 1:63–78, 1985

Skynner ACR: Group therapy with adolescents: the treatment of a group of young adolescent boys. Annual Review of the Residential Child Care Association 18:16–32, 1971

Slater PE: Microcosm: Structural, Psychological and Religious Evolution in Groups. New York, Wiley, 1966

Spinner D, Pfeifer G: Group psychotherapy with ego impaired children: the significance of peer group culture in the evolution of a holding environment. Int J Group Psychother 36:427–446, 1986

Sugar M: Group therapy for pubescent boys with absent fathers. Journal of the American Academy of Child Psychiatry 6:478–498, 1967

Thorpe JJ, Smith B: Operational sequence in group therapy with young offenders. Int J Group Psychother 2:24–33, 1952

Tuckman BW: Developmental sequence in small groups. Psychol Bull 63:384–399, 1965

Tuckman BW, Jensen MAC: Stages of small-group development revisited. Group and Organization Studies 2:419–427, 1977

Verdi AF, Wheelan SA: Developmental patterns in same-sex and mixed-sex groups. Small Group Research 23:356–378, 1992

Wayne J, Weeks KK: Groupwork with abused adolescent girls: a special challenge. Social Work With Groups 7:83–104, 1984

# SECTION II

# Diagnostic and Practical Issues

# CHAPTER 5

# Diagnostic Groups for School-Age Children: Group Behavior and DSM-IV Diagnosis

*Mala R. Gupta, M.D.,*
*Jo Rosenberg Hariton, Ph.D., and*
*Paulina F. Kernberg, M.D.*

The current format of child psychiatric evaluations involves obtaining historical information as well as interviewing and observing the child directly. A valuable assessment strategy may have been overlooked. Direct observations of peer group phenomena can take place in a diagnostic group and have the potential for enhancing diagnostic accuracy. This kind of group provides a setting that allows systematic assessment of the capabilities and limitations of children with their peers. The information is of value in corroborating and clarifying diagnosis, thereby enhancing the validity of the assessment. The relative obscurity of diagnostic groups in evaluation settings seems to reflect limited data regarding applicability as opposed to a consensus regarding lack of utility.

When children are evaluated, historical information must be gathered from all sources, including primary caretakers, teachers, and the children themselves. There are limits to the reliability of the information obtained from these informants. The adults in the child's life who are in frequent contact with him or her may be biased by their intimacy with the child. In many of the cases that present for assessment, the child does not initiate the evaluation; and in the role of unwilling or uncertain participant, he or she is not likely to be an adequate reporter.

Direct observation of the child, although vital in providing an integrated view, has its limits as well. The format of the clinical interview is such that it lies outside the usual range of experience for a child. Hence, it constitutes a contextual oddity. Furthermore, the evaluation process is encumbered by the presence of at least one strange adult and complicated by the presence of the parents just beyond the office door. The evaluation is fairly structured to allow the interviewer time to observe as well as to question, which imposes a limit on the type of behavior elicited. Finally and foremost, the child stands alone in the glare of scrutiny, isolated from the examiner by a gap of many years.

The normative setting of the diagnostic group serves to enhance the validity of the data by allowing direct observation of and focused attention on vital aspects of functioning: peer relations and social competency. Used in conjunction with existing assessment procedures for children, these groups may augment discrimination among childhood psychiatric disorders.

The importance of peer group phenomena was stressed by various authors in the 1940s and 1950s (Anthony 1965; Redl 1944; Slavson 1943). The role of the diagnostic group received renewed attention by Gratton and Pope (1972), Liebowitz and Kernberg (1986), and Scheidlinger (1982). Despite ongoing work on development of observational systems, there has been little focus on linking group behavior to differential diagnosis.

Liebowitz and Kernberg (1986) reported on their use of a diagnostic peer group in the evaluation of school-age children in an outpatient clinic. A format similar to that described in their report was used to observe peer relations in vivo with linkages to diagnostic categories. All school-age children being evaluated on an outpatient basis were seen together in a playroom. The children were dropped off and picked up by the evaluating therapist along with any adult who had accompanied the child to the evaluation. To minimize observer bias, the group leaders were not told the children's presenting complaints.

The group evaluation consisted of two 45-minute sessions on separate days. The sessions took place in a large playroom equipped with a variety of toys and games that allowed inventive play and facilitated group play. The children were permitted to play freely; structure was limited to a cleanup period at the end of the group. The children were directed only in being told that they were not to hurt themselves or others or damage property. The groups were videotaped through a one-way mirror to allow the authors to review the group sessions later.

Various authors have commented on guidelines for the observation of children in diagnostic groups (Kernberg 1978; Redl 1944; Schiffer 1986), and we have drawn on their work in our evaluations. Our assessment took place on three levels: notation of the attributes of each specific group, observations of the individual child, and interactions between group members. In this chapter, we outline the observational system and describe specific behavioral patterns by diagnostic category:

A. Situational assessment
　　1. Group setting
　　　　a. Size of room
　　　　b. Toys available
　　　　c. Evidence of taping or recording equipment
　　　　d. Presence of participant-observers (group leaders)
　　2. Composition of group
　　　　a. Familiarity with other members
　　　　b. Chronological age and development level of members
　　　　c. Gender distribution

B. Individual assessment
　　1. Mental status findings
　　　　a. Physical anomalies or other features that set the child apart from peers

      b.  Hearing impairment, visual impairment, or other sensory or motor deficits

      c.  Prominent defense mechanisms

      d.  Regressive potential

2.  Ability to separate from parent or familiar adult

      a.  Enters playroom independently and eagerly

      b.  Separates at door with brief reassurance

      c.  Insists on parent's presence initially; once involved with an activity or peer, allows parent to leave

      d.  Will enter room with parent but refuses to remain without parent

      e.  Will not enter room at all

3.  Relation to play material

      a.  Uses materials in a manner appropriate for age and as intended

      b.  Attempts to take toys apart

      c.  Destroys toys (note whether willfully or unintentionally)

      d.  Uses toys as weapons

      e.  Attempts to take toys from playroom

4.  Themes in solitary play

      a.  Extent of elaboration of themes

      b.  Thematic content

C.  Interactional assessment

    1.  Relationship to other children

      a.  Methods of approach and degree of avoidance

        (1)  Enters group activity readily and becomes an active participant

        (2)  Enters group activity but remains at periphery

        (3)  Initiates and maintains contact with individual children only

        (4)  Resists peer advances initially; then participates

        (5)  Fleeting, unsustained contact with one or more peers

(6) Resists and avoids all contact
  b. Quality of interactions
    (1) Predominantly positive contact (shares, shows, takes turns, etc.)
    (2) Predominantly negative contact or reaction to contact (cries, shouts, etc.)
    (3) Verbal or physical aggression
  c. Expectations of peers
    (1) Makes requests
    (2) Makes demands or is coercive
  d. Resolution of conflict
    (1) Collaborates and reaches a fair resolution
    (2) Retreats from conflictual interactions
    (3) Makes threats or is manipulative
    (4) Exhibits inappropriate affective response (runs out of playroom, pushes other child, etc.)
  e. Terminating social exchanges
    (1) Leaves after completion of activity
    (2) Leaves abruptly

2. Relationship with group leaders
  a. Ignores or avoids leaders
  b. Requests help or intervention
  c. Gravitates to leader or is clingy
  d. Responds positively to suggestions and demands
  e. Defies or is oppositional

3. Impact of child on group
  a. Assumption of group role (leader or follower)
  b. Introduces new themes or elaborates themes
  c. Disrupts group activities

4. Impact of group on child
  a. Adheres to group rules or norms
  b. Responds positively to group's attempts to change behavior
  c. Defies group rules
  d. Flees or retreats when group demands coherence

## ◆ Situational Assessment

The provision of a good enough physical environment (Schamess 1986) as a fundamental prerequisite of group therapy is applied as a principle to diagnostic groups. As long as the setting is adequate for the needs of the group and remains constant, its impact on group behavior is minimal. Even the presence of a microphone in the group room used for our observations was not problematic because it was a constant feature. Initially, most children expressed curiosity, and on occasion some children used the microphone as a prop in their play.

Our clinical experience indicates that the therapist's presence as a participant-observer is the most important structural element of the group. A visible observer has little impact on group behavior (Abikoff et al. 1977; Weinrott et al. 1978), but as the therapist moves along the continuum of participation his or her impact on group behavior increases. Because the leader was defined as an observer in our groups, the degree to which she became involved as a participant in the group was essentially a reflection of the group process. Such interventions were necessary to enforce limits, encourage interaction, and assist with activities because of the inability of one or more children to perform these functions.

The specific composition of each group session varied in terms of gender distribution, chronological age, and developmental level of each of the members, as well as the familiarity of the members with each other. Preliminary work on the effects of these elements on group behavior was done with preschool children (Doyle et al. 1980; Guralnick 1981) but not with this age group.

## ◆ Individual Assessment

As would be expected, the information obtained by observing each child on an individual basis often replicates the findings of the mental status exam and thus may corroborate the initial diagnostic impression. Children do, however, present differently in different settings, so additional information becomes available by altering the situation in which the child is evaluated. What may appear to be a stable finding when the child is seen alone may be influenced by the presence of the child's peers. For instance, the manner in which a child separates from caretakers is highlighted by a situation in which the child must not only leave the caretaker but also must enter a room where social demands will be made of him or her. Whether the child reacts to this situation as an opportunity or as a problem can be revealing. The various ways in which the child may negotiate this task are presented in the outline above.

Fluctuating ego states are expressed in the group partially as a function of the naturalistic setting and are also accentuated by the variation in group composition and content. Character traits and mechanisms of defense are more easily assessed when the opportunity exists for a multitude of interactions with a number of children with unique characteristics.

In other instances, regression has been noted in children who are stressed by peer interactions. A child who is assessed as developmentally on course may exhibit behavior such as thumb sucking or baby talk in the group. The demands imposed by the group exert a regressive pull that has allowed the observation of psychotic features that had previously gone unsuspected.

Children often play alone at the onset of the group as a prelude to joining group activity. This is appropriate in school-age children. When a child is unable to move beyond solitary play to cooperative play on more than one occasion, more widespread deficits in social competence may be indicated. The child's manner of using play material should be noted, as well as thematic content. Children may be more inventive in their play and more likely to divulge fantasy material in this setting, in which playing is the primary occupation of those present.

The glimpses into the child's psychic life are often invaluable. We evaluated a girl who in portraying a situation-comedy type of family seemed to drop the mother doll an inadvertent number of times. When questioned about this behavior by her play partner, she denied that these episodes occurred. This denial prompted further exploration of the child's history, and a history of ongoing spouse abuse in the family was discovered. The family secret around this issue prevented disclosure in the individual and family interviews. However, within the context of group play, evidence of the traumatic experience was spontaneously enacted.

# ◆ Interactional Assessment

In evaluating the interactions of the various children in the group, we are able to assess aspects of functioning that are not accessible to the clinician through the individual interview. The interchanges between the members of the group highlight the strengths and weaknesses of each child in regard to social relatedness. In addition, there is the elaboration of the child's world view, with the child assuming a position in the group reflective of his or her perceived position in life.

The opportunity to assess the positive attributes of the child as he or she sets about the task of getting along is another potential advantage of observation in a diagnostic group. Clinicians who received feedback on our evaluation of the child's strengths in the peer group frequently reported that this information was useful because it had not been obtained from informants or elicited in the individual interview.

For instance, a child who was reported by teachers and parents to be aggressive with peers did indeed threaten and torment group members on a day when he was evaluated with children in his age range. Our estimation of the boy's social competence was expanded on another occasion when only one other child attended the group. This younger boy was reluctant to enter the group room and stayed only on condition that his father remain. His timidity might easily have been targeted by the aggressive child. As the group leader took a more active than usual role in making the younger boy feel secure, she noted that the older boy gravitated toward the play table and easily joined the activity. He modeled his behavior after the leader while they played together and then was able to successfully engage the younger child in mutual play. Here then was a child who did indeed have the ability to make a friend, although under limited circumstances. Our diagnostic formulation for the boy was enriched from the observations of interactions in the group.

Thus for the interactional assessment, the major areas of focus are the relationship of the child with peers and group leaders, the impact of the group on the individual, and the ways in which each child puts his or her unique mark on the group. It is in observing the social dialogue in group process that we begin to see the child more clearly as the person he or she is. Our initial observations suggest that there is a relation between patterns of group behavior and DSM-IV (American Psychiatric Association 1994) diagnostic categories.

# ◆ Anxiety Disorders

Anxiety is an expected response to the situation in which the child who is being evaluated is placed. Uneasiness about entering a group of strangers is fairly stable across all diagnostic categories, yet for children with anxiety disorders these concerns are resistant to modification by reassurance or experiences in the group.

Although many children come to the group accompanied by their parents, children with significant anxiety have difficulty leaving their parents to enter the group. Some of these children are unable to separate at all. For example, a 10-year-old girl who came to the group was unable to stay despite the fact that her mother stood just outside the playroom at the open door. The following week she returned with two younger siblings and was able to stay for the entire 45 minutes. The children used each other as buffers from the rest of the group as they played in a tent, refusing entry to other members of the group. Attempts to engage the children in the tent met with commands to "get out and stay out." From time to time, toys were thrown out to ward off intruders. When the tent was removed, the three children retreated to a portion of the room where they played for short periods with various toys. They engaged in little verbal interchange, even among themselves, and their play was desultory and thematically impoverished.

Children in this diagnostic category use the leader, the only adult present, to make the transition from solitary activity to more interactive play. Once involved with the group, they still seek the group leader at times of stress for reassurance or for protection. These children are unlikely to confront their peers who bend rules in games or try to cheat. One 12-year-old boy with overanxious disorder actually assisted another boy in changing the rules in a baseball game to his advantage whenever the other boy appeared to be falling behind in the game. This was an attempt to avoid the anxiety engendered by conflict in a child already overwhelmed by the demands of social interaction. This same boy was also oversensitive to the opinions of others and sought to earn praise and protection through compliant behavior. In our groups, these features have been consistently observed in the group behavior of children with anxiety disorders.

Once actively involved in play, these children are able to engage in long play sequences with peers, partially because of their relatively docile behavior. Aggressive play drives them to the periphery of the group or to seek the comfort of the group leader.

As with children who are depressed, we rarely encounter difficulty having these children follow directions; at cleanup time, they are quite eager to be helpful. A tendency toward obsessive defenses is observed in the precision with which they replace play materials.

These children often return to their initial withdrawn stance at the end of the group, when the adults arrive to pick them up. In their eagerness to return to their parents, they may leave the group with a muted good-bye that is not directed to anyone in particular. In response to our usual invitation to return to the group on the second evaluation day, they say they would like to return but tend to require reassurance that the now familiar group leader will be present.

## ◆ Depressive Disorders

Children with major depression, dysthymic disorder, and adjustment disorder with depressed mood present to us for evaluation, and they have some aspects of group behavior in common. These children are often reluctant to enter the playroom but generally are not vocal in their protests. Once they have ventured across the threshold, they tend to remain separate from the others in the group by their demeanor as well as by maintaining physical distance. This phase is often temporary and is overcome by the demands of the other children to "come play."

After this reluctant entry, these children appear to be swept along by the group. They often enter play sequences in progress and may add creatively to the theme but rarely initiate thematic shifts within the play. The ability to adapt to a completely different activity is markedly limited in this group of children. They are often left alone with the discarded play materials when the others follow a more active child in his or her next round of play.

Aggressive play is more likely than not to be a deterrent to depressed children's participation. These children do not demand much of the other members and may in fact succumb to the wishes of others too easily. For example, such children readily give up play materials with little or no protest. They also offer little resistance to cleanup despite disappointment that the group has ended.

We usually find that these children are the cooperative ones in an otherwise difficult group and so have trained ourselves to attend to the quietness in the room as well as to the disruptiveness. When we have not done so, we find ourselves with little to write in the group note about these children. This situation is suggestive of the lack of impact depressed children have on the group or possibly a reflection of the lack of impact the group has had on these children.

# ◆ Disruptive Behavior Disorders

## Attention-Deficit/Hyperactivity Disorder

Children with attentional deficits and the related features of attention-deficit/hyperactivity disorder (ADHD) usually find their way to the evaluation clinic by school referral. Although a number of excellent diagnostic measures are available (Achenbach 1978; Achenbach and Edelbrock 1979; Connors 1969; Goyette et al. 1978), we believe that teacher and parent reports should be supplemented by observation in the peer group. Group evaluation is useful in a number of ways. These children present differently depending on the setting in which they are observed; most often, they have significant problems in unstructured settings (Loney 1980). The features of the disorder cause marked impairment in the ability to interact with other children. These children are often not liked or accepted by their peers, and the development of self-esteem is affected by this rejection. Peer reactions to children with these difficulties and their counterresponses are well assessed in the diagnostic group.

Children with ADHD frequently enter the room immediately on being brought to the group and often exhibit an urgency to explore the contents of the room. The other children in the room usually do not interest these children until they have acquainted themselves with the play material. They may reject a number of toys before their attention is caught by one, and at this point they may turn to their peer group. Our observations reveal that these children do not like to play alone.

In the presence of their peers, children with ADHD can enact DSM-IV criteria for this disorder. It is difficult for them to follow the rules of play or to wait their turn; they tend to intrude verbally or may physically interject themselves. They may also present a danger to others and themselves based on an inability to attend to the consequences of their actions.

These children may be able to elaborate themes in play when mildly to moderately overactive, but in more severe cases they can do so only when the theme of play is conducive to high levels of physical activity. When two or more subgroups are enacting different play scenarios, these children often evidence failure to confine their activity to one portion of the room. Their play spills over either as a function of their inability to limit the space in which they play or as a more willful intrusion on the quieter play of their peers. When these children find playmates who are able to tolerate or even to be engaged by a high level of activity, they leave feeling secure about their role in the group.

However, the group composition sometimes will not sustain a high level of activity. This situation occurs when there are more girls than boys in the group or when the tendency of the individual children is to play quietly and rather less adventurously. At these times, the rejection to which children with ADHD are subjected becomes apparent. We often see that the efforts of overactive children to add to the play are ignored because of the abruptness with which they attempt to enter play sequences. Distractibility and lack of attentiveness do not protect these children from the recognition that they are failing in their attempts to be accepted by the group.

Cleanup time is difficult for children with ADHD because they are distracted by the toys and the actions of other children as they go about this chore. For the same reason, termination from the session is also difficult for these children. Assistance from the group leader may be necessary for them to leave the room.

## Conduct Disorder and Oppositional Defiant Disorder

Children with conduct difficulties and disobedient behavior present in the group in a manner similar to that of children with deficits in attention and hyperactivity. However, some features of these two disorders set them apart not only from other diagnostic categories but also from ADHD.

Like children with ADHD, these children enter the playroom readily, often in a manner that attracts or demands attention. However, children with conduct difficulties and defiant behavior quickly display aggressive behavior. They often use play material inappropriately; toys are taken apart or destroyed and sometimes are used as weapons. Interventions are met with anger, and these children respond on a behavioral continuum between detachment and defiance.

Generally, these children do not enter their peer group gracefully. They tend to be impatient with other children; either they cajole the other child to "hurry up" or attempt to bypass the system of taking turns. They respond to suggestions of peers with devaluing comments such as "that's stupid," as opposed to more adaptive statements that would allow the play to continue. There is a tendency to brag and boast and to disregard the already established group hierarchy. These children display the desire to immediately command the group, as opposed to waiting until they earn the leadership role. They may resort to threats or belittling to achieve their ends in play. Sulking and moodiness are common when these children are compelled to compromise. This behavior seems consistent with the vulnerability to rejection often encountered in these children.

Another attribute we often observe is swift retaliation when these children feel slighted or when they are asked to accommodate another child's needs. The group leader's interventions as the authority figure may precipitate this misbehavior because the children interpret the intervention to mean they are being treated unfairly.

Leaving the group poses a problem for these children, who may not feel satisfied with the amount of time allowed in the room. They are prone to believe that the time limit is a punitive measure, and it is difficult to convince them otherwise. It is in this group of children that we have most often encountered the demand to take a toy home or an attempt to leave the playroom with toys despite our rules against this.

## ◆ Psychotic Disorders

During the process of evaluation, psychotic features may be observed for the first time in the setting of the diagnostic group. The high level of stimulation generated by peer interactions, the relative lack of structure, and the stress of social exchanges are unique aspects of the group situation that may cause children with psychotic disorders to decompensate. Not all psychotic children are equally susceptible to these factors. In fact, among all the children we evaluated, this group presented the widest variability in social competence. Although the reason for this variability is unclear, one consideration is the ability of some of these children to limit social contact, which serves to minimize emergence of symptoms.

Many of these children had a tendency to engage in long episodes of solitary play. Sometimes we noticed bizarre or inappropriate use of toys. For example, one girl repeatedly inserted the ear of a plastic rabbit into her nose. Avoidance of social contact could be attributed to the child's need to limit stimuli or could be secondary to internal preoccupation.

When children with psychotic disorders played with peers, they made tentative forays into the group, were driven to the periphery easily, and showed a preference for dyadic interchanges. Few episodes of play were initiated, and there was a tendency to follow play sequences with little contribution of fantasy material. A few children did, however, become disorganized in response to the group activity. In these instances, their contributions were so divergent from the ongoing theme of the session that the other children lost interest and began to exclude them. The psychotic children often seemed unaware of this rejection by their peers and so were unable to modify their behavior to promote acceptance. At the other extreme, paranoid children were oversensitive and perceived themselves as disliked when this was clearly not so. A few of these children left the group abruptly without explanation or an identifiable precipitant.

## ◆ Specific Developmental Disorders

Developmental disorders are frequently part of the diagnostic picture of children referred to the clinic for behavioral problems. In the diagnostic group, psychological sequelae such as impaired self-esteem may become apparent as the children play with their peers.

Children with expressive or mixed receptive-expressive language disorder can have difficulties joining other children. For the school-age child, social adaptation depends on facility with verbal communication. Play themes are embellished by the use of language. Children with mild language disorders can compensate for them. However, when the disorders are severe, these children often resort to tactics that can lead to disruption as opposed to the intended joining. Such a child may interpose himself or herself physically because he or she is incapable of making a verbal entry as a way of establishing social contact. Children with expressive language disorders may express frustration with aggressive outbursts because they cannot easily articulate their needs and feelings. Children with receptive language problems may seem oppositional because they are unable to clearly understand the group rules. They may have a more difficult time picking up the nuances of verbal communication and thus misinterpret the social cues of others. This misinterpretation can lead to their being ostracized in the group.

Specific cognitive difficulties such as memory deficits and problems with sequencing, spatial relations, or coding may be detected as children play games with their peers in the group. Following directions, remembering the score, doing things in order, and filtering out extraneous stimuli are all necessary skills for playing board games or similar activities. When children have trouble with these tasks, the group therapist is alerted to possible learning disabilities. Psychological testing can then be suggested to confirm the diagnosis.

## ◆ Conclusion

Initial observations on the group behavior of children indicate the presence of diagnosis-specific patterns of peer interaction. Data about peer relations that are observed directly during the evaluation process can confirm an initial diagnostic impression or clarify a diagnosis that is in question. There is a need for the development of an observational instrument capable of classifying children on the basis of social interactions. A formal assessment tool predicated on the use of diagnostic groups in assessment would have widespread clinical utility. The social profile of a child thus generated would aid in differentiation of diagnostic syndromes and underscore areas of social skills deficit. Interventions could then be targeted at these specific areas of deficit, and treatment response could be assessed by following the child over time in diagnostic groups.

Although we focused our observations on Axis I psychopathology, we believe that information regarding interpersonal behaviors that form the substrate for Axis II character pathology could be obtained in the group setting. This area should be investigated further.

Some diagnostic entities were not well represented in our yearlong observation. This chapter does not contain comments on children with mental retardation, pervasive developmental disorders, and bipolar disorders for this reason. Children with these diagnoses, as well as children with specific character pathology or traumatic experiences such as sexual or physical abuse, also require further study.

The data generated from diagnostic groups combined with historical information may in themselves be sufficient to make a reasonable diagnosis. Such a system would be particularly useful in triaging patients toward appropriate treatment modalities in settings where time and funds are limited.

# ◆ References

Abikoff H, Gittelmen-Klein R, Klein D: Validation of a classroom observation code for hyperactive children. J Consult Clin Psychol 45:772–783, 1977

Achenbach TM: The Child Behavior Profile, I: boys aged 6–11. J Consult Clin Psychol 46:478–488, 1978

Achenbach TM, Edelbrock CS: The Child Behavior Profile, II: boys aged 12–16 and girls 6–11 and 12–16. J Consult Clin Psychol 41:223–233, 1979

American Psychiatric Association: Diagnostic and Statistical Manual of Mental Disorders, 4th Edition. Washington, DC, American Psychiatric Association, 1994

Anthony EJ: Group-analytic psychotherapy with children and adolescents, in Group Psychotherapy. Edited by Foulkes SH, Anthony EJ. Baltimore, MD, Penguin, 1965, pp 186–232

Conners CK: A teacher rating scale for use in drug studies with children. Am J Psychiatry 126:884–888, 1969

Doyle A, Connolly J, Rivest L: The effect of playmate familiarity on the social interactions of young children. Child Dev 51:217–223, 1980

Goyette CH, Conners CK, Ulrich RF: Normative data on Revised Conners Parent and Teacher Rating Scales. J Abnorm Child Psychol 6:221–236, 1978

Gratton U, Pope L: Group diagnosis and therapy for young school children. Hosp Community Psychiatry 23:188–190, 1972

Guralnick MJ: The social behavior of preschool children at different development levels: effects of group composition. J Exp Child Psychol 31:115–130, 1981

Grunebaum H, Solomon L: Peer relationships, self esteem, and the self. Int J Group Psychother 37:475–513, 1987

Kernberg PF: Use of latency-age groups in the training of child psychiatry. Int J Group Psychother 28:95–108, 1978

Liebowitz JH, Kernberg PF: Diagnostic play groups for children: their role in assessment and treatment, in Child Group Psychotherapy: Future Tense. Edited by Riester AE, Kraft IA. Madison, CT, International Universities Press, 1986, pp 71–79

Loney J: Child hyperactivity, in Encyclopedia of Clinical Assessment, Vol 1. Edited by Woody RH. San Francisco, CA, Jossey-Bass, 1980, pp 265–285

Redl F: Diagnostic group work. Am J Orthopsychiatry 14:53–67, 1944

Schamess G: Differential diagnosis and group structure in the outpatient treatment of latency age children, in Child Group Psychotherapy: Future Tense. Edited by Riester AE, Kraft IA. Madison, CT, International Universities Press, 1986, pp 29–68

Scheidlinger S: Focus on Group Psychotherapy. New York, International Universities Press, 1982

Schiffer MS: Activity group therapy revisited, in Child Group Psychotherapy: Future Tense. Edited by Riester AE, Kraft IA. Madison, CT, International Universities Press, 1986, 223–262

Slavson SR: An Introduction to Group Therapy. New York, International Universities Press, 1943

Weinrott MR, Garrett B, Todd N: The influence of observer presence on classroom behavior. Behav Ther 9:900–911, 1978

# CHAPTER 6

# Children in Groups: Indications and Contexts

*Arthur J. Swanson, Ph.D.*

The group is a natural setting for children. Youngsters are taught in groups, live in groups, and often play in groups. The group offers opportunities for learning not afforded by an individual relationship with an adult. These opportunities include the chance to learn empathy and cooperation and to deal with such difficult issues as envy, competition, and aggression. In a group setting, children make social comparisons to determine how their thoughts and behaviors compare with those of their peers. They look to others, particularly older peers, for guidance in negotiating their lives.

Given the natural fit of children in groups, the popularity of group therapy for children in need is not surprising. Unlike adults, who generally prefer individual therapy (Budman et al. 1988), children often appear more comfortable in a group. Despite these obvious advantages, there are circumstances in which group is not the preferred treatment. In addition, as clinicians, we are often prone to refer a child to group without due consideration for the specific goals of the treatment and the type of group that would be most appropriate. In the current chapter, I review historical indications and contraindications for group treatment and the concept of assigning children to groups according to the characteristics of the group and the individual needs of the child. Because of the dearth of research in this area, what follows is based primarily on the clinical experience and wisdom of those in the field who have used this approach in the treatment of preadolescent children.

## ◆ Indications and Contraindications

In an article on nursery school education, Anna Freud (1949) stated, "If infants are insecure and lacking in response owing to a basic weakness in their first attachment to mother, they will not gain confidence from being sent to a nursery group. Such deficiencies need attention from a single adult and are aggravated, not relieved, by the strain of group life" (p. 35). Although this statement referred to infants, it also holds true for older children who have not completed this primary task. Such children tend to be disruptive to group process because they lack what Slavson (1943) referred to as social hunger, a need to be accepted by one's peers and to attain status in the group. These children tend to monopolize the group and seek individual attention from the group leader without regard for the needs of other children.

Children who are in crisis or who have experienced a severe trauma such as death or divorce have also been considered poor candidates for group. Presumably, such children would not receive the necessary support and guidance in the group that could be afforded them in individual therapy. With the advent of topic-focused groups, however, the needs of such children can often be met in a group format.

Although Ginott (1961) recommended the general inclusion of children with conduct disorder, he tended to exclude those who steal or who show little conscience. Because of the extent of their character pathology, these children can be very disruptive to the group process. Nevertheless, when they can be maintained in group, such children can profit from the positive peer pressure and modeling effects that occur in a well-orchestrated group.

Children who experience intense sibling rivalry have also been considered poor candidates for group. Such children are likely to reenact in group the rivalries that exist in their family of origin. Although it could be argued that such working through is a useful goal for group, it is often more helpful to address such issues first in individual or family therapy.

Finally, group therapy is not indicated in those circumstances where the designated therapists are either unfamiliar with or insufficiently trained in its use. Ginott (1968) suggested that the potential for help or harm is greater in a group. Children rarely refer themselves for treatment. Rather, they are typically brought for treatment by their parents, often at the recommendation of a professional. Nor are children given a choice about the form or duration of treatment that they receive. As such, the neglect or rejection of a child by his or her peers in a group will only serve to heighten the child's poor self-image. The proper training of group therapists is essential to creating an environment that is safe for all group members.

Contraindications notwithstanding, there is much to recommend group therapy for children. Children who are either isolated or aggressive are frequently recommended for group treatment. Their common denominator is an inability to engage in age-appropriate behavior, resulting in difficulties acquiring friends. For such children, group therapy offers the opportunity to try new behaviors in an atmosphere of relative safety. Unlike the playground, where a child may be systematically excluded from the activities of his or her peers, group makes such interactions a focus of treatment.

Many children find individual therapy difficult to tolerate. They are in a low-status position relative to their therapist. The presence of group members reduces this difference in status, thus allowing children to express themselves more freely. Another obvious advantage is the capability of the group to treat several children at one time. Given the scarce resources in some mental health settings, this consideration is important in providing comprehensive clinical services.

## ◆ Effectiveness of Group Treatment

Research on the efficacy of group treatment for children is relatively inconclusive. In a review by Abramowitz (1976), approximately one-third of the studies yielded positive results, one third yielded mixed results, and one third yielded no significant change. Parloff and Dies (1977) reported that group treatment was found to be effective for the postinstitutional adjustment of juvenile delinquents in only two of seven studies. Similarly, Wood (1978) reported that delinquent adolescents had better outcomes with individual than with group treatment, although her conclusions were based on admittedly "less than rigorous studies" (p. 440).

In a compilation of 13 studies comparing group with individual treatment, Luborsky et al. (1975) concluded they were equally effective: two studies favored individual treatment, two favored group treatment, and nine reported no significant differences in the two modalities. Finally, Toseland and Siporin (1986) reviewed the best designed studies available in this area and found group treatment to be as effective as individual treatment in 75% of the studies and more effective in the remaining 25%. In no study was individual treatment found to be more effective than group treatment. In the three studies involving preadolescent children, no significant differences were found between the individual and group treatment formats.

Toseland and Siporin (1986) concluded that patients should be referred regularly for group treatment because it is at least as effective as individual therapy and clearly more efficient. In a commentary on the Toseland article, MacKenzie (1986) argued that the authors need not justify the use of group treatment. Rather, the choice of individual therapy needs to be clinically defended given the results of this review.

Overall, the existing research suggests that group therapy works and that it is as effective as individual treatment. That said, the focus of future research and clinical efforts ought to be delineation of what type of group works with what kinds of patients. The model offered by Beutler and Clarkin (1990) regarding systematic treatment selection for adult patients can provide a framework for examining similar processes in the treatment of young children.

## ◆ Systematic Treatment Selection

In a landmark book, Beutler and Clarkin (1990) proposed that a fine-grained and interactive analysis of patient, therapist, and treatment procedures is necessary to optimize treatment outcome. They propose an integrative model containing four classes of variables: 1) patient predisposing variables, 2) treatment context, 3) relationship variables, and 4) strategies and techniques. The portion of the book describing treatment context pertains most directly to the issue of when to recommend group treatment and for whom it should be recommended.

## Treatment Context

Beutler and Clarkin (1990) viewed group therapy as one of three formats available in the psychosocial mode of treatment, the other two being individual and family/marital therapy. In this schema, several variables are important in the selection of treatment format:

1. Symptomatic or conflictual complexity of the chief complaint
2. Mediating goals of treatment
3. Life stage context
4. Phase of disorder
5. Treatment efficiency
6. Patient preferences

**1. Symptomatic or conflictual complexity of the chief complaint.** When a patient's symptom or conflict is manifested primarily in the home environment, family or marital therapy is often recommended. If, however, the individual's difficulties extend beyond the family context, are observed to be destructive in group interactions, and are largely ego-syntonic, group therapy may be a preferred format. If the conflict is ego-dystonic and less easily observed in social interactions, individual treatment is often recommended.

Given children's dependence on their families, it is rare that their problems exist exclusively outside of the home. Children who are having difficulties relating to their peers are also often estranged from their siblings. This does not apply, of course, to only children or children who are much older or younger than their siblings. Similarly, although a brother may have a good relationship with his similar-age sister, he may still experience difficulties with same-sex peers who present different developmental challenges for him. With children, especially young ones, it seems preferable to address social difficulties on both fronts: family treatment to help parents create a fair and flexible home environment and group therapy to address developmental tasks not typically encountered in the home.

**2. Mediating goals of treatment.** Beutler and Clarkin (1990) proposed a direct relationship between the format of a treatment and the mediating goals of that treatment. Individual therapy engenders the most intense identification of the patient with the therapist. Although such identification is often quite helpful for patients who can withstand this degree of intimacy, other patients may act out in therapy much as they would in other intimate relationships. For such patients, group therapy has been recommended to diffuse the intensity of the relationship with the therapist. Identification does occur in group, but not as much with the therapist as with one's peers.

Many children attach easily in individual therapy and use it to change the way they think and behave in the outside world. These tend to be better-adjusted children who live in an environment that supports their psychological and behavioral change. Other children, however, find themselves uncomfortable in a one-to-one relationship with an adult, particularly one who is not their parent. Such children either drop out or are so well defended they profit little from the experience. For other children, the potential conflict of viewing the therapist as the "good parent" and the actual parent as the "bad parent" is too much to bear. Similarly, when parents are ambivalent about their child's engaging in an intimate therapeutic relationship, this ambivalence can be an obstacle to effective treatment. In such instances, group therapy for the child and direct treatment of the parent-child relationship would be less threatening to the family. To the extent that the family is comfortable with the choice of treatment format, the therapeutic alliance is increased. Beutler and Clarkin (1990) reported that this alliance accounts for more of the variance in good outcome than does the choice of any particular treatment format or strategy.

**3. Life stage context.** Individuals who are especially dependent on their families are considered to be good candidates for a family treatment format. Such individuals include children, young adolescents, and severely disturbed or elderly persons who live within a family setting. Certainly, a child needs other family members to be involved so they can support the treatment process. However, family therapy is not always in the best interests of the child. Many times, parents are experiencing marital difficulties that are manifested in complaints about their problematic son or daughter. As a result, children in family treatment can be subjected to conflicts that are only indirectly related to them. Although it could be argued that these children are routinely subjected to these conflicts at home, perhaps in an even more raw form, the choice to separate marital issues from the child's individual issues does much to clarify responsibility for the existing problems.

In such instances, children are often referred for either individual or group therapy. Group therapy can be particularly useful if the child is in a group of youngsters with similar problems. This format has been especially effective for children whose parents are undergoing separation or divorce.

As children reach their latency and adolescent years, their involvement in family treatment becomes more critical. Not only are they aware of the problem areas, but they also contribute to these problems. Although not always deserving of the family label as the identified patient, neither are they innocent in the family's dysfunction.

**4. Phase of disorder.** Adults with disorders such as schizophrenia and bipolar affective disorder often experience acute episodes interspersed with periods of relative calm. Different treatment interventions are recommended according to the phase of the disorder. Given that children's psychiatric symptomatology is rarely as consistent or predictable as that seen in adults, the issue of determining treatment according to the phase of the disorder seems less germane to children. It is true, however, that some children need a psychopharmacological intervention before they can make use of any treatment format.

**5. Treatment efficiency.** Beutler and Clarkin (1990) argued that group therapy is the most efficient and individual therapy is the least efficient type of treatment. Group not only allows one therapist to help many patients at once, but the patients can be an important source of advice and support to one another. As such, the group has the potential to have synergistic effects on all of its members.

Group treatment would also appear to be the most efficient format for children. However, the selection of children for group is even more imperative than it is for adults, lest youngsters are included who are not developmentally able to meet its demands. Children who do not fit in can not only be hurt by the group; their presence also can be a detriment to other group members. Unlike adults, who are able to quit a group, children are more likely to be removed, further perpetuating their feelings of rejection and failure.

**6. Patient preferences.** As stated earlier, adult patients tend to prefer individual to group treatment, even though the research suggests that the two formats result in roughly equal outcomes. To my knowledge, no one has asked children what format they prefer. This issue is confounded by the fact that it is the parents who usually seek, as well as pay for, clinical services for their children. It seems likely that parents who have a predilection toward a particular format of treatment are likely to want that format for their children. However, if asked, children might tend to prefer the most efficient approach.

The reluctance of adults to enter group treatment is partly due to inadequate preparation for entry into group (Budman et al. 1988). Individuals should be told what to expect from group and what will be expected of them. The fact that they may not like all of the other group members should be discussed, but it should be viewed in the context of being an opportunity to work through interpersonal conflict. In more structured groups, sometimes a contract is written to further clarify treatment expectations. Such preparation for group often does much to allay patients' reservations about such an approach and increases the likelihood of a positive outcome. In the case of children, it is important that both the child and the parents be given such preparation so that all members of the family can support the treatment process.

In the adult literature, it has been recommended that patients first enter individual therapy and then, when appropriate, be assigned to group treatment either concurrently or on termination of individual therapy (Stone and Rutan 1984). The belief is that individual therapy provides the individual attention most adults seek when entering therapy while also developing a psychological mind-set that will ultimately facilitate group treatment. In an interesting twist, it may be that group treatment provides a good base for individual therapy of children, particularly when the group and individual treatment can occur with the same therapist. Perhaps the less intensive relationship with a group therapist would embolden a child ultimately to enter individual therapy when this format is indicated.

# ◆ Types of Groups

In group therapy literature an important distinction exists between homogeneous and heterogeneous groups (Frances et al. 1980). Homogeneous groups contain members who share a common condition. In the case of children, that condition could be social skills problems, chronic illness, grief over a significant loss, and so forth. Homogeneous groups tend to be more didactic; role modeling and advice are combined with active support.

In heterogeneous groups, individual members do not necessarily share a common problem. Members may vary widely in their problems and personal characteristics. These groups are more open ended; the group members set the agenda, and the therapist facilitates the process. There is less reliance on advice and role modeling and more reliance on insight and character change.

## Homogeneous Groups

With preschool-age children, homogeneous groups are rare. These groups typically rely on a preset protocol that necessitates a high degree of structure in the group. Many young children, particularly those of preschool age, do not have the requisite skills to profit from such structure. When such groups are designed, it is important to introduce a higher degree of flexibility in the approach to meet the attentional abilities of young children. For example, combining didactic instruction with play and rewards is often helpful. In some instances, small items can be used to reward the successful completion of various tasks of the treatment process. For example, individual children could be given stickers for participating in role-playing exercises. In addition, it is often quite helpful for the whole group to be given a reward on completion of a task by all of its members. This group contingency often facilitates members' helping one another for the benefit of all. Because of the developmental needs of preschoolers and the emphasis on a more structured approach, homogeneous groups should consist of three to five members, and sessions should be no longer than 30 minutes. Longer periods of time lead to behavioral regression, a process not typically addressed by this approach.

Many school-age children can profit from homogeneous groups. These groups provide children with the opportunity of meeting and working with peers who share a common problem. As with adults, the children's experience of commonality with other group members regarding a specific problem is a key element in effective group process. Though children need to share the common factor that brings them to group, they can differ on other variables such as sex, race, and socioeconomic status.

Given the rapid developmental changes that occur in young children, it is generally recommended that children in a group not differ by more than 2 chronological years (Slavson 1950). Of course, there are exceptions: young but precocious children might fit into a group of older children, and same-age children may not be suitable for an age-appropriate group because of low intelligence or extreme immaturity. One contraindication to assignment to a homogeneous group occurs when a child's pathology is so pervasive that focus on a specific problem area is impossible. Such children might be better served in a heterogeneous group where a variety of issues can be addressed, or, barring that, in individual or family therapy.

## Heterogeneous Groups

For preschoolers, heterogeneous groups may be more appropriate. The focus on providing an open atmosphere in which children are free to express themselves through their words and their behavior places less external demand on them. Nevertheless, internal demands exist as children seek ways of getting their needs met in group without violating the rights of others. Issues around competition and aggression are often prominent. The group leader attempts to intervene as little as possible with the goal of helping children experience conflict and be active in its resolution. By engaging in this working-through process with other group members, children begin to make changes in their out-of-group behavior. With these young children, the group therapist makes more use of reflecting on individual and group behaviors and on structuring the group. Interpretation is of limited use with this age group.

Heterogeneous groups are quite prevalent in the treatment of school-age children. The most common cause for referral to such groups is faulty interpersonal relationships. How these deficits are manifested may vary greatly, however; some children are passive and withdrawn, and others are overactive and aggressive. It is generally recommended that these groups contain children who show a range of behaviors so that a balance can be found between active and passive and verbal and nonverbal participants (Rose and Edleson 1987). It is hoped that each child's strengths can be used to benefit other group members. That is, a passive child may model self-control, whereas an active child may demonstrate appropriate assertiveness.

Leaders of heterogeneous groups for school-age children offer less structuring of activities than that which occurs with groups of preschoolers. More use is made of children's developing abilities to structure their own world and make their own rules. Because of the goals of these groups, they are often more long term than homogeneous ones. Frequently, an open-ended format is used, where new members are added midcourse to make up for children who have either achieved their goals or dropped out. With greater focus on the process of the group, the introduction of new members becomes less problematic than it might be in a content-focused homogeneous group. Nevertheless, issues do arise when new members are added, particularly when departed members will be missed. It has been recommended that two or three children be added at one time to relieve the pressure on the incoming members (Rose and Edleson 1987). In total, a group of five or six members is recommended (Mayer and Baker 1967).

## ◆ Settings

To the extent that homogeneous groups tend to be more time limited and psychoeducational in nature, they are often experienced by children and their parents as less threatening. Such groups do not typically require the same time commitment as heterogeneous groups, nor are they aimed at character change. As such, they are quite popular in settings that are primarily nonclinical, such as schools, day care centers, and community centers. However, their appeal is not limited to these settings. Outpatient clinics and private practitioners find it easier to market topic-focused groups than more experiential ones. Hospitals, too, use such groups, typically as an adjunct to heterogeneous groups. As mentioned previously, the more disturbed the individual, the less likely that a homogeneous group would be used exclusively.

Though heterogeneous groups can be used anywhere, they are often limited to clinical settings containing more disturbed children. The assumption is that such youngsters will need longer-term, process-oriented treatment. For these children, remediation of a problem behavior may not be sufficient to improve functioning in the outside world. At the same time, because there is less emphasis on content, leaders of heterogeneous groups need to be quite skilled in interpreting process and in responding therapeutically to the group's many demands. A therapist who is poorly trained to do such work or who lacks a theoretical framework is likely to have little success with the group; in an extreme case, he or she could potentially harm the persons involved. Conversely, a well-run group can promote an atmosphere of trust and affiliation and in the process provide out-of-group benefits for its members.

## ◆ A Comparison Study

Few attempts have been made to compare homogeneous to heterogeneous groups in children. One known study compared a behavior modification group to a self-concept group (Berry et al. 1980). Twenty-six children, ranging in age from 6 to 9 years, were matched on intelligence, age, and sex and assigned equally to the two groups. At posttest, neither group showed significant improvement on the Coopersmith Self-Esteem Inventory (Coopersmith 1967); and, contrary to expectation, the self-concept group showed significant improvements in both deviant behaviors and task behaviors, whereas the behavior modification group did not. These findings were confounded, however, by the fact that the authors served as therapists in the self-concept therapy group, but not in the behavior modification group, which was conducted by a teacher and an aide. The differences in experience and training of the group leaders or the expectations of the authors, or both, could have influenced the results in favor of the self-concept group.

Clearly, more research is needed comparing homogeneous to heterogeneous groups in children. Obstacles to such research include gathering enough patients to implement such studies and designing groups that are similar in duration and quality of treatment so as to be comparable. In addition, it is necessary to identify outcome measures that will accurately assess the goals of each type of group.

In this chapter, I have reviewed the relative indications and contraindications of group therapy for children, incorporating Beutler and Clarkin's framework (1990) for selection of the treatment format. Homogeneous and heterogeneous groups have been compared, and the types of children who might be referred to each have been indicated. Although some research has been reviewed, the majority of the findings are based on the clinical experiences of those in the field. Some progress has been made; however, research in child group therapy is still faced with the more general challenge of answering these questions (Paul 1969): What treatment, by which therapist, will be most effective for a person with a specific problem? Under what kind of circumstances? How does it come about?

## ◆ References

Abramowitz CV: The effectiveness of group psychotherapy with children. Arch Gen Psychiatry 33:320–326, 1976

Berry KK, Turone RJ, Hardt P: Comparison of group therapy and behavioral modification with children. Psychol Rep 46:975–978, 1980

Beutler LE, Clarkin JF: Systematic Treatment Selection: Toward Targeted Therapeutic Interventions. New York, Brunner/Mazel, 1990

Budman SH, Demby A, Redondo JP, et al: Comparative outcome in time-limited individual and group psychotherapy. Int J Group Psychother 38:277–292, 1988

Coopersmith S: The Antecedents of Self-Esteem. San Francisco, CA, Freeman, 1967

Frances A, Clarkin JF, Marachi JP: Selection criteria for outpatient group psychotherapy. Hosp Community Psychiatry 31:245–250, 1980

Freud A: Nursery school education: its use and dangers. Child Study 26:35, 1949

Ginott HG: Group Psychotherapy With Children. New York, McGraw-Hill, 1961

Ginott HG: Group therapy with children, in Basic Approaches to Group Psychotherapy and Group Counseling. Edited by Gazda GM. Charles C Thomas, Springfield, IL, 1968, pp 176–194

Luborsky L, Singer B, Luborsky L: Comparative studies of psychotherapies. Arch Gen Psychiatry 32:995–1008, 1975

MacKenzie KR: Commentary: when to recommend group treatment. Int J Group Psychother 36:207–210, 1986

Mayer GR, Baker P: Group counseling with elementary school children: a look at group size. Elementary School Guidance and Counseling Journal 1:140–145, 1967

Parloff MB, Dies RR: Group psychotherapy outcome research 1966–1975. Int J Group Psychother 27:281–319, 1977

Paul GL: Behavior modification research: design and tactics, in Behavior Therapy: Appraisal and Status. Edited by Franks CM. New York, McGraw-Hill, 1969, pp 29–62.

Rose SD, Edleson JL: Working With Children and Adolescents in Groups. San Francisco, CA, Jossey-Bass, 1987

Slavson SR: Introduction to Group Therapy. New York, Commonwealth Fund and Harvard University Press, 1943

Slavson SR: Analytic Group Psychotherapy. New York, Columbia University Press, 1950

Stone WN, Rutan JS: Duration of treatment in group psychotherapy. Int J Group Psychother 34:93–110, 1984

Toseland RW, Siporin M: When to recommend group treatment: a review of the clinical and the research literature. Int J Group Psychother 36:171–201, 1986

Wood K: Casework effectiveness: a new look at the research evidence. Social Work 23:437–459, 1978

# CHAPTER 7

# Supervision

*Edward S. Soo, M.S.*

Dyadic supervision has been the primary mode of practice in the field of psychotherapy. It has continued into child and adolescent group psychotherapy. Until recently, there has been scant reporting on supervision and training of child and adolescent group therapists (Kymissis 1991; Riester 1992; Soo 1986).

Slavson and Schiffer (1975) stressed individual supervision and weekly conferences with the supervisor to review and discuss the protocols of each session. An informal group discussion with therapists was added and was led by the supervisor. The emphasis was on the pattern and meaning of group members' behavior with respect to their problems. Discussions were about the therapists' responses to the members and the group as a whole ("but no effort must be made to identify the therapist's psychological reactions and attitudes. The supervisor should be pragmatic ... not involving the therapist's own feelings," pp. 267–268).

In Dies's (1980) review of more than 200 reports on adult group therapy training methods, he found agreement on four general categories: academic, observation, experiential, and supervision. The academic component consists of selected reading, presentation of didactic material, films, and role-playing. Observation is direct observation of

---

I wish to thank Dr. Alvin H. Richmond and the many therapists and patients whose work in group made this chapter possible.

groups. The use of experiential groups includes therapy, T-group, and personal group experiences. Supervision consists of various supervisory methods such as the dyad, cotherapists, group discussions, and the use of video and one-way mirrors. He found the most common problem of novice group therapists to be their difficulty with the group model. Training should emphasize group process in order to experience the group as a modality.

In a 1987 survey reported by Kymissis et al. (1991), 125 questionnaires were sent to all training directors of child and adolescent psychiatry. The response was 42.2%. They found the directors' orientation was primarily eclectic or dynamic, although there were a few analytic models and one behavioral model. An important question revealed that most group coordinators and group therapists were not M.D.'s. About 4% did research in child and adolescent group psychotherapy. Under the question "What type of supervision was offered?" no data were provided.

Kymissis (1991) reviewed his development of a training program in a teaching hospital for child and adolescent group therapy. He reported it as part of an overall training program for the child and adolescent psychiatric fellows. In addition to the program for the training of child and adolescent psychiatry, the fellows participated in a didactic seminar on child and adolescent group therapy.

In the first year's rotation, the fellows led their own inpatient groups on the child and adolescent units. In the second year, the fellows were assigned to outpatient groups. The patients ranged from kindergarten age through early and late latency to young and late adolescence. Parallel groups with the parents of the kindergarten and latency-age children were conducted by staff members. In their second year, the fellows participated in group supervision with mutual presentation of their groups. Kymissis (1991) found an adequate balance of cognitive offerings and experiential group participation that made possible valuable learning for trainees.

Riester (1992) reported on collaboration between a university and a community mental health facility to provide training in and supervision of child and adolescent group therapy. Social work graduate students and psychiatry residents participated in the program. They combined their resources, academic facilities, and on-site facilities to develop a training program. Their cooperation was found to benefit both institutions in enhancement of standards of practice and provision of quality service to the patient population. The program was able to incorporate the four factors of Dies's study (1980).

# ◆ Supervisory Format

The supervisory model suggested by Slavson and Schiffer was expanded by the author. A combined format of individual and group supervision included the following as training objectives: selection and formation of a patient group, understanding group formation and dynamics, subgroup and group resistance, and use of countertransference reactions in the management of individual and group resistance.

The therapist must have an excellent ability to relate to children and adolescents. His or her ability to accept and empathize with their mode of emotional expression is important in establishing relationships with them. The task of the novice group therapist is the comprehension of his or her patients' life histories, developmental needs, and psychopathology. Rosenthal (1977) affirmed that it is important that the group therapist understand the individual's dynamics within the group. The capacity to handle the group as an entity, the therapist's awareness of his or her own feelings in response to the group's interaction, and the recognition of group resistance are necessary for the group therapist to learn through the supervisory process.

The supervisory process for the novice group therapist should address these issues through the combination of individual and group formats. The combination of individual and group processes provides flexibility to target the specific learning needs of the novice group therapist. Learning is reinforced through the integration of didactic and experiential group experiences. The combined method of supervision offers a comprehensive approach to learning group psychotherapy with children and adolescents. This method does not exclude academic and other ancillary learning experiences offered as options outside of the supervisory format (Dies 1980).

## Individual Supervision

Although novice group therapists participate in a supervisory group, they are supervised individually regarding the formation of their groups. Individual supervision offers a didactic learning experience through a dyadic relationship with the supervisor. The dyadic process focuses on the novices' specific learning needs with respect to understanding the child or adolescent in group psychotherapy. In forming a group, the novice learns—through the process of selection—group balance, differential diagnosis, and the role and task of a group psychotherapist. The choice of an appropriate model is based on the children's and adolescents' age groups: preschool, latency age, preadolescent, young adolescent, middle adolescent, or older adolescent. The model chosen should address emotional needs, the structure of the group, and the problems of the specific age group. The role of a group therapist is discussed. The use of screening interviews with the parents or caretakers and group members should increase the novice's understanding of diagnosis, dynamics, and resistance. The interviews provide insights into precursors of premature termination in children and adolescents receiving group psychotherapy (Soo 1977).

The novice becomes familiar with children's and adolescents' developmental levels, emotional deficits, psychopathology, and potential resistances. He or she learns and understands each member's life history and dynamics and how these factors contribute to the transferences in the group. From the protocol of clinical material, the issues of transference, countertransference, and the novice therapist's activity are discussed. As the beginner becomes more knowledgeable about each of his or her group members, he or she becomes less anxious while conducting the group.

## Cotherapists

Cotherapy is a mutually supportive learning experience for novice group therapists. It is used as an apprentice training method in some psychiatric hospitals and mental health agencies. An experienced group therapist is coupled with a novice to help the novice learn how to conduct group therapy. As novices become more experienced, they are assigned to a new group, graduate, or become trainers for other novice group therapists. Some uses of cotherapists are designed for special populations and the specific problems of children or adolescents in groups. Other uses of cotherapy are for structure and mutual support. Male and female cotherapists are used as role models for corrective emotional experiences in object relations.

The format of individual and group supervision applies to cotherapists. The cotherapists are supervised as a couple in individual supervision and together as members of a supervisory group. In addition to the process of supervision, the supervisor should focus on the developing working relationship between the cotherapists. Their impact on their group should be viewed both as individual and dual relationships to the group. To complete his or her training as a group psychotherapist, each should lead his or her own group.

# ◆ Group Format and Structure

MacLennan (1977) and Schamess (1976) observed that various models of children's group psychotherapy have different formats. The structure of the group and the role and activity of the group psychotherapist differ according to the different tasks and goals of the models. The wide spectrum of emotional disorders in children and adolescents receiving treatment in various settings requires a variety of group therapy models. The objective is to address the different treatment needs and goals (Kraft 1980).

In an extensive survey of the literature on children's groups, Schamess (1986) addressed the issue of differential diagnosis and group structure in the placement of children in group psychotherapy. He used DSM-III typology (American Psychiatric Association 1980) and formulated three major diagnostic categories for children: developmental or personality disorders, psychosis, and neurosis. He used differential diagnosis as a conceptual framework to select a specific group structure for an age-specific group from the models used. An appropriate group structure provides a facilitating environment for group treatment, including the material and physical environment, to achieve optimum treatment goals. Group structure is critically important for treatment of impulse-ridden, borderline, and psychotic children and least important for children with higher-level intrapsychic functioning. Neurotic children make positive use of groups that promote affective expression and insights. Similarly, thoughtful considerations regarding differential diagnosis of adolescents and their need for group structure are applied when adolescents are selected for group treatment.

The choice of group format and structure is based on the age-specific developmental stages and diagnoses of the children or adolescents. On the basis of diagnostic and dynamic understanding of the children, various models have been developed for different age groups. Preschool play groups, latency-age activity groups, and activity-discussion groups are designed for preschoolers, latency-age, and preadolescent children, respectively. Interview-discussion groups are appropriate for middle adolescents, and interpretative group psychotherapy is appropriate for older adolescents. Each model has a specific format for each age group. In addition to group format and structure, another consideration is the amount of regression necessary to create a group treatment milieu. To provide an appropriate therapeutic atmosphere in a group, regression must be managed. The group psychotherapist regulates the amount of permissiveness and structure to allow for effective group treatment.

The short-term group provides task-oriented treatment that uses a structured format to deal with specific problems. The group is designed for problem solving. Goals are set for decision making and task completion. The life of the group is time limited, with a beginning, middle, and termination process. Differential diagnosis and appropriate age range of group members should be considered when assigning children and adolescents to short-term group treatment.

# ◆ Selection

Slavson and Schiffer (1975) and Schamess (1986) placed special emphasis on selection to achieve appropriate placement of children and adolescents. Therapists use diagnostic and dynamic understanding of patients to match them to groups according to age appropriateness, developmental needs, and therapeutic tasks. They also consider whether the group environment can be structured to meet the patients' needs. Not all children or adolescents are appropriate for group treatment. Some children or adolescents are excluded because of their inability to sustain a group experience or because of a primary need for a one-to-one relationship. Psychotic or brain-damaged children do very poorly in unstructured groups. They have no inner resources and limited controls. They risk emotional inundation, and their fragile egos become overwhelmed. If a group is indicated for atypical children, a group setting is organized to provide the necessary structure to meet the members' therapeutic needs (Trafimow and Pattak 1981, 1982).

A thoughtless selective process that neglects consideration of a balanced membership dooms a group to failure (Soo 1991). For instance, a group composed of highly aggressive and impulsive adolescents with conduct disorder creates turmoil. Such a group leaves the group therapist feeling helpless and struggling for control. The group becomes destructive and fails to achieve therapeutic results. Another example is a group of very depressed and withdrawn children. Instead of creating a therapeutic atmosphere, the group is emotionally dead. The group members becomes resistant to the group psychotherapist's efforts to revive the group.

An overbalanced or imbalanced group establishes a specific dynamic toward an emotional valence that becomes destructive to the group's treatment.

Groups that have similar core issues, symptom pictures, and dynamics should be balanced according to diagnosis, age, and sex. Children and adolescents who have had similar traumatic experiences, such as alcoholism, divorce, bereavement, or sexual abuse, can find commonality in a mutually supportive, homogeneous group.

Balanced grouping of children and adolescents moves the group toward equilibrium. Balance involves the placement of members with varying degrees of adaptive and defensive mechanisms to promote a broad spectrum of interaction, behavior, and feelings. The contrasting relationships and behavioral patterns will create various levels of conflict in object relationships. These conflicts arise out of group interaction in the process of group treatment. A well-balanced group will develop its internal mechanism to permit and limit the boundary of regressive activity. The group will self-regulate the amounts of anxiety related to aggressive and libidinal drives according to what it can safely tolerate.

The sex of the group therapist influences the group formed (Scheidlinger 1992). Inappropriate placement of a group therapist and members by sex disregards the developmental sexual issues of children and young adolescents. Groups composed of preschoolers through young adolescents are usually single sex and are led by a group therapist of the same sex. Time-limited homogeneous groups in which members have similar issues can be coeducational and led by group therapists of either or both sexes. Middle and older adolescent groups are usually coeducational and are led by either sex.

## Screening Interview

After each patient is reviewed as a potential candidate for group membership, he or she is screened to validate the selection. The purpose of the screening interview is to observe the patient's and the parents' presentations of their problems. Their attitudes toward group membership, their requests, and their expectations provide the group psychotherapist with insights into resistance that could arise in the group. The induced feelings conveyed in the screening interview help the group therapist to anticipate how the patient will function in the therapist's group. It provides clues as to how the novice therapist needs to relate to each member therapeutically. His or her therapeutic stance toward each member is based on diagnosis, the patient's emotional and developmental needs, and dynamic understanding of the patient's life history. The novice can determine his or her overall perception of the group and can discuss concerns about his or her role as a group psychotherapist. Questions can be raised about the potential dynamics and resistance reenacted in group treatment.

The training in selection and the screening interviews allow assessment of the novice's learning needs with respect to diagnosis, understanding dynamics, and resistance. The novice learns about his or her role as group therapist in relation to each member and to the group as a whole. His or her countertransference reactions (Soo 1980) to the selective and screening processes are part of the training process. The novice's awareness of countertransference feelings is necessary to minimize the unconscious bias that contributes to premature termination and resistance in group treatment (Soo 1977).

### Case Example

Two 13-year-old girls were referred to group psychotherapy. Both youngsters were from broken homes, had a history of poor school-work, and had chronic difficulties with peer relationships. Each of the girls had severe problems in relationships with her mother at home.

Sharon was a product of an unknown father and a teenage drug-addicted mother. She was raised by her maternal grandmother, who was strict and punitive. Sharon was described in school as highly disruptive, with a bad mouth. She invited negative attention. She was often scapegoated by her classmates.

Cheryl had witnessed fighting between her mother and an alcoholic father. In a state of drunkenness, he had often physically abused her mother. After the father separated from the family, the mother complained that Cheryl was abusive toward her. She acted helpless toward Cheryl and felt victimized by her daughter. In school, Cheryl was argumentative with her teachers. She fought and intimidated her classmates and had gained a reputation as a bully.

Initially, the novice thought that both girls were ideal for her group. Both Sharon and Cheryl had problems with peers. She felt that the group's interaction would address their conflicts in relationships. On further examination, however, their character problems were too severe. They would immediately become engrossed in a sadomasochistic relationship. Their conflict would turn the group process into a secondary-gain behavior, which would become destructive to the group.

A child's tendency to be scapegoated or to bully can be helped in a group where the members are able to confront their character problems. Scapegoating is often part of the process of group formation. A member may provoke scapegoating as a role in a group or as a symptom of group resistance. However, if a pathological scapegoater and a scapegoat were in the same group, they would only entrench the group and the novice group psychotherapist in their pathology.

# ◆ Countertransference

Included in the supervisory process are issues regarding countertransference reactions that emanate from the clinical material. The novice group psychotherapist learns that countertransference reactions can be used as an instrument of treatment.

Rosenthal (1953) reported on countertransference that typically arises in activity group therapy. He observed that group psychotherapists who begin with group psychotherapy of children must endure the reawakening of repressed conflicts caused by feelings about their childhood and familial life experiences.

Inherent in the process of child and adolescent group psychotherapy are individual and multiple transferences and the group psychotherapist's reactions to the feelings caused by these transferences. Child and adolescent transferences, though similar to adult transferences, are not identical to them. Child and adolescent transferences demonstrate a combination of current life experiences and maturational needs, as well as the reenactment of conflicts resulting from emotional deprivations and family pathologies.

If the interaction derived from countertransference reactions continues to be unrecognized, these unconscious feelings will solidify the group into a state of group transference resistance. The group will be established on the emotional level of the novice group therapist's unresolved conflicts. Left unattended, the group will experience no movement in treatment. Such a group is in a state of treatment resistance that will destroy the group.

The supervisor prepares the novice for the inevitable eventuality of countertransference. He or she assists the novice to understand the dynamic operation of individual and multiple transferences in the group. The novice's recognition of his or her reactions to the individual and multiple transferences can be used constructively to clarify the dynamics of ongoing transferences. If the novice learns to differentiate his or her subjective countertransference reactions from objective ones, he or she will be in touch with these feelings. The novice learns to be sensitized emotionally to his or her patient group. Identification of the objective countertransference reactions that emerge from the group treatment process, as opposed to the subjective countertransference reactions, becomes the focus in the supervisory process.

The subjective countertransference reactions provide clues to the level of psychic conflict that the transference generates. The control of subjective countertransference feelings is the novice's responsibility. Analysis of objective countertransference reactions helps develop insights into the dynamics of member and group transference. When the novice understands the objective countertransference reactions, he or she can use the induced feelings from the interaction to communicate appropriately. An intervention is developed that is appropriate to the content in the context of the transference resistance. Use of countertransference reactions as an instrument to resolve transference resistance enhances the group therapist's skill and adds a valuable dimension to his or her treatment repertoire. Using himself or herself to monitor the induced emotional communication from the transference, the novice becomes an effective instrument for the management of transference in child and adolescent group psychotherapy (Soo 1980).

## ◆ Supervisor's Task

The supervision of group psychotherapy involves a triangular relationship of supervisor, novice group therapist, and patient group. The symbolic role of the supervisor as an authority and parental figure must be considered in the learning experience with the novices. The relationship between the supervisor and novice influences the novice's role as a group therapist through identification. The supervisor's individualization of the novice's learning needs and assessment of his or her capacity for learning places the supervisor in a vulnerable position. The supervisor's reactions to the expression of acceptance, approval, dependency, and various other feelings of compliance by the novice must be recognized in the supervisory process. Obstacles to learning may be created from the underlying emotional components in the relationship.

A major part of the supervisor's task is to create a receptive atmosphere of trust. This atmosphere assures the novice that his or her revelation of feelings and vulnerabilities is held in confidence. The novice's feelings toward the patient group are subject to analysis as a constructive means of understanding the group. The novice's feelings toward the supervisor and the supervisory group are clarified to support his or her learning. The supervisor's task is to maintain the narrow line between supervision and treatment. The supervisory and training process may have therapeutic value, but it is not group psychotherapy.

Another task of the supervisor is to create a receptive atmosphere for learning. How the supervisor handles the novice's developing resistance to the supervisory process becomes integral to the novice's training. Novices can readily become defensive about the clinical material. The anxieties provoked by the children and adolescents from the novice's patient group are exposed. The supervisory group is designed to ensure that the novice's presentation of clinical material is examined constructively.

The supervisor's handling of the developing resistance in supervision becomes integral to the training process.

Novice group therapists have little or no experience with groups. In their presentations of material about their groups, novices rely mostly on their experience as individual psychotherapists. Novices tend to relate to the individuals in the group rather than to the group as a whole. They report their observations of and relationships to the group members from the individual perspective. Novices need help with the transition from an individual perspective to a group one. They need to attend to individual dynamics in the context of the group's dynamics.

As novices accept the group as a whole, they begin to recognize issues involving group dynamics. The dynamics of group formation are studied from a developmental point of view. The process of equalization of power among the peer group members and the development of individual, subgroup, and group transference resistance can be examined from the perspective of the novices' groups. The application of object-relations concepts is identified, studied, and discussed on the basis of the clinical presentation (Soo 1992).

# ◆ Novice's Reaction

Novices can deal with the loss of their first patient more adequately than they can with the loss of their first group. The loss of a group can be the most demoralizing experience that a potential group therapist can have with child and adolescent group psychotherapy. It is equivalent to a loss of a family. Therapists have abstained from use of the group modality because of the enduring negative imprint left by their loss of a first group. The experience damaged their feeling of competence as group psychotherapists.

Conducting a group with a support system of training and supervision is an anxious situation for all novice group therapists. If novices undertake a group without training and supervision, they do themselves a professional disservice and provide destructive treatment to their patients. They contribute to their own incompetence as group therapists.

When the composition of his or her group is completed, the novice faces a period of anxiety during which he or she is initially exposed to group. A beginning individual psychotherapist can maintain a higher degree of control over a patient than a novice group psychotherapist can over a group of patients. How many patients will show up—all, some, or none? In the novice's first session, he or she is confronted with eight patients observing and testing him or her as a leader. The novice experiences a sense of loss of control, uncertainty, and unpredictability.

The combined format of supervision predisposes novices to another anxiety situation. They are expected to present material about their group to fellow colleagues for supervision. This can generate for the novices a spectrum of feelings, defenses, and behavioral attitudes that are reflected in the learning situation. They are more vulnerable in the supervisory group. As learners with colleagues, they risk exposure of their mistakes and threats to their self-esteem and self-image. Positive recognition of the attitudes and behavior that each novice contributes to the supervisory process is important. Understanding the effects that the underlying process has on the novice's learning helps remove individual and group obstacles to learning group treatment.

## ◆ Supervisory Group Process

The supervisory group is composed of novice group therapists as participant members and the supervisor as leader of the group. Prerequisite for membership in the supervisory group is that members have a patient group of children, adolescents, or their parents. A member who is in the process of completing a group is eligible. No exceptions are allowed.

An agreement is made with the novice therapists that the supervisory group's task is to help members to be better group therapists. They are to present material about their patient groups for supervisory assistance. The role of the supervisor is to facilitate that agreement. The goals of the agreement are achieved through mutual assistance and shared learning based on the novices' presentation of material about their groups. The supervisor explains that the novices will experience feelings of being members of a group. This experience is achieved through members' interaction and participation in the supervisory group. The supervisor studies the members' deviation from the agreement to help each other become better group therapists as signals of resistance. The group sessions start promptly and end as scheduled.

Late arrivals to sessions are common manifestations of resistance. In every instance of lateness, the leader attempts to explore whether it may be an individual or a group resistance. Typical explanations are "I had a session that ran over" and "I was delayed because of a case conference."

It is crucial to explore the importance of lateness or absences as symbols of resistance. Lateness may be a precursor to testing limits and the leader's role in the supervisory group. Behind the resistance are concerns about safety, trust, confidentiality, and management of aggression. Members challenge the leader's competence to deal with their concerns and learning. Individual and group resistance arises from the group's process. How the leader handles the resistance provides an example of how he or she performs the role as leader. A more pertinent question is paramount in the minds of the members. Is group psychotherapy a legitimate modality of psychotherapy? The leader's appropriate handling of the presenting resistance facilitates the group toward the next phase of group formation.

## Initial Supervisory Group Experiences

In the beginning of the supervisory group, the novices believed that their groups were not completely formed and that they lacked material to present to the group. The leader offered the supervisory group the choice of deciding on a topic and format until their patient groups were formed and ready for presentation. When the supervisory group was given the choice to decide, the members began to struggle with divergent views for an agenda. The regressive pull of the group influenced some members to ask the leader for direction; other members, asserting their independence, wanted to establish their own agenda. A power struggle developed as a result of the members' attempts to impose their views on each other. The struggle brought out conflicts, anxieties, frustration, and anger in the members.

For many of the members, the power struggle reactivated previous emotional struggles and roles in familial and peer relationships. These were displaced and projected on the supervisory group in the form of splitting into subgroups. There were hostile confrontations between members, a tendency toward scapegoating, and childish or adolescent-like behavior. Complaints about authority and members' being confused were all expressions of individual and group resistance toward the regressive forces of the group's process. The impasse that the group developed was the group's resistance to arriving at an agenda.

The supervisory group's inability to resolve the impasse required the leader's intervention. The leader explored the impasse by inquiring whether he had contributed to the group's immobility. The inquiry brought on a series of complaints: "There are too many arguments," "We can't agree on anything," "This is a crazy group," "It's too much like group therapy."

The leader agreed that the supervisory group appeared confused, frustrated, and at an impasse, but the group was not contracted for group psychotherapy. The novices were reminded of the agreement, and no agreement was made for them to reveal their life history, dreams, or problems. It was legitimate for the novices to discuss their feelings as members of the group and their observations about the leader's role and handling of the group.

The leader's role was scrutinized: "You're too laid back," "You should be more active instead of being passive," "All you are concerned with is us being on time." The leader was blamed for letting the group get out of control: "You should have shown more preparation and provided an agenda."

Some supervisory group members wanted to continue with the present course of the group's process. They felt the experiential method was a positive learning experience. The group was not able to reach consensus. The leader accommodated the subgroup that preferred a more didactic approach.

A bibliography with required reading was proposed, and the members were to report their assignments to the group for discussion. The group expressed reluctance to report the assignments, protesting that they were overwhelmed by paperwork and that the leader's demands were unrealistic. They preferred the leader to lecture.

The Slavson film on activity group therapy [1] was shown. Several other topics relating to diagnosis, selection, and various models of child and adolescent group psychotherapy were examined. As the lectures proceeded, it became evident to the leader that the group was bored with the didactic material. He observed that the group was oversaturated with the leader's lectures.

A member suggested that material about one of their patient therapy groups be presented. The supervisory group agreed, but expressed reluctance about presenting this material. Members felt vulnerable to the risk of exposing themselves to the group's aggression and hostility. They were explicit with each other as to what would prevent them from presenting material: they anticipated painful reactions to their colleagues' potential criticism. The members' concerns were recognized and accepted as realistic. The group thoroughly discussed the need for an atmosphere of mutual trust before any member could fully participate in cooperative learning.

---

[1] *Activity Group Therapy,* obtainable through American Group Psychotherapy Association, 25 East 21st Street, 6th Floor, New York, NY 10010

# ◆ Supervisory Group Goals

The experiential-process group accomplishes two goals. First, the novices are involved in a group as members rather than leaders. Their participation in the process of group formation, their exposure to regressive interaction and behavior, and the development of individual and group resistance simulates the atmosphere and emotional impact of a dynamic group. The group process creates sensitivity to the multitudes of feelings encountered. This enables the novices to develop some emotional insulation to tolerate the impact of feelings induced by children and adolescents in group treatment.

The second goal is the evolution of a training group into a supervisory group. It is essential that the training group effectively overcome the obstacles to this evolution to achieve a group atmosphere of trust and cooperation. Any novices require a cooperative group to expose their work to scrutiny and learn to use countertransference reactions in the management of individual and group resistance. The goal of the supervisor as leader is to develop an appropriate group atmosphere of trust and cooperation. By dealing with distrust as a manifestation of resistance in supervisory group, members become more receptive to learning to be better group therapists in child and adolescent group psychotherapy.

## Supervisory Group Experience With Presentations

The novices were presenting vignettes about their groups without revealing too much clinical material that required supervisory comments from the group. This pattern of presentation was recognized by a member. He stated that the presenters left much to be desired and the group agreed. The leader suggested that perhaps the novices no longer needed supervisory help. Laughter ensued. The members' reluctance to present fully was recognized. They revealed their concerns about adequacy, feelings of incompetence, and questions of confidentiality. The members were uncomfortable that their work with groups might be discussed outside of the supervisory group. When their concerns were addressed, the novices were more comfortable in presenting material about their groups openly.

Hilarity and teasing of a member by two other members were exciting the supervisory group. The leader commented on the excitement of the group. He wondered whether he should interrupt the members when they were having such a good time. The teased member said laughingly that she was being picked on by the guys. The other members said that she did not mind and enjoyed the attention. The leader asked who was next in line to gain the benefits of the group's teasing?

The sexual undertones of the excitement were discussed by the members. This discussion led the teased member to acknowledge that there was sexual acting out in her adolescent girls' group. This sexual acting out produced sexual excitement similar to that in the supervisory group. The excitement was analyzed as a manifestation of group resistance in her group. The novice therapist acknowledged that she was concerned about the sexual escapades of the girls in her group. She had become interested, and her group obliged her by expounding their exploits. She displayed the feelings of sexual excitement induced by her therapy group in the supervisory group. She realized from the induced countertransference reactions that she was seduced by the reports of their exploits. Because she was intrigued by the group members' sexual encounters, the group's resistance persisted. Once the resistance was understood, the supervisory group helped develop an appropriate intervention.

The novices' avoidance of presentation was symbolic of resistance. To encourage more open presentation of material about the therapy groups, the supervisory group needed to investigate and understand the resistance. The manifestations of individual and group resistance in a supervisory group are frequently disguised. The latent content induced by the transference resistance in the novices' groups is revealed in the manifested interaction of the supervisory group.

Focusing prematurely on the novice's activity before understanding his or her group's dynamics only draws attention to the novice. It invites the novice to be more preoccupied with his or her self-image, self-esteem, and defenses. He or she becomes emotionally less available to be in touch with the dynamics of his or her group. The novice's reactions to the feelings induced by his or her group are deferred. The novice becomes defensive and ceases to learn group treatment.

The material presented in supervisory group induces reactions and behavior from the novices. Observation of the supervisory group's reactive behavior often provides insights into the dynamics of the patient groups. Analysis of the parallel behavior in the supervisory group helps novices to understand and manage transference and countertransference resistance within their patient groups.

The supervisory group should focus on understanding the dynamics of the patient group about whom material is being presented. History of the patient members, reenactment of the dynamics on their individual and multiple transferences, and the impact of these transferences on the novices as manifested in induced countertransference reactions are explored by supervisory group members. The exploration facilitates cooperation. Countertransference reactions of the novices are accepted as providing insights into their reactions to the transference. An appropriate intervention is developed based on the supervisory group's understanding of the dynamics demonstrated by the group's interaction. The intervention is developed cooperatively by the novices in the supervisory group.

## ◆ Summary

The didactic approach to supervision is essentially geared toward reinforcing the cognitive learning and technical abilities of the novice. The didactic approach is limited in its ability to incorporate observations of group phenomena. The combination of individual and group supervision transcends the dyadic approach to supervising child and adolescent group psychotherapists. The combined supervisory format in the form of a training and experiential group supports the integration of cognitive learning with clinical practice. Through the novice's participation as a member of a group, he or she experiences the process of group formation and engages in the development of individual and group resistance. He or she observes how the supervisor handles the group. The novice learns how to apply didactic material by way of the group experience.

It provides the flexibility for learning group treatment. In going through the learning process of forming their groups, novices comprehend developmental and emotional needs of children and adolescents. The novices learn from the screening and selection process to form a balanced group and to understand diagnostic and pathological issues. The process enables them to experience some of the impact of dynamics and resistance. They understand the need to choose a specific group modality that is matched appropriately to the age of the child or adolescent.

The use of an experiential supervisory group enables novice group therapists to become familiar with group treatment. As members, novices participate in group formation. They become more sensitive to group dynamics through observation and participation. They interact with other members in a process of development of individual, subgroup, and group resistance. Through the process of working through the basic distrust among members, novices become more receptive to supervision. Their participation as members of the supervisory group enhances their skill in understanding group process. They can identify with the members of their patient group as a result of their experience as members of a supervisory group. They gain security in the use of the group modality.

The evolution of the novice as a member from an experiential training group to a supervisory group marks a positive transition for cooperative learning. The combined method of individual and supervisory group maximizes training and supervision in children's and adolescents' group psychotherapy.

The challenge for the supervisor is to facilitate the learning experience of the novice group psychotherapists. Maintaining the quality of the standards is the task of the supervisor in training and supervision. It aids the novice group psychotherapists in becoming competent professionals in group psychotherapy with children and adolescents.

Reactivation of the child and adolescent committee of the American Group Psychotherapy Association has led to revising previous guidelines to establish standards of qualification for child and adolescent group psychotherapists.

Psychiatric hospitals, mental health clinics, residential treatment centers, and schools serving children and adolescents with group modalities that operate on good intentions achieve at best a poor beginning and encouragement for an unsuccessful outcome. Administrators and therapists who lack knowledge and experience in group therapy make inappropriate use of groups. These persons reveal an inadequate understanding of children, adolescents, and parents in diagnosis, psychopathology, and treatment needs and goals. Their naivete does great disservice to treatment programs, professional staff, and the patient population. The lack of understanding of standards and the lack of a support system of training and supervision deny a group therapist constructive use of a treatment modality. Untrained group therapists depreciate the value of group therapy as a modality and fail to provide the proven, quality service they could provide to their patient group of children, adolescents, and parents.

## ◆ References

American Psychiatric Association: Diagnostic and Statistical Manual of Mental Disorders, 3rd Edition. Washington, DC, American Psychiatric Association, 1980

Dies R: Current practice in the training of group psychotherapists. Int J Group Psychother 30:169–185, 1980

Kraft IA: Group therapy with children and adolescents, in Treatment of Emotional Disorders in Children and Adolescents: Medical and Psychological Approaches to Treatment, Edited by Benson RM, Blinder BJ, Sholevar GF. New York, Spectrum, 1980, pp 109–132

Kymissis P: Training in adolescent group psychotherapy. Journal of Child and Adolescent Group Psychotherapy 1(4):237–242, 1991

Kymissis P, Licamele W, Boots S, et al: Training in child and adolescent group therapy: two surveys and a model. Group 15(3):163–167, 1991

MacLennan BW: Modification of activity group therapy for children. Int J Group Psychother 27:85–96, 1977

Riester AE: Partnering to train group therapist. Journal of Child and Adolescent Group Therapy 2(1):53–60, 1992

Rosenthal L: Countertransference in activity group therapy. Int J Group Psychother 3:431–440, 1953

Rosenthal L: Qualifications and tasks of the therapist in group therapy with children. Clinical Social Work Journal 5:191–199, 1977

Schamess GH: Group treatment modalities for latency age children. Int J Group Psychother 26:455–475, 1976

Schamess GH: Differential diagnosis and group structure in outpatient treatment of latency age children, in Child Group Psychotherapy: Future Tense. Edited by Riester AE, Kraft IA. Madison, CT, International Universities Press, 1986, pp 29–68

Scheidlinger S: Therapist gender in child-adolescent treatment groups. Journal of Child and Adolescent Group Therapy 2:105–108, 1992

Slavson SR, Schiffer M: Group Psychotherapies for Children: A Textbook. New York, International Universities Press, 1975

Soo ES: The impact of collaborative treatment on premature termination in activity group therapy. Group 1(4):222–234, 1977

Soo ES: The impact of transference and countertransference in activity group therapy. Group 4(4):27–41, 1980

Soo ES: Training and supervision in child and adolescent group psychotherapy, in Child Group Psychotherapy: Future Tense. Edited by Riester AE, Kraft IA. Madison, CT, International Universities Press, 1986, pp 157–171

Soo ES: Strategies for success for the beginning group therapist with child and adolescent groups. Journal of Child and Adolescent Group Therapy 1(2):95–106, 1991

Soo ES: The management of resistance in the application of object relations concepts in children and adolescents group psychotherapy. Journal of Child and Adolescent Group Therapy 2(2):77–92, 1992

Trafimow E, Pattak S: Group psychotherapy and object development in children. Int J Group Psychother 31:193–204, 1981

Trafimow E, Pattak S: Group treatment of primitively fixated children. Int J Group Psychother 32:445–452, 1982

# CHAPTER 8

# Anatomy of Exits From Inpatient Adolescent Therapy

*Harvey Roy Greenberg, M.D.*

The greater potential for turbulent behavior in adolescent groups compared with their adult counterparts is well known. An adolescent group therapist regularly encounters physical and verbal displays ranging from amusing high jinks to alarming actions directed at property or person—including the therapist's person (e.g., see Cerda et al. 1991; Corder et al. 1981; Crowdes 1975; Fluet et al. 1980; Friedman et al. 1975; Lange 1980; Ramos and Richmond 1991).

Even neurotic teenagers or youngsters with relatively mild character pathology may become surprisingly unruly in group. However, the more disturbed group members are correspondingly more likely to act out. In this chapter, I address a particularly disruptive group therapy occurrence: leaving sessions either by choice or on demand (subsequently referred to as *elective* or *compelled* exiting). Despite the frequency of such exiting, there is no substantive English literature on this phenomenon.

In this chapter, I explore a number of exit scenarios encountered in several inpatient adolescent settings and describe the diagnostic and character types involved. I also discuss group dynamics and influences extrinsic to the group that foment exits, describe behavior after exiting, and discuss the impact of exiting on those remaining behind. Pertinent management issues are addressed.

Although my remarks are based on work with inpatient groups, I hope they prove helpful to therapists grappling with the less common, but no less troublesome, exits from outpatient adolescent group therapy.

# ◆ Settings

Observations are based on my experience from 1965 through 1985 as an attending or supervising psychiatrist in several different adolescent treatment programs.[1] The stay in these settings ranged from 6 weeks to several months on one acute-care unit and from several months to years on two long-term units.

The patients' ages ranged from 12 to 17 years, with the sexes about equally represented. Socioeconomic backgrounds ranged from maximally impoverished to lower middle class; African American and Hispanic clients predominated over whites, with a few Asian Americans. Predominant diagnostic categories were schizophrenia, major depression, borderline states, and conduct disturbances in which one of the preceding diagnoses usually underpinned (and often influenced) the disordered conduct. Relatively few patients had mental retardation, anxiety states, or neurotic or personality disorders uncontaminated by more serious pathology.

# ◆ Group Therapy Structure

Group therapy was part of an intensive milieu program, with other modalities running concurrently (e.g., individual, occupational, and recreational therapy and school). Groups were composed of 8–10 patients of both sexes and were balanced as well as circumstances

---

[1] Successively, these adolescent treatment programs were the Inpatient Adolescent Service, Bronx Municipal Hospital Center, 1965–1967; the Inpatient Adolescent Program, Training Wards, Bronx Psychiatric Center, 1967–1971; and the Inpatient Service, Bronx Children's Psychiatric Center, 1972 through the present. All are under the auspices of the Department of Psychiatry, Albert Einstein College of Medicine, The Bronx, New York.

permitted regarding age, sex, social background, diagnosis, level of functioning, and personal style (e.g., extraversion versus introversion, verbalization skills).

Groups were led by cotherapists drawn from the various milieu disciplines; psychiatrists, psychologists, and psychiatric social workers predominated. Whenever possible, cotherapy teams were male and female and contained at least one member with considerable group experience.

Group therapy was talk oriented, as opposed to task oriented, and was psychoanalytically inflected according to the leaders' various theoretical backgrounds. Generally, grappling with immediate experiences within the group and on the ward led to the healing experiences of group (see, for example, Slavson 1964 and Yalom 1975; studies that specifically concern adolescent groups include Bekrowitz 1972, Brandes 1973, Chase 1991, and Scheidlinger 1985). Family and family-related transferential issues were less likely to be dwelt on by patients and were less an interpretive focus for therapists. However, groups that ran longer and contained better-functioning youngsters did allow for interpretive work of greater depth.

Although the benefits of group participation were stressed, patients were never compelled to join a group if they continued to raise objections that could not be worked through in individual therapy or by other means. Once in group, patients were not forced to attend a session if they were judged by themselves or others to be too troubled to do so, although this issue was not always easily assessed.

Initial guidelines for group members included coming on time, maintaining confidentiality, and allowing each other to speak without interruption. Patients were told they could leave a session when they wished, after presenting their reasons to the group (a rule often broken). It was emphasized that harm or threat of harm to person or property would not be tolerated and would constitute grounds for being taken out of group temporarily or permanently. Some therapists presented further reasons for removal such as excessive high jinks, teasing, sexual play, and behavior otherwise disruptive to effective group functioning. Others chose to discuss removal for such problems when the need arose, lest the leadership appear too heavy-handed or excessively preoccupied with rules.

## ◆ Exit Categories

Exit scenarios are legion, and I submit that *any* adolescent group member can become an exiter. The following list, drawn from my clinical experience, is notably selective. Common categories mingle with idiosyncratic ones.

Some exits were precipitated by intrapsychic pathology or events in the patient's life outside the hospital, or both. Others chiefly evolved out of group process. Still others arose from the impact of ward events on the group. However, there was rarely only one reason for most exits. Usually, several precipitating factors were present.

### Exits of Patients With Conduct Disorders

Not unexpectedly, the largest number of exits involved youngsters who ran the gamut of conduct disorder pathology. In various mixtures and to various degrees, these patients exhibited behavior that was impulsive, aggressive, delinquent, dyssocial (i.e., unsocialized, odd, or offputting), or frankly antisocial (usually in the setting of substantive Axis I pathology, as noted above). They were often highly resistant to entering group in the first place:

> A 14-year-old boy with a history of truancy and petty theft repeatedly ran away from home and then ran away from an impressive roster of placements. Eventually, his entire identity came to devolve around his skills at elopement. On the ward, he boasted that "the place hasn't been built that can hold me!" He protested against joining a group and then changed his mind. In the middle of his first session, he stated "this is total bullshit!" and exited. Shortly thereafter, he ran off the unit and was never heard from again. (This case was the most notable of several in which exiting constituted a trial run for full-fledged elopement.)

Even when reasonably engaged in therapy, youngsters with conduct disorder still exited as a function of the same impulsivity and aggressivity they manifested elsewhere:

Two 16-year-old boys with a history of serious antisocial behavior and depression had been active participants in group for several months. Earlier on the day of a session, they fought over a girl on the unit. Their quarrel erupted anew shortly after entering the session. Despite attempted interventions by other members, they hurled escalating insults at each other, dared each other to "take it outside," grappled, tumbled out the door, and continued their struggle with each other in the hall.

Youngsters with conduct disturbance, who often defended themselves against painful affect through acting out, were particularly prone to exit when a hurtful issue was raised in group:

After her parents died in an auto accident, a 15-year-old girl had been expelled from a succession of foster placements because of behavior difficulties. She was eventually hospitalized after a serious suicide attempt.

During a session in which several group members spoke feelingly about absent or deceased parents, the patient began giggling, interrupting with tangential stories, and generally making a thorough nuisance of herself. Attempts to interpret the source of her anxiety or quiet her down proved fruitless. She was eventually asked to leave.

Other compelled exits of youngsters with conduct disorder were precipitated by disruptive clowning or aggressive behavior that seemed obscurely motivated at the time, but that in retrospect appeared to reflect anxiety about the pressure of intimacy caused by greater group cohesion. Disruptions on this basis often decreased as the patient became more firmly bonded to the group.

## Exits of Psychotic Patients

Psychotic youngsters were not placed in group until their condition was deemed sufficiently improved to enable effective participation. However, on several occasions a recompensated patient temporarily erupted into psychotic behavior that led to exiting. Sometimes, psychotic symptoms were clearly related to the group's impact:

When her group embarked on a spirited discussion of teenage pregnancy, a 16-year-old schizophrenic girl recovering from an episode of acute schizophrenia grew increasingly withdrawn and agitated and had to be escorted out of the session. The patient came from an extremely religious background. Just before her psychosis, she had begun dating a boy over her family's objections. She developed strong sexual feelings, which caused intolerable anxiety. The group discussion apparently had reawakened erotic longings (including a wish to become pregnant herself), as well as overwhelming guilt.

In other instances, psychotic behavior that led to exiting was related more to an intrinsic disease process than to the group process:

A 17-year-old boy who seemed well on his way to recovering from a hypomanic episode entered his first group session. Immediately, he began to talk giddily at the top of his voice and shouted down attempts to quiet him. The members were amused, then irritated, and then frightened. He was finally taken back to the ward.

Whether more attentiveness to the first patient's emerging agitation would have prevented eruption of her symptoms is moot. It was clear in retrospect that the boy with bipolar disorder was not nearly as prepared to join group as several optimistic team members had thought.

## Exits Due to Teasing or Scapegoating

Teasing is a ubiquitous activity among children and adolescents. It is the bane of adult attempts to preserve group cohesion, whether in a class or on a camping trip. Virtually any vocal or physical trait, any feature of behavior or dress, or any aspect of family, social, or religious background can become a source of teasing, given the presence of a "gettable" teasee.

Teasing may be based on fondness for the person being teased. But at its worst it can be a public flaying, motivated by a conflation of sadistic, competitive, and narcissistic wishes to belittle, humiliate, and even destroy the teasee. Pathological teasers may have fragile self-esteem and may seek to alleviate a profound sense of deficit; they may actually share with the teasee the very characteristics they mock. The similarities between the psychodynamics of localized teasing and more generic examples of prejudice are obvious.

Teasing may be ineluctably contagious. The limited toxicity of a one-on-one teasing situation can escalate into generalized scapegoating, with far more devastating impact on the targeted youngster. Youngsters who might not otherwise have been inclined toward teasing can join such dubious "fun" as a response to peer pressure, in order to fit in, or to avoid being teased themselves. Loosening of superego strictures is a hallmark of these circumstances; single members of adolescent cliques or groups allow themselves to be seduced into deeding over responsibility for teasing, and worse, to the group as a whole—or to a charismatic leader (Erikson 1942).

Teasing is a perennial problem on adolescent inpatient services. It arises from a yeasty mix of potential teasers and teasees who live in close quarters, manifest a spectrum of serious pathologies, and have limited, skewed social skills together with ill-contained aggression.

Although virtually any patient can be teased for any reason, particularly virulent teasing or scapegoating was directed at 1) certain schizophrenic youngsters with bizarre hallucinations, delusions, and no notable violent behavior; 2) extremely effeminate, unaggressive, openly homosexual boys; 3) mentally retarded youngsters who were also depressed, passive-dependent, and painfully eager to please.

These three types shared an undefended vulnerability capable of inciting intense repulsion and fear in peers (especially in male patients vis-à-vis the effeminate homosexual patient). The disturbed schizophrenic patient's unabashed "craziness" could acutely mirror an adolescent's own worries about being crazy, just as the specter of the mentally retarded patient could invoke a sense of "dummyhood" close to the concerns of many of our patients. The offending crazy or dumb Other became a target for disavowed inner disease, just as the faintest perception of personal homoeroticism was undone by scapegoating the "faggot" who evoked it by his mere presence.

In our adolescent groups, teasing predictably ran the gamut of possibilities from mild initiatory hazing to merciless minimizing. Even with the most robust counteractive measures, serious teasing was arguably the most significant cause of exits, next to aggressive acting out by youngsters with conduct disturbance:

> A 16-year-old boy with schizoid personality and major depressive disorders was persistently teased by several girls in the group about his crush on another girl, who did not reciprocate his interest. The rest of the group and the therapist remonstrated with them to no avail, and the boy rushed out of the session in tears.

The fewer the teasers, the easier it is to head off teasing. Generalized scapegoating, an infrequent occurrence in a well-run group, presents greater management difficulties:

> A 15-year-old boy with attention-deficit disorder, mixed personality difficulties, and mild retardation came from an extremely unsocialized home. His deficient personal grooming and table manners were a focus for intense ward criticism. He consistently turned peers and staff off with unamusing clowning and bumptious behavior. Over several weeks, his presence in group was barely tolerated. When he took off his shoes at the beginning of a session, the air quickly filled with noxious vapors from his terrible case of athlete's foot. Howls of protest over the stench were succeeded by an avalanche of objections to other examples of his "disgusting" persona by virtually every member.
>
> The therapists agreed that there were realistic grounds for complaint, but they stressed that the patient had never had the opportunity to learn more adaptive habits until now and insisted that "rat packing" would never foster change. The group dismissed these "shrink excuses" and continued their relentless criticism until the patient indignantly stalked out of the room.

Both these patients subsequently returned. Their respective groups were able to work through the issues that caused their exits. The asocial boy's group became more cohesive immediately after his exit, a phenomenon encountered with some frequency. Enhancement of group process after a member's departure may be genuine if he or she was consistently undermining the group's functioning. However, an unwary therapist can be lulled into validating the solidarity temporarily purchased at the expense of sacrificing a useful member (see "More on Exiting Aftermaths," below).

## Exits as a Function of (Reenacted?) Symbiotic Conflict

Patients who made symbiotic exits had severe borderline pathology, accompanied by narcissistic and histrionic character traits. Their lives seemed to be spent in crisis. Relationships were pervaded by symbiotically charged hostile dependency and severe splitting, inevitably recapitulated in the hospital setting:

> Shortly after joining the group, a 16-year-old girl with a history of impulsive suicide attempts began monopolizing sessions with tearful accounts of manifold injustices meted out to her at home and in the hospital. She bitterly resented any suggestion she might bear a bit of responsibility for her difficulties. She would beg poignantly for advice and then become scathingly critical of the group, complaining that "nothing here is doing me any good!"
>
> Her grievances were presented articulately enough to enlist some support. When she commenced threatening to leave sessions, the membership split between those pleading with her to stay and those angrily telling her to go. She moved her seat near the door and frequently made motions to leave. One of the therapists finally stated that her behavior mirrored her demands on her exhausted family; that only she could decide whether the group could be useful to her or not; and that if she did decide to stay, it would be very helpful for her to learn how to share the group's attention with others. She promptly exited, vowing never to return.

This patient's virulent claims on an intrusively doting mother had virtually excluded her siblings. Her ambivalent behavior in group reinvented the overwhelming neediness and need for escape enacted in her relationship with her mother. Individual therapy and other milieu interventions ultimately proved more productive, if intermittently stormy, venues for working out her difficulties. It is conceivable that she could have been accepted back into group if her narcissism had been less militant.

## Exits Precipitated by Collective Group Disturbance

Exits precipitated by collective group disturbance always involved several patients and sometimes involved a majority of the group members. They were usually preceded by multifocal waves of discontent that seemed to gather momentum and usually defied intervention. Collective exits were more common in groups whose "texture" was informed by members with conduct disturbance. Some were mainly caused by intragroup tension:

> Two coleaders who had just started working together with a largely delinquent, belligerent group developed major disagreements about limit setting and other issues. From the start, sessions were fragmented and marked by unfriendly horsing around, belittling, and challenging. The leaders separately pursued opposing strategies: rigid and tough versus easygoing. The group finally exploded in a chain of vituperative ethnic confrontations that concluded with the ejection of three members.

Other exits dictated by collective group tension occurred during ward crises that affected staff as well as patients, brought on by census problems, alterations in the chain of command, unpopular policies imposed on the unit from elsewhere, and so forth:

> A unit had been over maximum census for several weeks because of an unanticipated influx of court cases. At the same time, an unusual number of patients were on one-on-one status because of psychotic and suicidal behavior. The door had recently been locked around the clock because of a rash of elopements. Staff morale declined, evidenced by increased absenteeism, clique formation, and covert and open blaming of leadership. During a turbulent unit meeting at this time, patients teased and squabbled with each other, and complaints were voiced about a broken ward television, bad food, thievery, overcrowding with "crazy kids," and so forth.
>
> A group session immediately afterward continued in the same vein. An air of generalized restlessness prevailed. Arguments broke out; as soon as one was quelled, another began. Patients expressed disgust with various aspects of ward life. The coleaders were criticized, and the worth of the group was dismissed. Two boys accused

each other at length of stealing and started sparring. They were removed; then two girls promptly declared they were "too upset to stay" and ran out the door. The remaining three members sat in glum near-silence until the session ended.

An intriguing "10 little Indians" collective exit—the only one encountered—unfolded in a similarly overheated milieu. Inchoate patient anxiety and complex staff emotion swirled around the imminent departure of an admired, strong head nurse because of pregnancy, in the midst of other ward difficulties. At a session of a group usually uninclined toward acting out, members ruminated over what would happen with the nurse leaving while "everything was such a mess."

Expressions of fear and sadness were punctuated by anger at unnamed staff "who just come in to pick up their checks and don't care." Despair spread until one girl asked to be excused to go to the bathroom. Then another member wanted to get a drink of water. Then a boy said he needed to lie down in his room because his stomach ached. Finally, every member but one (a phobic, passive-dependent young man) had trudged out of the room. The ordinarily effective coleaders found themselves curiously paralyzed before this forlorn exodus.

A collective exit is painful for members and leadership alike. But grasping its underlying causes can be immensely helpful for advancing group process. In the first example, abrasive interactions of a new, unruly group could not be properly addressed because of faulty communication between leaders who were also new to each other. The collective exit spurred the leaders to examine their stylistic and theoretical differences. Their enhanced harmony—and the permanent removal of the most disruptive youngster—helped members to move past their initial wrangling and to begin relating empathically to each other.

The microcosm of group reflects the larger world of the adolescent unit. Stanton and Schwartz (1954) observed that a collective disturbance not only is expectable but also can be an extremely beneficial event, highlighting crucial group, individual, and administrative issues for the entire unit. An effective resolution can stir new vitality into a bogged-down milieu.

The second and third examples cited above indicate the sensitivity of an adolescent group to unit and extraunit tensions (Setterberg 1991). Ward pressures eventually subsided in both cases because of specific interventions (e.g., tightening up the criteria for court admissions) and with the simple passage of time (e.g., time needed to mourn the pregnant nurse's departure and get to know her replacement). Corollary to the unit's improvement, the respective adolescent groups pulled together.

What seemed to be a summary disintegrative experience in both cases ultimately proved integrative. With members now willing to stay in place, the troubling outside issues that had sparked group internal dissension and precipitated collective exiting could be worked through. The group members who abandoned the leaders during the 10 little Indians incident—as they themselves were afraid to be abandoned—learned to deal with hurtful loss through communicating their emotional distress instead of fleeing it.

## ◆ More on Elective Versus Compelled Exits

A thin line may separate electing to quit a session and being told to leave. Why some patients get removed from group while others opt to remove themselves is a vexing question. The answer would seem to reside in each exit episode's unique blend of contributing factors, the group's thrust toward containment or expulsion, and the exiter's diagnosis and dynamics. Space does not permit unraveling this intricate weave at much length. I am specifically intrigued by patients who insist on remaining in session while they enable their inevitable expulsion, rather than bolt on their own or calm down.

Many of these adolescents seem driven by a conflation of exhibitionistic, narcissistic, sadistic, and masochistic wishes, such as the desire for attention; the desire to torment or punish the group as a whole, its leaders, or particular members; the obscure *frisson* of rejection by expulsion; and even the clouded hope that genuine benefit might yet come from the group despite (or precisely because of) their provocations. Such dynamics may recapitulate a conflicted pattern of gratification derived from previous family experience (see the case example in the section "Exits as a Function of (Reenacted?) Symbiotic Conflict," above).

A few disturbed and disturbing psychotic patients were simply too disorganized or confused to leave on their own. One hesitates to overinterpret this phenomenon dynamically. Overpsychologizing (e.g., about regression to obtain oral nurturance from the group's symbolic family) can ignore the tumultuous biological disturbances of a schizophrenic or manic diathesis.

## ◆ More on Exiting Aftermaths

Directly after the fact, exits were rarely indifferent events to those left behind. Some exits were highly traumatic. They compromised group cohesion because of devastating feelings of despair over the exiter's loss, as well as guilt and anger over not offering the departed one effective help. The anger was sometimes expressed within the membership, but it was more often directed at the leaders. Other exits were initially perceived as helpful, particularly when an extremely disruptive, threatening member was removed. Cohesion then often seemed enhanced, but the rapprochement could ultimately prove to be dubious, as in pseudotogetherness after a scapegoated exit.

As for the exiters' immediate fate, some (mainly those removed from group) were returned to the unit accompanied by a staff member. Others were brought back to the unit after various degrees of on-site resistance or pursuit; some went back to the unit on their own. Once the exiters were back on the unit, the majority of them usually quieted down and quickly returned to the daily group program. A minority—mostly fragile borderline or psychotic youngsters—continued to be sufficiently troubled to require exclusion from the group program for variable periods, observation, medication, seclusion, a visit with a therapist, and so forth. No instances of suicidal behavior after exit were encountered in this cohort (or elsewhere).

Yet another group of elective exiters were ambivalent after the fact. These youngsters hung around the area outside the therapy room. Here they would pace, clown, rage, weep, or diffidently chat up staff members and patients passing by until they were brought back to the unit or returned under their own steam. It was not unusual for them to attempt reentry into the group, with variable success. Their chances of being allowed back were greater when their mode of exit had not been markedly disruptive and when the group entertained positive feelings toward them and wanted to help with whatever problem had led to their exit.

On a few occasions, youngsters who had exited sequentially or simultaneously formed an impromptu group outside the therapy room rather than scattering. Accounts of interactions in these intriguing gatherings on the margin of the parent group are fragmentary. I know of at least one instance where patients continued to heatedly discuss issues the group had been considering at the time of their exit.

The long-term consequences of exiting are arguably more important than the short-term impact. An overwhelming majority of exiters were able to return to their groups, usually by the next session. However problematic they were at the time, many exits had little significance not long afterward. When significant personal or group issues were involved in exiting, these were usually worked through in combined individual and group therapy, with the overall benefits for group cohesiveness noted above.

Patients deemed unsuitable for the group from which they exited were eventually placed in more appropriate groups or were treated individually without notable deleterious effects. However, several youngsters who had been scapegoated into exiting were a specific exception to the generally neutral or frankly positive outcome of exiting. They were either gun-shy about returning or flatly refused to participate further in group.

## ◆ More on Management Issues

Exits are an inevitable attribute of adolescent groups, especially those with more troubled members. Hope for absolute control of exiting must therefore be deemed illusory.

A major step in exit prevention occurs before a group ever meets—through a comprehensive selection process that ensures that a youngster is truly ready to enter group and then places the youngster in a group appropriate to age, sex, psychopathology, level of functioning, and so forth.

The evaluation should also inventory previous group therapy experience, paying particular attention to disruptive activity, including prior exiting behavior and the circumstances precipitating an exit. If possible, former group therapists should be contacted to flesh out the patient's account. The youngster should then be well counseled as to the aims and actualities of group therapy.

The extent to which exiting should be addressed in explaining rules to a new group or a new member is moot. At the very onset of group, one does not wish to burden members with excessive information or to worry or incite them. I do think it helpful to explain briefly that exiting does occasionally occur, to provide a few guidelines, and to indicate that these can be amplified and modified by the group if the situation arises.

Once the group is under way, the leader should be aware of group members' testing various requests as ways of exiting. Requests to use the bathroom, get a drink of water, and the like are best viewed as emblematic of limit testing, resistance, anxiety, and so forth. These often pathetic pleas can be somewhat reduced at first by reminding group members to attend to thirst or latrine needs before entering a session. Thereafter, leaders should use gentle but firm dissuasion, unless there is a genuine sense of urgency. All too often, what begins as a plausible call of nature can end up as an exit by a resistant youngster.

Adolescent groups vary impressively in their ability to contain a youngster who wants to exit and in their propensity to expel a difficult youngster. If exiting behavior suddenly erupts, keeping your head while all about you are losing theirs is no easy task. A besieged leader does well to consider these disparate possibilities:

1. A youngster is being retained when the group—and frequently the patient as well—would do better if he or she were taken out of the session. This stage has been reached when a potential exiter remains totally impervious to effective interventions and when group time is being inappropriately monopolized.

2. A youngster who is in danger of leaving or being removed might be retained with appropriate intervention. This situation is harder to evaluate. It tends to arise in groups where keeping order is an important aspect of the group's agenda (often referable to the tighter style of the group's leaders).

Preventable exits may also be a function of group scapegoating, occasionally with the leadership's witting or unwitting participation. As a rule, group members openly express the wish to be rid of an unpopular member. A leader's collusive aversion, however, is more likely to go unrecognized. One must maintain vigilance lest the group herd a constituent out the door; the other side of this vigilance is the ability to perform a quick countertransference checkout in aid of ascertaining whether one is abetting a collective thrust toward expulsion.

Leadership techniques for keeping a potential exiter in session include devoting a reasonable portion of the group's time to working on the problem spurring the exit; emphasizing the youngster's importance to the group; rallying members to the would-be exiter's support, particularly if such help is not readily forthcoming; and standing up for the patient's right to be in the group in the face of inappropriate opposition.

Offering food or drink, if already part of the group's routine, can be helpful on a case-by-case basis. How "physical" to be beyond this is problematic. I believe forcibly restraining a youngster from leaving a session is antitherapeutic, and group leaders should likewise dissuade members from the practice. Physically comforting an extremely troubled paranoid, psychotic, or other potentially violent preexiter also can create more difficulties than it solves. But in selected instances some type of appropriate, nonintrusive contact can help provide a benevolent holding environment, particularly when a pat on the back or hand-holding is administered by a valued group member.

Whether for altruistic or suspect reasons, some group members will want to retrieve an exiter (such fetchers may themselves be motivated by a yen to exit!). They should be discouraged by a gentle statement that ascertaining the exiter's location and welfare is properly the leaders' job. The importance of keeping the remaining membership intact and in place should also be underscored.

With sufficient experience, one develops a sixth sense about when a troubled youngster must be taken from group. Ignoring the signals to indulge in shilly-shallying will only undermine the group process even further. Leadership's ambivalence here may be especially subversive of the adolescent's confidence in the adult capacity to care competently.

When there are good reasons for removal, they should be succinctly stated in language the patient, or at least the group, can grasp. Leaders should emphasize that removal is not a punishment; rather, it is being undertaken for the benefit of the patient and the group. If circumstances warrant, a youngster can be reassured that he or she will be able to return at another time. When this judgment cannot in all honesty be made, such reassurance should not be given.

In the best of all possible worlds, taking a youngster from group would be accomplished with a minimum of compulsion and disruption—an ideal often notable for its incomplete attainment. In the end, most patients do allow themselves to be escorted out the door with little fuss. Indeed, they may be greatly relieved to go.

Inevitably, however, more than token resistance is going to be encountered, whether dictated by masochism, psychosis, or nonpsychotic oppositional behavior. If force must be used with a youngster unwilling to leave, I again deem it best not to involve group members unless a reasonable certainty of serious harm to someone exists. Unless other staff members are available, the main responsibility for taking an uncooperative adolescent out of group properly resides with the leaders. Coleadership is a tremendous asset here. Two people at the helm can exert more control over the youngster when necessary; under less dramatic circumstances, one leader can keep the group running while the other performs whatever escort duty is necessary.

When groups had strong acting-out potential, a nursing staff member occasionally sat in to help remove recalcitrant patients, as well as assist with other problems. Even if this person was officially a nonparticipant, his or her presence could hardly be considered neutral and inevitably affected the members—if only to remind them that they were perceived as sufficiently unstable, obstreperous, or special to require such intervention.

In my opinion, the least intrusive, most helpful addition to a group is a staff member stationed just outside the door who 1) can be called into the group to assist with difficult preexiting behavior and other problems and 2) can deal with a freshly bolted exiter. In the latter case, a youngster can be immediately ushered back to the unit or—depending on the judgment of the leadership and the staff member—can be kept on location until he or she is calm enough to reenter the session. Personnel shortages often do not permit such a luxury. Any viable alternative—reaching a unit on-call staff member by phone from the session or even alerting secretaries in nearby offices that a group is being run—is better than nothing.

## ◆ Afterword

Sex and death are said to be the ultimate ambiguous experiences, symbolizing just about anything to the unconscious. Exiting may not be quite as overdetermined, but the more this fascinating phenomenon is studied, the more meanings it yields up. I have pondered only a few of these meanings and hope that this chapter provides a springboard for future investigations.

Finally, I wish to stress how important it is to appreciate the positive aspects of exiting, rather than merely dwell on the dark side. Like the eloping described in my earlier study (Greenberg et al. 1968), exiting may paradoxically be the first sign of productive engagement with the therapeutic milieu. It is a signification easily ignored amid the exiter's sound and fury.

## ◆ References

Bekrowitz I (ed): Adolescents Grow in Groups. New York, Brunner/Mazel, 1972

Brandes N: Group Therapy With Adolescents. New York, Jason Aronson, 1973

Cerda RA, Wolarsky-Nemiroff HJ, Richmond AH: Therapeutic group approaches in an inpatient facility for children and adolescents: a 15 year perspective. Child and Adolescent Psychotherapy 20:71–80, 1991 (special issue)

Chase JL: Inpatient adolescent and latency-age children's perspectives on the curative factors in group psychotherapy. Child and Adolescent Group Psychotherapy 20:95–108, 1991 (special issue)

Corder BF, Whiteside R, Koehne P, et al: Structured techniques for handling loss and addition of members in adolescent psychotherapy groups. Journal of Early Adolescence 1:413–421, 1981

Crowdes NE: Group therapy for pre-adolescent boys. Am J Nursing 75:92–95, 1975

Erikson E: Hitler's imagery and German youth. Psychiatry 5:475–493, 1942

Fluet NR, Holmes GR, Gordon LC: Adolescent group psychotherapy: a modified fishbowl format. Adolescence 15:75–82, 1980

Friedman S, Schlise S, Seligman S: Issues involved in the treatment of an adolescent group. Adolescence 10:357–368, 1975

Greenberg, HR, Blank HR, Argrett SA: The anatomy of elopement from an acute adolescent service: escape from engagement. Psychiatr Q 42:28–47, 1968

Lange G: Sexually provocative behavior of older male, acting out adolescents within a multimedia group setting. Pratt Institute Creative Arts Therapy Review 1:18–24, 1980

Ramos N, Richmond AH: Adolescent group therapy in an inpatient facility. Child and Adolescent Group Psychotherapy 20:81–88, 1991 (special issue)

Scheidlinger S: Group treatment of adolescents: an overview. Am J Orthopsychiatry 55:102–111, 1985

Setterberg SR: Inpatient child and adolescent therapy groups: boundary maintenance and group function. Child and Adolescent Group Psychotherapy 20:89–94, 1991 (special issue)

Slavson S: A Textbook in Analytic Group Psychotherapy. New York, International Universities Press, 1964

Stanton AH, Schwartz MS: The Mental Hospital. New York, Basic Books, 1954

Yalom I: The Theory and Practice of Group Psychotherapy. New York, Basic Books, 1975

# SECTION III

# Groups in Specialized Settings and Special Populations

CHAPTER 9

# Analyst Self-Disclosure in Adolescent Groups

*Arnold Wm. Rachman, Ph.D., and*
*Velleda C. Ceccoli, Ph.D.*

## ◆ Ego Identity Development in Adolescence: Erikson's Fifth Stage of the Life Cycle

### Role of Theory in Adolescent Group Psychotherapy

About 20 years ago, Rachman (1972, 1974, 1975) first presented his theory of adolescent group psychotherapy. An earlier article had presented these ideas in embryonic form (Rachman 1969); later, an expanded version of the case study that illustrated the theory was published (Rachman 1975, Chapter 1). We thought then, as we do now, that the greatest shortcoming in the field of adolescent group psychotherapy is the absence of coherent theoretical frameworks.

Application of the theoretical concepts and clinical techniques first described as "identity group psychotherapy" (Rachman 1972, 1974, 1975) has withstood the test of the present decade. Continued application of these ideas and methods by other clinicians has verified their significance and broadened their application (Rachman 1989; Rachman and Heller 1974, 1976; Raubolt 1982, 1983; Sabusky and Kymissis 1983).

A meaningful and relevant theory is indispensable to, and cannot be divorced from, meaningful and relevant clinical practice. In fact, without such an underpinning, clinical practice with adolescents can be a haphazard, disorganized, difficult, and confusing enterprise. Practitioners of adolescent psychotherapy have a particular mandate to be organized, consistent, and clear in their method, technique, and mode of therapeutic intervention. Adolescents need and want direction, organization, consistency, and clarity in their attempts at identity crisis resolution. As the *confusion of tongues theory* makes clear (see "The Confusion of Tongues Theory," below), it is imperative that an adult's behavior encourage clarity, directness, and, above all, honesty.

Erikson's conception of the individual's distinct developmental struggles in the life cycle provides a useful backdrop for the understanding of the therapeutic issues that arise in adolescent group analysis. The major theoretical construct in Erikson's fifth stage of the life cycle is the concept of ego identity (Erikson 1958, 1959, 1968). Ego identity has three distinct aspects: an intrapsychic or personal identity, an interpersonal or group identity, and an ideological or philosophical identity.

The development of ego identity is an intrapsychic process that occurs within a relational matrix. Identity in an adolescent is crystallized by meaningful experiences with adults as well as peers.

## Personal Identity

The intrapsychic aspects of ego identity refer to an adequate sense of oneself as a separate, functioning, positive person with a sense of destiny and goal directedness. Colloquially speaking, ego identity refers to this state of mind:

> You know who you are; where you want to go and how you are going to get there. Somewhere in the middle of you, you have a good feeling about yourself, and no one can take it away from you. (Rachman 1989, p. 22)

Identity formation is the process of discovering who one is as a separate, distinct person and becoming aware of and valuing one's distinct assets as well as shortcomings. This identity search can be exemplified by a creative period of self-discovery, as in George Bernard Shaw's withdrawal from society as a young adult (Erikson 1959), or by a protracted, severe identity crisis, as in Martin Luther's agonizing young adulthood (Erikson 1958). Adolescent therapists are also susceptible to identity crises (Coles 1970; Rachman 1977).

Individuals need to have a period of creative retreat in the service of self-exploration. As social structures that reinforce withdrawal and introspection in our culture change, opportunities for retreats of self-actualization become scarcer for youth. Psychotherapy can become a significant social structure in which young people can have an opportunity for creative withdrawal in the service of personal identity formation.

## Philosophical Identity

Identity formation has the implicit notion of self-actualization—the individual's capacity for becoming fully what he or she is capable of being as a person.

> As we have indicated, fidelity is that virtue and quality of adolescent ego strength which belongs to man's evolutionary heritage, but which—like all the basic virtues—can arise only in the interplay of a life stage with the individuals and the social forces of a true community. (Erikson 1968, p. 235)

Fidelity is faithfulness to an ideological point of view. Without a philosophy of life—a cause for which to exist—to provide overall meaning to existence, one feels an existential vacuum. Identity formation helps define the meaning of one's existence, creating new value and direction.

Fidelity can also refer to valuing oneself, being secure in knowing who one is, and being faithful to this sameness. It is a feeling of psychic balance and predictability—that one will be the same person tomorrow that one is today. This stage in human development is beyond object constancy. The individual develops a sense of himself or herself as a constant object, allowing him or her to be less dependent on another person.

A sense of sameness does not refer to a rigid, inflexible, compulsively oriented intrapsychic and interpersonal stance. The sameness is experienced as a good feeling; individuals know who they are and who they are becoming.

Adults need to provide adolescents with meaningful, positive ideologies with which to identify. A psychotherapist needs to have a meaningful, positive, consistent, personal and professional frame of reference with which adolescents can identify. A psychotherapist who works with adolescents must stand for something and make his or her stand known.

## Group Identity

The process of identity formation is also an interpersonal one. It occurs not only within the individual but also between the individual and the group:

> The growing child must, at every step, derive a vitalizing sense of reality from the awareness that this indvidual way of mastering experience is a successful variant of the way other people around him master experience and recognize such mastery. (Erikson 1959, p. 89)

Adolescence is also characterized by the psychosocial mandate to form positive, meaningful peer relationships. An individual's peer group experience throughout childhood can aid or hinder his or her capacity as an adolescent to resolve issues of group identity. Identity formation is not complete without such an encounter.

At all stages of the life cycle, ego identity is more than personal identity. Peer group affiliation is a psychological need of human beings:

> The conscious feeling of having a personal identity is based on two simultaneous observations: the perception of the selfsameness and continuity of one's existence in time and space and the perception of the fact that others recognize one's sameness and continuity. . . . Ego identity . . . is the awareness . . . that there is a selfsameness and continuity . . . [a] *style of one's individuality* . . . [which] coincides with the

> sameness and continuity of one's *meaning for significant others* in the
> immediate community. (Erikson 1968, p. 50)

Such a view recognized people's inherent social nature. An individual's growth and development are directly related to his or her interaction with significant others throughout the life cycle (Mead 1934). The most pathological identity problems occur when individuals have been seriously deprived of meaningful human contact—for example, the so-called feral children reared in isolation from human contact (Bettelheim 1954). Feral-like behavior has been observed in the senior author's clinical observations with urban youth from disadvantaged backgrounds.

## ◆ Identity Confusion and the Psychopathology of Adolescence

### Identity Confusion

The psychological danger of the adolescent stage of development is identity confusion, the negative stage of the identity crisis:

> A state of acute identity confusion usually becomes manifest at a
> time when the young individual finds himself exposed to a combina-
> tion of experiences which demand his simultaneous commitment to
> physical intimacy (not by any means always overtly sexual), to
> decisive occupational choice, to energetic competition, and to psy-
> chosocial self-definition. (Erikson 1968, p. 166)

Although identity confusion is the negative stage of the identity crisis, it can be normative. All adolescents pass through a period when inconsistency, lack of commitment, and feelings of confusion, disorganization, and impulsiveness- predominate in their thinking and behaving. Therefore, adolescent confusion is not an affliction or disease, but a "normal phase of increased conflict characterized by a seeming fluctuation in ego strength as well as by a high growth potential" (Erikson 1968, p. 163).

It must be emphasized, however, that such a normative crisis has the inherent potential for either psychopathology or self-actualization. Which direction the adolescent takes depends on his or her previous personality development (perhaps especially the development of ego strength), as well as his or her interaction with adults and society.

Besides personal pathology, social conditions can lead to identity confusion, a lack of positive and meaningful adult leadership, absence of meaningful ideologies with which to identify, and little or no opportunity for free role experimentation. It is when identity confusion predominates and is continuous that psychotherapeutic intervention is crucial and mandatory. Group psychotherapy, in particular, can offer the adolescent an opportunity to experiment with and crystallize an identity via his or her interactions with other group members and the group leader(s).

## ◆ The Confusion of Tongues Theory: Ferenczi's Observations on Childhood Trauma

Ferenczi's last clinical presentation (1933/1955) was entitled, "The Confusion of Tongues Between Children and Adults: The Language of Tenderness and Passion." This article raised enormous professional, personal, and social issues for Ferenczi, psychoanalysis, and the psychoanalytic community. It signaled Ferenczi's final difficulty with Freud and the analytic establishment, as well as an indication, as some think (Masson 1984), of emotional upheaval. In this article, Ferenczi crystallized a new method of psychoanalysis, reintroduced the seduction hypothesis, urged professional focus on the acceptance of sexual abuse in children, and demonstrated the emotional demands on the analyst when treating difficult cases.

There are several dimensions to the metaphor of the "confusion of tongues":

1. The child is confused (traumatized) by the adult (parent or parental surrogate) when the adult seduces the child sexually (or emotionally).

2. The child wants tenderness, not sexual passion.
3. The adult is intruding his/her sexual needs into the innocent longings of a child for love and tenderness.
4. The child is tongue-tied, confusing sexuality for love but unable to speak of the confusion. (Rachman 1995a, b)

The experience is not only the physical abuse of the child, but an ensuing psychological trauma.

The child develops a series of pathological defenses to maintain the fiction of tender contact with the adult. These defense mechanisms (many of which Ferenczi described for the first time) include dissociation, splitting, identification with the aggressor, fragmentation of the self, blunted affect, and schizoid withdrawal. They lay the emotional groundwork for adult perversions, disturbed object relations, and a narcissistic, borderline, or psychotic disorder. The child becomes tongue tied and unable to give voice to his or her feelings of confusion, rage, and violation. He or she lives in a semiconscious state, like a robot, protecting the fragmented self from further psychological disintegration and assault. The adult abuser, overcome with guilt, also becomes mute. He or she compensates with excessive moralistic behavior. The nonabusive but coconspiring parent becomes deaf to any attempts to break the bind of confusion of tongues, attributing the child's verbalizations of abuse to "hysterical lying."

Second, Ferenczi described the confusion of tongues that a patient can experience when being treated by an analyst who maintains the stance of a cold, detached, neutral, and nonparticipating observer. By removing oneself from the emotional experience of the analysis and evoking the concept of resistance when the patient expresses negative feelings toward the analyst, the analyst unwittingly recreates the childhood trauma. The analyst confuses the analysand by this communication and interaction. Ferenczi named this position "professional hypocrisy."

Third, Ferenczi described the situation of the analysand's speaking in genuinely emotional terms regarding the feelings of coolness and detachment, but the analyst's responding with additional coolness and detachment by evoking the notion of resistance rather than examining his or her feelings. Ferenczi argued for a more genuinely emotional encounter, where the analyst examined his or her countertransference to rock bottom to create a corrective emotional experience that would aid in the uncovering of the childhood trauma of sexual seduction and emotional abuse.

## ◆ Confusion of Tongues in Adolescence: Judicious Self-Disclosure in Adolescent Psychotherapy

When we use confusion of tongues as a central concept in understanding adolescent treatment, we acknowledge that there is a fundamental issue in adolescent and adult interactions that must be addressed as Ferenczi addressed it in his original formulations.

The confusion of tongues between adolescents and adults centers on the trauma of blaming the child. By blaming the difficulties in the adult's relationship with the adolescent solely on the adolescent, the adult traumatizes the teenager. It becomes a trauma because it reevokes the confusion of tongues experience of childhood, when the child felt confused and inadequate, blamed himself or herself, and could not determine whether the parent(s) had contributed to his or her difficulties. In essence, an altered sense of reality developed, based on a false self (Winnicott 1971) or a submerged self (Kutash and Wolf 1992), which was created to acquiesce to the needs and wishes of the parent. Besides the reactivation of the childhood trauma, adolescent-adult relationships encourage the trauma of blaming the child by not owning their personal contribution to the emotional and interpersonal difficulty. When there is a difficulty in the relationship, the adult blames the adolescent for the difficulty. The adult does not practice the Ferenczian idea that all relationships are two-person relationships. In this instance, the adult does not examine his or her contribution to the difficulty, thus excluding himself or herself from the interaction and putting the burden of resolution on the adolescent.

In a two-person interaction, the adult would not only examine his or her contribution to the particular difficulty, but would also share it openly, directly, and judiciously with the adolescent. We consider the inability to view adolescent-adult relationships as two-person experiences and the inability of the adult to share his or her contribution to that experience as fundamental causes of emotional crisis in adolescence. Our approach to the group treatment of adolescents thus focuses on the therapist's ability to remain aware of, and directly and judiciously acknowledge, his or her contribution to the relationship.

## Typology of Judicious Self-Disclosure

We view analyst self-disclosure as a meaningful and, at times, necessary dimension of the treatment of adolescents. It is a deliberate, conscious intervention whereby the analyst reveals a personal feeling, thought, or any other aspect of his or her behavior. The intention is to aid the therapeutic process by answering a need the group or individual member has for authenticity. Individuals who have had traumas that center on parental deception, unresponsiveness, and emotional neglect are especially needy for authentic emotional interaction with a parental figure (Ferenczi 1932/1988, 1933/1955).

We distinguish this deliberate, conscious self-disclosure from the variety of ways an analyst reveals him or herself in a less conscious, more indirect way. An analyst's office, manner of dress, style of relating, and types of intervention all reveal personal elements (Balint 1968). Therapists really cannot present a "blank screen." Freud practiced in his home; his patients were greeted by his housekeeper, and the odor of food cooking wafted through the waiting room. This situation did not provide anonymity. Rather, it disclosed a warm family atmosphere (Roazen 1975). Freud's office proper was the opposite of a blank screen. His favorite pieces of antiquity were prominently displayed on his desk; his Chow dog sat at his feet; and the office was rich in appointments of Oriental rugs, tapestry, and Victorian furniture.

Judicious self-disclosure by the analyst has several basic characteristics. What follows is an expansion of an original attempt at definition (Rachman 1982):

1. The disclosure is geared to responding to the analysand's need for authentic communication.

2.  The disclosure is part of a matrix of empathic responsiveness before, during, and after the intervention.
3.  Only material that will aid the therapeutic process is revealed.
4.  The sharing of information should not represent a counter-transference reaction, unless such a reaction comes under the scrutiny of the group.
5.  The most appropriate sharing of personal functioning should come from a conflict-free area of the analyst's personality. Secondarily, one could judiciously share material in areas where one is in the process of resolving an issue.
6.  The content of what is revealed should meet the expressed needs of the analysand. It is not necessary to go beyond the request. All the intimate details of the issue in question need not be revealed.
7.  Discretion should be exercised in the wording and emotional intensity of the self-disclosure. Particularly vivid language, dramatic exclamations, and emotionally laden behavior can traumatize rather than soothe the analysand's need for authenticity.
8.  Self-disclosure is best practiced during a period of positive relationship or transference to the group analyst.
9.  An analysis of the impact of the self-disclosure should occur afterward. The analyst needs to be sensitive to individual differences in experiencing the disclosure and to help all group members work through their particular emotional reactions.
10. The analyst can decline to reveal himself or herself, but in doing so, he or she must embed the response in an empathic stance, taking care not to convey rejection, annoyance, or indignation about the request. The analyst should be emotionally and interpersonally comfortable with what is revealed; this comfort level can vary from clinician to clinician.

## Conspicuous Self-Disclosure

Just as judicious self-disclosure is therapeutic and growth enhancing, conspicuous self-disclosure is antitherapeutic and can be emotionally injurious to the analysand. Rather than meeting the needs of the analysand, it serves the narcissistic needs of the analyst. Some of the characteristics of this type of intervention follow:

1. The analyst is acting out in the transference.
2. A countertransference reaction is operative.
3. The disclosure goes beyond what is needed to meet the analysand's needs.
4. The content and style of the presentation traumatize, rather than soothe, the analysand.
5. Analyst and analysand are not in genuine emotional contact.
6. The disclosure is an indication of manipulation, emotional pressure, or intrusiveness.
7. An unresolved need of the analyst is expressed in the disclosure.
8. The analyst uses the group to work on personal problems.
9. The disclosure is an attack or an assault rather than an invitation to engage in an authentic relationship.
10. The disclosure reflects a lack of respect for the analysand's sense of self.

An important point must be emphasized regarding analyst self-disclosure and the method of group analysis. This type of intervention is only meaningful when the analyst uses a method that places central emphasis on the role of empathy. The empathic method can serve the treatment process during the relationship-building, uncovering, and working-through phases of treatment (Ferenczi 1928/1955, 1932/1988, 1933/1955; Kohut 1971, 1977, 1984; Rogers 1951, 1959, 1961). An analysis that emphasizes the empathic method should precede the analyst's self-disclosure. When the analyst decides to self-disclose, it should not be experienced as a shock to the therapeutic interaction system. Rather, it should be a special instance of empathic responsiveness, which has been preceded by other attempts to understand and respond to the subjective experience of the analysand. The self-disclosure can have meaning only in the context of the overall attempts at empathic attunement and responsiveness. If the analyst's self-disclosure is experienced as a shock to the system, it may have been an inappropriate way of responding (e.g., conspicuous self-disclosure). In addition, responsiveness after analyst self-disclosure should also be in the empathic mode.

## Judicious Self-Disclosure in Adolescent Groups

Adolescent psychotherapy has a dimension of interaction where there is a push for genuineness. Because adolescents are preoccupied with self-definition, they bring to the therapeutic interchange a need for a role model. Thus, adolescents often bombard therapists with questions about their own values, feelings, behavior, and experiences. We view these questions as expressions of identity needs and as crucial for formation of ego identity, rather than as resistances to the treatment. The therapist who is willing to respond judiciously to these questions allows the adolescent to try on the thoughts and feelings of a significant adult. This free role experimentation helps to create a new sense of self.

Adolescents need and want to be involved in meaningful emotional contact with significant others who are open, authentic, and direct. Their identity concerns require the presence of adults who stand for something—who communicate a sense of values, a philosophy, and a belief system. By interacting with adults, adolescents struggle to define their own emerging values, philosophies, and beliefs.

An adolescent group can often feel like a trial by fire for the group therapist because of the intense emotional climate that can spread through the group by emotional contagion. Such an experience causes intense countertransference reactions in the group analyst. Sharing these feelings often becomes necessary because the adolescent either observes the therapist's emotional reaction or inquires about it directly. Retreating to a resistance interpretation not only fails to address the identity needs of the adolescent, but it also recreates the trauma of being held responsible for the analyst's (i.e., the adult's or parent's) reaction. To be effective, resistance interpretations rely on the very thing that the adolescent struggles with—a solid ego identity. Therefore, these interpretations often fall on deaf ears. More important, they create a confusion of tongues between adolescent and adult.

In our experience, judicious self-disclosure of the countertransference in an interaction that involves sharing of feelings, thoughts, and values allows adolescents to experience a curative authority figure who responds by giving himself or herself in an empathic and compassionate way. Such disclosures provide an interpersonal context within which adolescents experience the adult authority's way of handling emotional reactions, the adult's capacity to deal with confrontations, and the value of vulnerability and openness in a relationship. When the leader reveals who he or she is and was in the past, the adolescents are able to accomplish this necessary ego development. The following are some of the judicious considerations involved in self-disclosure:

1. Self-disclosure should be done to enhance the group's functioning.
2. Self-disclosure can be offered voluntarily or in response to a request. Requests for self-disclosure are seen not as inherent resistance, but as a dimension of the identity search.
3. The therapist can and should set limits on the amount, content, and frequency of self-disclosure to protect his or her privacy.
4. Self-disclosure should be limited to appropriate material, in other words, to issues, conflicts, and feelings that are part of the expressed interest of the group (not a preoccupation of the therapist).

Self-disclosures that operate within this judicious framework have a significant therapeutic impact on adolescents. Because they revolve around the concept of a two-person interaction, they encourage each participant to assume responsibility for his or her behavior and actions. In so doing, they alleviate the focus on intrapsychic pathology, create an interpersonal context of empathy and honesty, and free the adolescent to develop insight gradually. Additionally, such disclosures firmly establish the group therapist as an adult who can be trusted and who can provide a realistic role model for identity formation and effective problem resolution. Last, judicious self-disclosures encourage creative experimentation with ways of being and relating to others and elevate the adolescents' self-esteem and confidence.

The following section provides some case examples of what we consider judicious self-disclosure and conspicuous self-disclosure.

## ◆ Case Examples of Analyst Self-Disclosure in Adolescent Group Psychotherapy

### Judicious Self-Disclosure

#### Case Example 1

The following example occurred in an inpatient, acute-care adolescent unit, where the group consisted of 10 adolescent girls, 13–16 years old, from varied socioeconomic backgrounds. It was conducted by a female therapist.

Before a group meeting, the therapist was seen dancing and playing an imaginary guitar to rock and roll music that was being played on the radio. The group therapist was unaware that her behavior was being observed by any of the adolescents; in essence, she was in a private reverie.

The group session began by focusing on several adolescents whose inappropriate behavior had caused them to lose unit privileges. There was much discussion around limit setting and what constitutes appropriate and inappropriate behavior. At this point, a member of the group addressed the therapist, telling her that she had seen her dancing and playing an imaginary guitar around the unit to music and that she thought that the therapist "was crazy and that was crazy behavior." The group therapist agreed with her and stated: "You are absolutely right. That was crazy, and I can be crazy sometimes. The trick is to know when it is OK to be crazy and when it is not. When you can do that, you will not have to be here anymore."

The first response to this self-disclosure was that the group burst into laughter and appeared relaxed and at ease with the therapist. Then, some of the group members began to talk about being perceived as crazy and the implications of being labeled this way by friends, family, and others. They were able to begin to articulate the difference between their *behavior* (acting crazy) and the *affective experience* (feeling crazy).

In this vignette, the group therapist's self-disclosure ameliorated the syndrome of confusion of tongues in the following ways:

■ The adult was open and honest when confronted with her behavior. She did not hide behind a clinical facade or become defensive. This openness created a direct emotional encounter in the here and now between the adolescents and the adult authority.

■ The adolescents verified that their perception of the reality—that is, seeing their group therapist behave in an unconventional way—was correct. When the behavior was called crazy, the therapist agreed that it was crazy in that it was unconventional and offbeat. The behavior was not what one usually expects from an authority figure; rather, it was what one expects from an adolescent.

■ The therapist's self-disclosure empowered the adolescents to believe in their observations and conclusions about the experience. Thus, their insight and psychological acumen, not just those of the adult, were verified.

■ The adolescents gained greater emotional and psychological contact with the group therapist and with each other. As a result, the pathology of the confusion of tongues (dissociation and repression) was arrested.

■ The adolescents' defensiveness was avoided because they became more self-revelatory themselves.

### Case Example 2

The following example occurred in a large outpatient psychiatric clinic in a major urban center. The group consisted of 14- to 17-year-olds of mixed ethnic backgrounds. One of the girls began to complain about her mother, which she had done many times before. She asked the coed, cotherapy team to respond by talking about their experiences with their mothers.

The male group therapist volunteered: "I can understand your wanting to know how adults handle the same problems you are struggling with. I did have difficulty with my mother when I was an adolescent. I feel she was controlling and had to have things her way. It was tough to grow up with a controlling mother. I was able to get help with this by talking to my friends. When I got older, I worked on it in therapy. Now I realize she was controlling because of her own personal problems. I can separate her problems from me."

The group was very appreciative and went on to discuss their relationships with their mothers.

In the preceding example we see that the therapist did the following:

- Addressed the identity need of the adolescent
- Did not go into all the gory details (e.g., did not mention that he thought his mother was cold or that she made him feel inferior)
- Functioned as an adult authority and gave hope to the next generation (Erikson 1968)

## Conspicuous Self-Disclosure

### Case Example 3

This example occurred in an outpatient, delinquent male adolescent group in an urban setting. The group began to confront the male group therapist regarding his homosexuality. The therapist did not respond in any direct way to the issue; rather, he interpreted the group's "need to know." The group became increasingly more agitated, first verbally attacking the group leader and then each other. Over the course of time, they began to bring weapons to the sessions. The group became unmanageable and was disbanded.

The group therapist was conspicuous in his confusion and in his inability to engage adolescents in an open dialogue regarding the issue of his homosexuality.

### Case Example 4

A female group analyst became very tense, defensive, and overly interpretive when asked about her sex life in an all-female adolescent group with disadvantaged youth in an outpatient clinic.

Instead of allowing group members to express their identity needs in the area of sexuality so they could more fully explore their own anxieties, the group therapist conspicuously disclosed her own anxieties about sexuality in her overly interpretive behavior. She attacked the group intellectually by interpreting their need to know, when in reality she was exposing her fear of discussing sexuality. She blamed the adolescent group for stimulating her anxiety and then attacked them for being resistant.

The group members were aware of the therapist's anxieties and felt attacked by her overly interpretive interventions. Rather than talk about the confusion, because the leader deemed she was not responsible for any of the difficulty, the group dropped the subject.

## ◆ Summary

We have examined the fundamental need in adolescence for crystallization of a sense of ego identity. Adult authority figures such as the group analyst provide a necessary figure with whom the adolescent can create a new beginning in the identity search. Adolescents need and want interaction with an adult who is empathic, honest, and direct. They need someone who can share his or her own struggles toward self-definition and is willing to own his or her contribution to any difficulties that arise in the adult-adolescent relationship. Through a review of the contribution made by Sandor Ferenczi in his development of the theory of the confusion of tongues, we hope to have demonstrated the importance of judicious self-disclosure in creating an honest and empathic atmosphere within a group setting, wherein the adolescent is free to use the leader's experience for his or her own identity development.

For group therapists who work with adolescents, the capacity to disclose themselves is both a liberating and an insightful experience. It frees the therapist to respond empathically to the special needs of adolescents struggling with their identity formation and with their experience of parental unresponsiveness and distrust. Rather than being bound by a tradition that emphasizes the need to interpret, the therapist can adopt a more person-centered approach that encourages risk taking and the therapist's attunement to the needs and frame of reference of the adolescents. Such an interaction creates a humanistic relationship that aids both the therapist and the group members. The therapist and the group members are thus freed to experience an authentic human relationship in the psychosocial context of the group.

# ◆ References

Balint M: The Basic Fault. London, Tavistock, 1968

Bettelheim B: Feral children and autistic children. American Journal of Orthopsychiatry, 11:56–66, 1954

Coles R: Erik H. Erikson: The Growth of His Work. Boston, Little Brown, 1970

Erikson E: Young Man Luther: A Study in Psychoanalysis and History. New York, WW Norton, 1958

Erikson E: Identity and the life cycle. Psychol Issues 1(1):1959, entire issue

Erikson E: Identity: Youth and Crisis. New York, WW Norton, 1968

Ferenczi S: The elasticity of psychoanalytic technique (1928), in Final Contributions to the Problems and Methods of Psychoanalysis, Vol 3. Edited by Balint M. New York, Basic Books, 1955, pp 87–102

Ferenczi S: Ferenczi's Clinical Diary (1932). Edited by Dupont J. Cambridge, MA, Harvard University Press, 1988

Ferenczi S: The confusion of tongues between adults and children: the language of tenderness and passion (1933), in Final Contributions to the Problems and Methods of Psychoanalysis, Vol 3. Edited by Balint M. New York, Basic Books, 1955, pp 156–167

Kohut H: The Analysis of The Self. New York, International Universities Press, 1971

Kohut H: The Restoration of the Self. New York, International Universities Press, 1977

Kohut H: How Does Analysis Cure? Edited by Goldberg A, Stepansky PE. Chicago, IL, University of Chicago Press, 1984

Kutash L, Wolf A: The Submerged Self. Northvale, NJ, Jason Aronson, 1992

Masson JM: The Assault on Truth. New York, Farrar, Strauss, Giroux, 1984

Mead GH: Mind, Self and Society. Edited by Morris CW. Chicago, IL, University of Chicago Press, 1934

Rachman AW: Talking it out rather than fighting it out: prevention of a delinquent gang war by group therapy intervention. Int J Group Psychother 19:518–521, 1969

Rachman AW: Group psychotherapy in treating the adolescent identity crisis. International Journal of Child Psychotherapy 1:97–119, 1972

Rachman AW: Identity group psychotherapy, in New Directions in Clinical Child Psychology. Edited by Gordon S, Williams G. New York, Human Science Press, 1974, pp 391–416

Rachman AW: Identity Group Psychotherapy With Adolescents. Springfield, IL, Charles C Thomas, 1975

Rachman AW: Identity conflicts of adolescent psychotherapists. Paper presented at the annual meeting of the American Psychological Association New Orleans, LA, August 1977

Rachman AW: Judicious self-disclosure in group psychotherapy. Paper presented at the annual meeting of the American Group Psychotherapy Association, New York, February 1982

Rachman AW: Identity group psychotherapy with adolescents: a reformulation, in Adolescent Group Psychotherapy. Edited by Azima FJ Cramer, Richmond LH. New York, International Universities Press, 1989, pp 21–41

Rachman AW: The confusion of tongues between adolescents and adults: communication and interaction in adolescent group psychotherapy. Paper presented at the annual meeting of the Missouri Group Psychotherapy Society, St. Louis, MO, April 1995a

Rachman AW: Sandor Ferenczi: The Psychotherapist of Tenderness and Passion. Northvale, NJ, Jason Aronson, 1995b

Rachman AW, Heller ME: Anti-therapeutic factors in therapeutic communities for drug rehabilitation. Journal of Drug Issues 4:393–403, 1974

Rachman AW, Heller ME: Peer group psychotherapy with adolescent drug abusers. Int J Group Psychother 26:373–383, 1976

Raubolt RR: Short term inpatient psychotherapy groups for adolescents, in Varieties of Short Term Therapy Groups. Edited by Rosenbaum M. New York, McGraw-Hill, 1983, pp 273–290

Raubolt RR: Brief, problem focused group psychotherapy with adolescents. Am J Orthopsychiatry 53:157–166, 1983

Roazen P: Freud and His Followers. New York, Knopf, 1975

Rogers C: Client Centered Therapy: Its Current Practice Implications and Theory. Boston, MA, Houghton Mifflin, 1951

Rogers C: A theory of therapy, personality, and interpersonal relationships as developed in the client centered framework, in Psychology: The Study of a Science, Vol. 3. Edited by Koch S. New York, McGraw-Hill, 1959, pp 184–256

Rogers C: On Becoming a Person. Boston, MA, Houghton Mifflin, 1961

Sabusky GS, Kymissis P: Identity group therapy: a transitional group for hospitalized adolescents. Int J Group Psychother 33:99–109, 1983

Winnicott CW: Playing and Reality. London, Tavistock, 1971

# CHAPTER 10

# A Structured, Educative Form of Adolescent Psychotherapy

*Sandra Swirsky Strome, C.S.W., B.C.D., and*
*Erica M. Loutsch, M.D.*

In this chapter, we describe the implementation of a structured, educative form of group therapy on an adolescent inpatient treatment unit, as well as characteristics of this different approach to group therapy. We address the therapist's role as facilitator, role model, and educator and the use of strategies such as cognitive restructuring, feedback, and problem solving in effecting therapeutic change. We also describe and discuss patients' responses to these methods and this form of group therapy.

Very little has been written about the techniques of group therapy for psychiatric inpatients, and even less has been written about the success or failure of existing techniques with adolescent inpatients. Currently, no specific or standardized guidelines are available to therapists for the treatment of the inpatient adolescent as a distinct target of group therapy.

The established therapeutic community generally agrees that psychotherapy of adolescents should focus on improving reality testing, maintaining defensive equilibrium, and promoting ego strengths specifically by focusing on present functioning as opposed to exploring the past. However, this key issue still remains: what mode of group therapy works best with adolescents?

Modifying the techniques of group therapy in general is not a new idea. An educative model was addressed (Maxmen 1978) long before the current study was independently conceived. Maxmen suggested that the primary goal of the group was to facilitate therapeutic interaction among the patients. This goal was achieved by allowing the therapist to motivate, determine group boundaries, train group members, and consistently reinforce group norms. By being somewhat active, the group leader could basically promote action from the patients themselves by positively reinforcing group members when they acted therapeutically. The assumption of Maxmen's model, although based on an adult study, was that the groups' value derived from the patients' perceiving themselves, rather than the leader, as the agents of change.

Endorsing judicious self-disclosure by the therapist as a way of modeling openness, Yalom (1983) found that the therapist could gain trust and encourage risk taking and self-disclosure among the patients by using this technique. Focusing again on the present, instead of exploring the past, Yalom questioned the old psychoanalytic opinion that the therapist must remain a blank screen to facilitate the therapeutic process.

Kibel (1981) also saw the therapist as a moderator, providing support and encouragement while clarifying the here and now of the milieu, as opposed to interpreting intrapsychic conflicts. Although the therapist still remained the object of transference, Kibel found that he or she could also take on an active role and promote interaction in the group while focusing it in the present.

Again, although more classical techniques involving neutrality may work well with adult inpatient groups, other authors (Hurst and Gladieux 1980) discovered that passivity and ambiguity on the part of the leader, coupled with an unstructured situation, produced high levels of anxiety and nonproductiveness in adolescents. The study also showed that this ineffectiveness stemmed from the fact that adolescents feel more defensive than adults when analyzed. Hurst and Gladieux concluded that by offering alternative suggestions as to why certain behaviors took place, the leaders opened the group up so that the adolescents could achieve a degree of actual self-exploration. Hurst and Gladieux also found that the leaders could feel comfortable in the occasional use of physical contact as a means of reassurance and even control, if necessary, when they remained firm in establishing and protecting group norms in this format.

Hannah (1984), on the other hand, warned against any technique that involves a great deal of activity on the part of the therapist. He believed this activity may encourage rationalized forms of countertransference. We question the use of such classical, unstructured techniques in the group treatment of adolescents.

The aforementioned literature (other than Hannah) attests to the fact that others have independently questioned the efficacy of classical group treatment. Because of concern that adolescents as a group have specific qualities that separate them from the overall adult population, it seemed very important to examine whether less traditional views could be put to the test in a model group.

The experiences of the group's leaders (see below) have shown that, despite any countertransference that may exist, the positive aspects of some carefully measured activity by the therapist outweigh the risks. The incorporation of structure, role modeling, facilitation, and education was deemed successful in increasing the levels of interest and participation among the patients in our model adolescent group. An idea for a new group format was thus conceived. After 18 months of these group sessions, results reinforced the views held by both the group leaders and the authors previously mentioned.

Before the implementation of this new group model, all adolescents admitted to the inpatient unit were assigned to group therapy without an assessment of whether or not group therapy was an appropriate treatment modality for them. The staff dealt with all adolescents according to a basic comprehensive treatment plan consisting of individual psychotherapy, group therapy, a therapeutic milieu, and psychotropic medications when indicated. The group format used classical psychoanalytic techniques.

The adolescents in the study were patients on a 24-bed unit at a large private psychiatric hospital in suburban New York. Most patients were between 16 and 25 years of age and carried a DSM-III-R

Axis I diagnosis of a major affective disorder and Axis II diagnoses of severe personality disorders with borderline and/or narcissistic features (American Psychiatric Association 1987).

Entry into the group generally occurred 2 months after admission to the hospital. As previously stated, requirements were based solely on age, without any assessment of individual appropriateness. A standard group consisted of nine members and was co-led by the unit psychology fellow and a social worker. The group met twice a week for 45 minutes. Attendance was required. With mandatory presence the rule, punitive measures followed when an adolescent failed to attend. For instance, when a patient was more than 5 minutes late for a session, the doors were locked and the adolescent's status was lowered for 24 hours.

The group's original model was based on the assumption that a relatively unstructured format where the patients could say anything was necessary to facilitate open discussion. The therapists found many difficulties in this approach, especially when coupled with the presence of rigid rules.

Within this format, group members were often silent and resisted participating. They did not seem to grasp what was expected of them in such an unstructured atmosphere. Comments such as "I don't have to talk, I just have to be here" were voiced regularly. The adolescents frequently challenged both the legitimacy of the treatment and the competency of the leadership. The group became an arena for acting-out behavior. It was thought that perhaps the implementation of less classical and rigid techniques might increase the overall participation of the group members. It was hoped that changes to both the admission process and the format would be therapeutically beneficial.

Restructuring began by changing the criteria for membership in the group. Because the current admission policy resulted in the presence of a number of poorly motivated, inattentive, or inappropriate patients, the therapists began to screen the adolescents on the basis of their ability to perform in group, their level of motivation, and their ability even to attend. The group leaders thought that this screening, coupled with a plan to develop a structured, task-oriented group with active and direct leadership, was more likely to provide a better therapeutic experience and a more robust level of interaction.

A unique aspect of this restructuring process was that the proposed changes were discussed with existing group members, thus engaging them to help determine the new group admission criteria. These changes included the following:

- Staff would determine whether group therapy was indicated for a particular patient, rather than admitting a patient based solely on his or her age.
- Membership would be voluntary instead of mandatory.
- There would be a contract between the group leaders and the patient that he or she would remain in the group for at least 4 weeks or eight consecutive sessions. If the patient chose not to attend after that time, there would be no negative consequences.

Another change implemented by the patients and staff was that members were responsible for bringing a topic for discussion at each session. The subject matter could be of their own choosing.

As a result of these modifications, the group members began gradually to experience themselves as well as the therapists as the principal agents of change. The therapists remained active and used techniques of self-disclosure. They also acted as role models, facilitators, and educators to promote group process.

In terms of self-disclosure and role modeling, the group leaders demonstrated effective strategies for problem solving and shared some personal experiences that facilitated empathy on the part of the patients. It must also be noted that this type of open intervention was carefully integrated at strategic moments and judiciously used.

> An example of self-disclosure by the leaders was seen in their interaction with Justin, who demanded constant attention by disrupting the group with inappropriate comments and jokes. When his efforts failed, he resorted to burping loudly or getting up to go to the bathroom. When one of the group leaders shared with Justin the fact that she often giggled as a result of feeling anxious or nervous, Justin said that he felt understood. He gradually calmed down and became a more interested and appropriately active participant in the group. He eventually began speaking of his feelings of sadness, depression, and anxiety. His acting-out behavior also subsided significantly.

Another example was Kate. She was a guarded, quiet girl with a great deal of hostility toward authority. She had a history of substance abuse and shared how difficult it was to give up this addiction. One of the group leaders shared how difficult it was for her to give up an addiction to three packs of cigarettes per day, which she had had since age 16. Kate was surprised at the openness of the therapist. From that day on, she functioned significantly better in the group. She stated that she felt closer to the group leadership. The very fact that the therapist had told her something personal had facilitated Kate's ability to express herself. Although this self-disclosure may have gone against the more traditional norms of therapeutic neutrality, it seemed to be effective.

As facilitators, the leaders set limits and actively intervened when necessary to maintain the smooth functioning of the group. They brought to consciousness many of the variables that affected group process. When these interventions occurred, they were openly discussed, and the purpose was always explained. Interpretive-like statements were offered as suggestions or as personal reactions to minimize the resistance of group members. For example, when a patient was silent, angry, or dominated the session, the leaders made comments leading to self-examination. Comments such as "Kate, you seem very quiet today" or "Justin, I noticed that you're talking very rapidly. Are you aware of that?" were very helpful to both the individual and the group as a whole. If the group member was unaware of why he or she was acting in such a manner, the group members were asked to offer suggestions as to what they thought might be going on. As important as, or even more important than, facilitating group process was the use of empathy and relating to others. Group members not only shared their impression of what might be going on with the other group member, but they were also encouraged to share similar feelings of their own.

Feedback was another facilitative tool frequently used to acknowledge instances of caring that were observed in group members. An intervention such as feedback was found to be especially important to this population of adolescents because most of their self-images tended to be negative and their self-esteem was unstable, depending very much on external reinforcement. Praise and acknowledgment of their contributions to the group proved to be very beneficial.

As educators, the group leaders taught social skills through role-playing exercises. Interactions between group members were encouraged at every step. Concepts of developmental differences between people, defense mechanisms, and the unconscious were introduced to the group members. Given the fact that many individuals in the group had a borderline range of ego organization, one defense frequently in evidence was splitting. Frequent educative interventions dealing with this defense focused on the maladaptive consequences of seeing things as black and white or good and bad. Open discussion of borderline defenses such as these increased the patients' understanding of such tendencies and enabled them to identify these patterns in themselves and in one another.

One important element that individual members had agreed on before joining the group was that they were to bring in a topic for discussion at each session. This topic could be anything from conflict with parents to difficulties on the treatment unit to tensions among themselves. This requirement provided a structure to deal with the inherent anxiety that is very common when the group is silent. Having the topics to fall back on provided both the leaders and the members with an agenda within which group process could evolve.

In addition to this structure, this group format also had a great deal of flexibility. Given the fact that this population had difficulty with impulse control and regulation of affect, it was often necessary to stop the group process and have a time-out for individual members. If a group member was having an especially difficult time sitting in the group, he or she was allowed to leave the room and was encouraged to return when feeling more in control. There would be no consequences if the group member failed to return. In most cases, the leaders found that the adolescent did return and was either able to share with the group what was going on or to tolerate sitting quietly until group was over.

An example of this technique can be seen in the case of Tammy. This physically unattractive adolescent had been adopted into a dysfunctional family that made her feel extremely negative about herself. Her physical appearance, which included obesity and a severe case of acne, only compounded her problems as the family scapegoat. Having become self-destructive to the point of slashing her wrists, Tammy also sought out abuse from those around her and eventually became the unit scapegoat. She was usually quite agitated and often left the group. When she returned, she could not articulate what was bothering her. After a period of time in the group and with the acceptance and empathy of her peers in a nonthreatening environment, she eventually opened up and began to talk about her home life and problems. No doubt, this was a totally new experience for her.

The flexibility of this model offered several advantages. It allowed for and encouraged the growth of the group's cohesiveness and also provided an opportunity to identify with the leaders, thereby modifying the group members' harsh and punitive superegos. This model also made room for a variety of intervention strategies that took into account the mood of the individual and the group, members' ego strengths and deficits, and the developmental level of the group members.

The results of the implementation of this new therapeutic model were overwhelmingly positive. The climate at sessions became pleasant and very cooperative. The level of trust and cohesiveness among members continually evolved. The frequency and duration of silent acting-out episodes were reduced, and there were fewer expressions of hostility to group leaders. There was more interaction (either supportive or appropriately confrontational) among group members and an increase in empathetic feelings toward each other. These adolescents' understanding and tolerance of the idiosyncrasies and behaviors of others increased markedly. Self-motivation was also observed by noting the frequency of attendance and the high participation rate. Group members began to identify and carry out the roles of the group leaders, acting as facilitators themselves and being more open with their own feelings and experiences. In fact, they began to use some of these new-found social skills to solve specific problems and to master certain tasks for themselves on the treatment unit.

Because the therapists repeatedly conveyed the notion that each member of the group was an important factor in the group's development as a whole, the roles of the therapists themselves were demystified. Because they were treated as responsible agents in the change and running of the group, the adolescents began to experience a sense of personal power and a stronger self-image. They felt important and vital—many for the first time in their lives.

There was also a gradual change in the kinds of topics the members brought into group. Whereas the topics of the previous sessions generally focused on issues such as being institutionalized, not feeling safe, and how to get a pass home, the new topics became more personalized and intimate. The group now spoke of their negative attention-seeking behavior and their maladaptive relationships with one another. They spoke about guilt, fears of intimacy, thoughts of suicide, and their dependency issues.

These shifts in topic content had a major impact on a patient named Sybil. Sybil was a 15-year-old black female in the 10th grade. She had an Axis I diagnosis of major depression and an Axis II diagnosis of borderline personality disorder. She came from a fragmented family that abandoned her at an early age. Trust was a heavily conflicted issue for this adolescent, and her initial entry into the group was characterized by isolation from her peers and an inability to express herself verbally. She externalized all her problems and would frequently leave the group when she sensed danger. Danger in Sybil's case meant that the group was dealing with issues of intimacy and closeness.

The group members, who had already become quite adept at modeling themselves after the therapists, were extremely supportive and empathic toward Sybil. Gently, they began to encourage her to express her feelings. After months of being withdrawn and socially isolated, Sybil began to express herself in the group. She stated that she felt that the group members accepted her and she experienced their support and concern.

Sybil was also one of two black adolescents on the ward. When the other black adolescent was discharged, she again became depressed and withdrawn. The therapists, acting as facilitators, asked her if it was difficult being the only black person on the unit. Her response was startling, as was the response of the group. Not only did she verbalize the strain and isolation of her situation, but the group also rallied around her and supported her totally. Reacting to her honesty, one group member stated, "We wouldn't care if you were blue, purple, or even green. We'd still love you." After that session, the staff observed Sybil interacting with Tammy. She empathized with Tammy's feelings of isolation and exclusion. The two adolescents became friends, and the scapegoating of Tammy ceased.

Although the therapists were delighted with the overwhelmingly positive reactions to this new group model, they thought it important to see what the patients themselves thought of the whole process. A questionnaire was distributed to the members of the group to gather their reactions. These reactions included not just whether they thought group therapy was helpful, but also how they felt about the new format and style of this type of group. They were also asked whether they would consider seeking outpatient group therapy after being released from the hospital. The unanimous response from the members was that they found the group extremely helpful because they learned that they weren't alone with their problems or feelings. Also unanimous and very encouraging was the fact that all who answered said they would seek outpatient group therapy if needed in the future.

Additionally, members expressed positive attitudes about the style of the group and its leadership. A case in point is that when one of the therapists celebrated a birthday, most of the members of the group got together and gave her a card. The card was filled with affectionate phrases and actual words of thank-you for what they considered a very beneficial experience in their lives.

The staff were asked for their comments in an informal attempt to ascertain whether or not the group had any impact on the treatment unit as a whole. All the impressions, based on day-to-day observations of the adolescents, were positive. Staff reported that group members seemed to take a more problem-solving approach to many of the issues concerning the unit. The adolescents originally involved in this project had initiated their own patient-run meetings on the unit and always prepared an agenda of their own before every community meeting. Members were more apt to be involved in patient government and had begun to seek out staff to address issues of concern to them. This was quite a contrast to the acting-out behavior before implementation of this group model.

Conducting a group of this type presented certain challenges to its developers because of the nature of adolescence itself, the treatment unit, and the teaching hospital environment in which it was established. The first concern was the integration of a membership that varied considerably along the dimensions of age and type and degree of pathology. Previously, it was thought that the commonality of the hospital experience created a feeling of unanimity among the patients, thereby reducing the negative effects ordinarily triggered by such heterogeneity. These differences, however, augmented by the fact that adolescence in general is a period of cognitive transition, led to inevitable developmental variations within the group at any given time and were a serious consideration in the development of the new group. For instance, the ability to think abstractly and the capacity to empathize are two important cognitive dimensions affected by these variations. The group members were taught to be aware of and supportive of the differing functional levels among themselves while gaining experience in noting their own intrapersonal variations in functioning.

Bringing in topics for discussion was used as a technique to realistically address the adolescents' developmental and diagnostic differences. The original format, based on the idea of just saying anything that comes to mind, placed unrealistic demands on a population that was developmentally delayed and unable to think abstractly. Group members took turns writing on a large blackboard the topics for discussion brought in by each group member on that particular day. Writing topics where they could be seen by all seemed to provide a constant, concrete representation of the day's work. This fostered broader participation in the process by the less cognitively mature members of the group.

The second challenge revolved around maintaining the group's ongoing process despite the flux in membership that is to be expected on an acute-care inpatient unit. The potential for interruptions in the therapeutic process was reduced by the efficiency with which new members were incorporated into the group. The stress of these transition periods lessened as the group's structure evolved. During these times, both the old and the new members were encouraged to express feelings related to either being a new member or accepting one. Expression of feelings about members of the group who had been discharged was encouraged, thereby providing the opportunity for these adolescents to develop object constancy.

Another issue that needs mentioning is the fact that the group was conducted in a teaching hospital where rotations took place. Every January and July, new leaders were assigned to this group. The difficulties these changes presented were minimized by the level of autonomy at which the group came to operate, as well as by the predictable framework of the sessions. The potential stresses on group cohesion and productivity lessened because new leaders were more easily integrated into the group.

In summation, it appears that the change to a structured, educative form of group therapy was responsible for the positive changes observed in the functioning of the group.

Voluntary membership, a decrease in rules, changes in structure and technique, and the focus on the here and now seem to be the basic ingredients that elevated the functioning level of the group members. The introduction of an agenda based on individual personal topics served as the catalyst in that it provided a structure for the sessions. This agenda proved to be a creative way to engage the adolescents involved in the group. This model appears to support Hurst and Gladieux's premise (1980) that a structured environment, as opposed to unstructured ambiguity, reduces an adolescent's anxiety level enough to increase his or her availability to be engaged in a productive group treatment program.

## ◆ References

American Psychiatric Association: Diagnostic and Statistical Manual of Mental Disorders, 3rd Edition, Revised. Washington, DC, American Psychiatric Association, 1987

Hannah S: Countertransference in inpatient group psychotherapy—implications for technique. Int J Group Psychother 32:257–272, 1984

Hurst G, Gladieux JD: Guideline for leading an adolescent therapy group, in Group and Family Therapy. Edited by Wolberg LR. New York, Brunner/Mazel, 1980, pp 151–163

Kibel HD: A conceptual model for short term inpatient group psychotherapy. Am J Psychiatry 138:74–80, 1981

Maxmen J: An educative model for inpatient group therapy. Int J Group Psychother 28:321–338, 1978

Yalom ID: Inpatient Group Psychotherapy. New York, Basic Books, 1983

# CHAPTER 11

# Therapeutic Use of Theater With Adolescents

*Emily Nash*

The desks line the sides of the classroom. In the center a group of junior high school students sit in a circle of chairs. Luis is dozing on Tania's shoulder. Risa sits sucking her thumb, holding the hand of Mario, this week's boyfriend. Alex, Tommy, and Carlos stare out into space, arms folded. Maria calls Alex stupid, and he rises, ready to strike. A team of theater professionals enter; they are workshop leaders with Creative Alternatives of New York. The mood in the classroom shifts: the actors have arrived. "Hey, what are we gonna do today?" "Where's the video?" "I want to be the judge in the scene this time."

Everyone speaks at once and it's hard to imagine how all this disparate energy will be focused. But the leaders of this group will ultimately transform a traditional classroom setting with learning-disabled students into an ensemble of young actors who will weave together their life experiences and hitherto untapped imaginative forces into drama.

"OK," the leader announces, "let's begin!"

Creative Alternatives of New York (CANY) theater workshops are designed to provide emotionally and psychologically disabled persons with a therapeutic experience. At the heart of the work is the belief that every person, no matter how dysfunctional, has a healthy self and within that self is the potential to create. CANY sees the creative process as a healing experience of self-discovery and renewal. Theater, in particular, has the power to transform—to act as a bridge from one world to the next and from one part of the self to another. Because drama reflects the full range of human experience, it becomes a natural discipline for those who may have no other avenue to express their inner selves.

For the past several years, CANY has been leading theater groups for learning-disabled students in a junior high school. These students have emotional, cognitive, and physical disabilities and do not respond well to traditional approaches to learning. They are considered academically slow and unable to focus, concentrate, or work well in groups. Most of them come from abusive, chaotic homes and have rarely, if ever, known a nurturing adult. Their sense of self is fragmented; most engage in antisocial, self-destructive behavior.

For these young people, the dramatic process offers a way to tap into their creative and intellectual energies. Freed from the expectations of standard academic achievement, they can engage in an activity in which they can excel if given the chance: creative expression.

In the theater workshops, the students are never approached in light of their "deficits." In a creative enterprise such a category does not exist. There is no right way or wrong way; no expectations are superimposed or standard goals set. "These workshops tap into a full set of skills the students have not failed at," is the succinct explanation offered by Steve Kahn, director of special education for the district involved in this school project (personal communication, May 1992).

In this framework, many behavioral problems otherwise viewed as negative and uncontrollable can be turned to positive use. Students who are illiterate or on the verge of suspension find themselves successfully writing, directing, and acting in their own one-act plays. Students who are unable to sit still and constantly demand attention become greatly appreciated for their willingness to jump into improvisations or freely offer creative ideas. Those who dominate and bully others can become brilliant directors. Shy, sensitive, insecure individuals may be profoundly insightful in developing story lines.

Thus, antisocial and self-destructive energies are redirected and given constructive form. As deficits turn to assets, the sense of self as "handicapped" begins to fade, and new feelings of competence, worth, and effectiveness emerge and can begin to be integrated. Through characterization and improvisation, these students gain a stronger, more integrated sense of self and awareness of others. CANY's work with adolescents reveals how creative metaphor can unlock dormant energies and facilitate new, more positive patterns of behavior, freeing participants from the actual circumstances of their lives and providing them with a means of expressing their imaginative powers and revealing their otherwise suppressed thoughts and feelings.

## ◆ History

The work of CANY was originally designed for psychiatric inpatients. Margaret Ladd, an actress, and Lyle Kessler, a playwright, pioneered the approach, developing a repertoire of structured exercises derived from their own theater training. Their intention was to free up blocked energies and engage patients in imaginative play.

It was discovered that through playing characters outside themselves (e.g., characters from mythology, fairy tales, history, and literature and characters inspired by hats, props, postcards, and paintings), patients were able to activate dormant creative energies. They began to express aspects of their personalities too threatening to disclose in real life; they could voice thoughts and feelings that were otherwise quite inaccessible. Through improvising fictitious scenes, patients found new abilities to interact with others in spontaneous and appropriate ways. The use of metaphor, as in acting a role, offered a protective guise that enabled even the most regressed nonverbal patients to engage themselves with others.

After several years of successful work with adult psychiatric populations, CANY was asked to work with hospitalized adolescents. Full of confidence that they would be equally effective with this population, a CANY team brought their repertoire of exercises to a group of 12 adolescent patients. To their surprise and dismay, attempts to engage these young people in the fanciful world of myths, fairy tales, and make-believe was met with enormous resistance, anger, and lack of interest. The patients clearly felt silly and infantilized; they were self-conscious—mortified by what they were being asked to do.

The team was bewildered. Adult patients of all ages had taken delight in playing Ulysses, Cinderella, and the Big Bad Wolf. Far from feeling self-conscious, they had felt protected. Through these archetypal characters, unconscious thoughts and feelings had found a way to conscious expression. It seemed to make sense that adolescents would reap the same benefits. But it soon became clear that whereas the goals and basic philosophy could remain the same, the exercises themselves needed vast revision to be applicable to adolescents.

The artistic team decided to listen carefully to what the kids were saying: they rejected the offered exercises but came up with ideas of their own. They wanted to do scenes about families, school, relationships, and unresolved conflicts between people—all the issues of their own lives. As they expressed these ideas, they were bursting with energy, enthusiasm, and determination. The young people and the CANY team had stumbled onto a way to provide a desperately needed outlet. If the artistic team could supply the framework, the kids were ready to play.

The group began developing scenes about conflicts between parents and children, siblings, peers, and teachers and students. No longer feeling childish, these soon-to-be grown-ups had opened the door themselves and found a way to make the group work. Although scenes remained fictitious and never included exact reenactments of actual events or real persons from their lives, the *themes* were clearly drawn from the teenagers' experiences and needs. This gave them a means of mobilizing, in more direct and socially appropriate ways, the deep well of emotional and creative energy locked inside them.

Thus, CANY's theater work with adolescents began. Since that time, the work has evolved considerably, along with a more complete understanding of the developmental tasks of this stage of life and how we can help facilitate these arduous labors of the adolescent years through the dramatic process.

## ◆ The Method

Fundamental to the successful evolution of a theater group is the artistic team's ability to create the necessary "facilitating environment"

(Winnicott 1971, p. 141): a caring, accepting, nonjudgmental climate in which group members can feel safe to express themselves. Building a working group and providing appropriate artistic and therapeutic interventions are key to this methodology. Skillful interventions engage individuals in the moment and facilitate their movement in new directions.

Theater artists who choose this work are carefully trained in a full range of intervention techniques designed to 1) create the facilitating environment, 2) respond to the dynamics of the group, and 3) skillfully guide participants through artistic metaphors (fictitious characters and situations that group members choose to enact). These interventions awaken spontaneity, affirm choices, present new possibilities, redirect negative energies, facilitate communications, and *join resistances.* In joining resistances, rather than trying to overcome or argue with a patient's negative expression toward the group, the leader verbally joins the patient, fully taking his or her position.

> "I hate this group," one group member, Carla, says. "I'm not coming!"
>
> "Oh come on," responds the leader, "tell us all the ways you hate it. We're very interested."
>
> Another young girl announces, "I'm Sonia, and I'm not going to participate. And that's what I'm going to tell everyone when we say our names!"
>
> "Wonderful," says the leader, "but I think you should say 'I'm not going to participate and my name is Sonia'—let's get the most important things out first. And why not find out who else is *not* going to participate?"
>
> Sonia finds out each person's name and asks each one if he or she intends to join in or not. By the time the session ends, Sonia has played the title role in a group improvisation.

The most appropriate intervention says to workshop members, "I understand you," "I'm on your side," "I enjoy your process," and "I believe in you." The depth, openness, and richness of the creative work rest on the leaders' awareness of the needs of every group participant at each stage of the process. A positive relationship with an adult authority figure is especially important for disadvantaged and learning-disabled adolescents (Rachman 1989, p. 30).

The leaders function as facilitators and participants, directors and players, and artists and therapists. They are there to discover, pursue, and delight in every contribution made by members of the group and to protect them from feeling attacked, humiliated, or isolated. The leader is a devoted ally, willing to remain engaged no matter how turbulent the process may at times become.

# ◆ The Structure of the Group

Group cohesion is built through the exercise process. During the initial stages of a new group, the leaders quickly establish the group contract by plunging immediately into creative exercises that include everyone, do not directly confront anyone, and are fun. All contributions made by group members are accepted, applauded, and taken seriously. Participants soon understand that they are involved in an activity with no expectations other than cooperative work. The rules of cooperation are established as the leader readily intervenes in all hurtful or destructive behavior: "No attacking in this group," "No dissing [showing disrespect]," "No hitting allowed in here." These interventions are frequently repeated. Eventually the group members start to monitor themselves: "Hey, man, no *dissing!*"

Every workshop session has three basic structural components: 1) the warm-up, 2) the "passing," and 3) dramatic improvisation. The first two components serve to unify the group in preparation for the third.

## The Warm-Up

Warm-up exercises are an essential ritual at the beginning of each session. They join individual energies into a common flow. They center and focus the group and launch it into the world of play. This nonverbal activity prepares members for more verbal interactive work. All warm-ups begin with breathing and stretching—ideally in the same format each time. Some members may giggle, balk, or sit on the sidelines, but eventually all join in with the secure feeling of a shared ritual.

Warm-up exercises are typically more difficult for adolescents than for any other group because adolescents are so vulnerable to feelings of self-consciousness; they are terrified of looking foolish in front of their peers. Leaders need to develop exercises that neither embarrass nor alienate group members, but rather energize them and draw them together. Successful warm-ups with adolescents accomplish the following:

1. They elicit attitude: each member greets the group with a physical gesture that says, "I'm cool," or "I don't care about anything," or "I'm a rock star [a cop, a teacher]."
2. They join the resistance: each member makes a sound and a movement that express boredom, anger, frustration, or other negative responses.
3. They use phrases linked to recognizable character types—for example, a strict teacher, a frightened child, or an angry mother.
4. They take the existential plight of teenagers seriously.

In one successful warm-up, a group created a dream tree. In this exercise, all members are asked to state a dream they have for themselves and to express the dream with a phrase (e.g., "I'm dreaming of my future," "I'm dreaming of love," "I'm dreaming of money"), together with a corresponding movement. As each member performs this task, he or she must physically connect to another member, until a treelike form takes shape.

## The Passing

Passings are vital links in developing group cohesion. They allow thoughts, feelings, ideas, and experiences to be verbalized in relation to a given theme. Passings that work best for adolescents elicit their opinions, anxieties, and thoughts about the future without exposing their vulnerabilities. Examples of useful themes are "What is something you would change about your community (New York City, the world)?" "What don't grown-ups understand about kids?" and "What would you like to be doing 10 years in the future?"

The responses group members have toward one another during the passing serve the group-building process as members, without realizing it, begin to relate to each other with a new kind of respect and awareness. They start to identify with one another in a positive way; they see reflected in one another what may be possible for themselves. The leader can facilitate this uniting of the group by "bridging" members. In this extremely effective technique, the leader draws group members out on every point, prompts them to respond specifically to each other's statements, and furthers their potential for reinforcing one another. "*Through bridging* they develop emotional connections where they did not exist before" (Ormont 1992, p. 15).

> The leader asks, "What would you like to be doing in 10 years?"
>
> One boy answers, "Play in the World Series." Another says, "Go to college, become a lawyer." A very angry, withdrawn girl, Diana—to the great surprise of the entire group—says that she, too, wants to be a lawyer.
>
> The leader, picking up on this, furthers the interaction.
>
> LEADER.   Two lawyers in the group! Great! Anyone else want to be a lawyer?
> JASON.   No, I want to be the mayor.
> LEADER *[providing a bridge]*.   Terrific, two lawyers and a mayor. Alex, what kind of lawyer do you think Jason would make?
> ALEX.   A great one. He's smart, he can talk!
> LEADER.   What about you, Susanna?
> SUSANNA.   I don't want to be anything like that. I'm going to be a singer, a famous rock star.
> LOUIS.   You should be, you have a beautiful voice.
> LEADER.   Would you like to hear her sing?
> LOUIS.   Hell, yeah!

As bridges begin to be built, members become more involved in the group flow, and positive connections begin to replace negative, provocative behavior. Interest in others starts to develop, paving the way for more active involvement in the passing and perhaps in other activities as well. These passings can often provide raw material for improvisations, where ideas are developed dramatically.

## Dramatic Improvisation

Improvisation provides group members with a playground in which to explore any number of given realities. Fictitious situations, while rooted in real life, are distanced enough to provide a comfort zone. In an improvisation the players can direct circumstances in any way they choose. Imagination interwoven with experience produces whatever story the participants wish to tell. Adolescents in search of identity need the chance to assume a number of different types of roles and sets of values—to try them on for size, according to Rachman (1989). Improvisation offers adolescents a safe setting for experimentation. "It is in playing and only in playing that the individual child or adult is able to be creative and to use the whole personality, and it is only in being creative that the individual discovers the self" (Winnicott 1971, p. 54).

The chosen metaphor (i.e., the fictitious character or situation) frees adolescents to explore parts of themselves and their experience too threatening to express in any other way. Personal traits not readily apparent in other parts of their lives surface. Individuals feel empowered as they reach beyond their fixed patterns of behavior, taking risks and exploring new possibilities.

More specifically, the aspects of improvisational work that proved particularly valuable in CANY's work with adolescents included

- The chance for group members to play a variety of roles—parts of themselves, figures in their lives, and possibilities for the future
- Empowerment, which means the adolescents' experiences are acknowledged; they are offered a chance to reenact frightening, enraging, or confusing events; their feelings and point of view are affirmed; and they discover some of the options available for meeting challenging situations and resolving conflicts
- The availability of corrective family experiences, which offer a reparative working through of difficult family dynamics and a chance to practice more functional behavior
- The opportunity to fill in significant maturational gaps through dramatization of experiences that may have been missing from the life cycle

■ The experience of success and accomplishment
■ The pleasure of imaginative play, which runs throughout the work

The following detailed examples show how in any given improvisation these various dynamics tend to overlap so that the group members simultaneously benefit from several of them. To illustrate the process, I isolated examples of all but the pleasure of imaginative play, which is self-explanatory and a cumulative result of the entire experience.

## Play: Acting Different Roles

According to Erik Erikson's theory of stages of the human life cycle, adolescence is a time of "identity confusion which is the inability to choose a viable set of roles. To settle one's identity confusion also means to abandon for good, or to reintegrate into a future role, that negative identity which is the sum of all that one has learned one is *not* supposed to be and which contains some of one's abandoned potential" (E. H. Erikson, quoted in J. M. Erikson 1976, p. 50).

In theater, one can play many roles that are not perceived as being part of the self. Members of a workshop group can pursue the necessary adolescent task of experiencing a range of identities without judgment or censorship. Within the dramatic structure, all types of persons and human experiences are worth our attention. All roles are equally interesting and human. Here, a group member could be a villain and a hero, a child and a parent, a criminal and a cop, the judge and the accused. For example, as group members play out both the bad mother and the good, forgiving mother, they begin unconsciously to make choices about what feels right to them and what fits best. Giving equal regard to all facets of the self without judgment frees them to honestly favor one over another without needing either to rebel or to please. There is full license to explore the darker, potentially destructive aspects of the self without consequence, thereby offering the possibility of understanding and resolution.

Jenny, a rather angry member of the group who often acts out, talks about her grandmother. Her mother, she tells us, died of AIDS and she has been left in the care of her grandmother. She describes this woman as restrictive, punitive, and often abusive. Jenny feels as though she lives with a "wicked old witch" who doesn't let her do any of the things she wants to do. She feels that when she is with her grandmother, she always has to be "good." She is furious and desperately unhappy.

The group sets up a scene in which Jenny plays a grandmother who cares for her three granddaughters. The sisters are frightened by her temper and abusive behavior, but they have decided on this day to stand up to her. They want very badly to go to a certain party, wear fancy dresses, and stay out later than the early curfew imposed on them by their caretaker.

The scene begins with the sisters asking if they can go to a party in the evening. When Jenny, as the grandmother, verbally assaults each sister for even contemplating making such a request, she reveals levels of venom, hatred, and disgust that could only have their source in the personal assaults she herself has experienced in her real home. Not for one moment does the grandmother in the scene listen to the girls, despite their various attempts to reach her. It is as if she had a whip she cracked each time one of them opened her mouth. She will not budge; the sisters are not allowed to go anywhere.

When the scene ends, the leader praises Jenny for the strength of her characterization and expresses understanding of her difficult situation. Then the leader asks Jenny how she, in her own life, would like her grandmother to react in such a situation. Jenny says she likes her grandmother's strictness but wishes she would listen and show more understanding and ability to compromise. The leader asks Jenny if she wants to reenact the scene incorporating these wished-for qualities in the grandmother. She does.

This time, Jenny as the grandmother asks the sisters where they are going, what they will be wearing, and what time they intend to be home. She listens, asks questions, and agrees to compromise on the outfits and curfew time. It is the first time she, Jenny, has shown any tenderness or flexibility. As the grandmother, Jenny even reveals a sense of humor as she recalls "my own youthful experiences."

The second enactment of the scene left Jenny feeling more in control because she was able to choose between being harsh and being understanding. She discovered some flexibility in her own emotional behavior instead of being possessed by one overpowering emotion.

As group members dramatized different aspects of themselves, they discovered strengths and capacities they had never before experienced. "We are so confined to who we think we are," said one member. Another commented, "Playing so many different characters has made me realize I have so many different parts of myself." As Joan Erikson (1976) noted, acting can help adolescents work toward resolving confusion. Their roles in improvisations model new roles and behaviors that they can then attempt to incorporate into their own lives.

Several group members request that the group do a scene in which a boy who is feeling hopeless about his life threatens to kill someone and then jump off a roof himself. "Yeah, yeah, let's do it," comes the echo of the others.

The group leader quickly tries to assess the underlying subtext in the request for such a scene and what metaphor she can use to allow the issue to be dramatically and safely explored.

She wonders aloud, "I hear you talking about a very angry kid who is feeling completely hopeless, and the only thing he can think of doing is to give it all up."

The group looks very interested. She asks, "What's going on that makes him feel this way?"

Responses come tumbling out: "He's all alone." "Nobody understands him." "His parents never spend any time with him." "Nobody listens to him."

The leader asks, "Why did he drop out of school?"

"Nobody helps him with his homework," someone answers.

"Okay," says the leader, "he feels abused, misunderstood, angry as hell. Let's imagine he's locked himself in his room and refuses to leave."

"Yeah," say some members, "and we can have different friends of his come try to talk to him."

"Yeah, and maybe his family, too," others say.

The leader asks, "Who from his family?"

"His father and his brother," someone says. "He gets to tell his father how mad he is at him."

"All right," says the leader. "Let's set up the scene."

The characters are cast and given fictitious names, ages, and individual characteristics. The group determines the order in which the other characters will come to talk to José, the main character. The scene begins with José alone in his room. The leader suggests that he begin by speaking aloud an inner monologue, putting his thoughts into words. An inner monologue lets buried thoughts and feelings come to the surface, allowing the character to understand more about himself or herself. In this way, unconscious motivations are more clearly understood and can be channeled consciously into the life of the scene.

José speaks of his sadness, his aloneness, and his feelings of being trapped. He speaks of his family's never being around, of the constant fighting when they are, of his need for his father, his wish to do better in school, and his anger at the guys who sell him drugs. Through verbalizing all this, José lets the other characters in on his inner life, and perhaps the actor is also sorting out the enmeshed strands of his own emotional confusion.

The characters enter the scene in turn. First comes the father, played by Richie, a very immature, insecure, withdrawn, thumb-sucking teenager:

FATHER.   Son, I want to speak with you.

SON.   Don't you have to go to work? You always have to go to work.

FATHER.   I'm worried about you. I'll take the day off if I have to. Please let me talk to you.

SON.   You never had any time before. Why now?

FATHER.   Because I see you're in trouble. I know I'm probably part of the problem. I've been blind, selfish. I just haven't realized what was going on.

SON.   Son (very cautiously): OK—let's talk.

FATHER.   What's going on? Why are you so upset? Did your girlfriend break up with you?

SON.   No. Everything is wrong. Nothing is working out. You never have time. You're never around to talk to.

FATHER.   You're right. I'm very sorry, son. I want to change, to work things out, to help you.

SON.   I dropped out of school, couldn't concentrate, didn't do my work. I feel angry all the time.

FATHER.   I see how I've neglected you, son. I do. I didn't know any differently. I just did what my father did. He was never there, and when he was he just yelled. I want to help you. I'll take more time off from work. Spend time doing your homework with you. We'll do things together.

SON.   I would like that. But how do I know it will happen?

FATHER.   I promise.

SON.   OK, I feel better that we talked.

After this scene, José's closest friends come to talk to him and tell him how special he is to them, how much he'll be missed, and how he needs to reach out and ask for help. They urge him to come out and make contact with people. His girlfriend enters and offers her faith in him, sharing with him how hard his hurting himself is on her. The brother enters with a more confrontational, but equally caring, attitude. José agrees to give his life another chance.

The participating students left this workshop session with the feeling of being more closely bound together as characters—and as people. The intimacy achieved through playing such a scene is one major value of this work. In character, the students or group members can open up emotionally to one another in ways they themselves are not yet ready for. For people generally so defended and on guard, these experiences are highly meaningful. "Interplay with others, often difficult in life, can offer a timebound intimacy and camaraderie" (E. H. Erikson, quoted in J. M. Erikson 1976, p. 102).

## Play: Acting Future Roles

For the young people in our workshops, as for all adolescents, these years are a time of transition—a rite of passage from exploration of self to definition of self. Yet for these adolescents the future is bleak. Given their social and economic status and the stigma of being learning disabled, even a vision of a meaningful future is beyond reach. Models for a positive set of values or a rewarding vocation are scant, and dreams of accomplishment seem unrealizable, thwarted by obstacles that appear impossible to overcome.

Therefore, it is quite meaningful to provide a supportive milieu that encourages these young people to form visions of the future and to experience their capabilities to think, feel, and behave as adults. In helping them imagine the future and become characters in that future, the theater workshops give them the chance, as one CANY consultant has said, to "think through and define goals, reach inside and find what's important to them—to sort out specific thoughts and feelings."

Erik Erikson pointed out the connections between discovering a value system, achieving a sense of community and cohesiveness, and being able to imagine a future growing out of the present: "Childhood proper ends when and where the young person can freely enter some commitment to a set of values and a course of activity. *Fidelity* is the capacity to pledge loyalties along with the capacity to follow a future course. . . . Fidelity thus becomes the cornerstone of a sense of identity. . . ." (E. H. Erikson, quoted in J. M. Erikson 1976, p. 49).

Diana, the withdrawn girl who expressed a desire to become a lawyer, provides an illustration of how the theater workshops can open up not only a vision of the future but also the possibility of a commitment to that vision. The leader recognized that Diana's revelation of her ambition was significant and asked Diana to come up with a situation in which she could act as a lawyer. Diana created a courtroom scene in which she was a district attorney in a child-abuse lawsuit.

For Diana, who viewed herself and was seen by others as "not very bright" and as a reluctant participant in the group, performing this scene was a turning point. A hidden self was revealed when she assumed the role of a professional: a self that had a superior intelligence, strong points of view, and a capacity for self-assertion. The rage that could be palpably felt through her silences and withdrawals had now been redirected with force and self-definition.

Diana was visibly proud of her work. She had activated a dormant potential, and the rest of the group now saw her in a new light. Diana gradually took on more of a leadership role, spontaneously offering new ideas, directing scenes, and becoming more willing to reveal other aspects of her personality: her vulnerability, her humor, and her flexibility.

Tony, a young adolescent in a short-term inpatient unit in a hospital, attended the theater workshop with uncharacteristic enthusiasm and commitment. His provocative, impulsive, and disruptive behavior had threatened to get him kicked out of almost every other group he had been in. As far as the artistic team could tell, the only exception to this pattern was his engagement in the theater group. He seemed to seize on the opportunity to reveal his better self—the self striving toward maturation and recognition. When he regressed to his disruptive behavior, he could be quite easily redirected back into the group if given some responsible, adult role, either as leader in the group process or as an important character in a scene.

During passings, for example, he was asked to elicit responses from other group members and often assumed the role of casting director or playwright, which served to sustain his interest in the improvisational work. In scenes, Tony consistently chose the roles of mature, responsible men in leadership positions.

> During a scene between a boy who was flunking out of school and his sympathetic schoolmate, Tony quickly volunteered to step in as the teacher. He assigned other group members to be part of the class and proceeded to lecture them on the merits of paying attention and working hard. He was gentle and understanding with the students in trouble, offering his suggestions and his help.
>
> On another occasion, Tony chose to play an important business-man making a trip with his wife to visit Bill and Hillary Clinton. He had "some important questions" to ask Bill in order to help further his own career. He also had some "important" things to tell him.
>
> The group leader asked him one day, "Tony, why is it that you are so cooperative in this group and in the other groups they are ready to kick you out? Why do we see the best of you here?" Tony replied, "Because I really like it. I like acting. It gets my energy out."

It got his energy out and made him feel competent, empowered, and rewarded with positive feedback. Tony experienced a positive bond *and* an identification with the artistic team. He responded to the unconditional acceptance of and respect for who he was.

As seen with Diana and Tony, taking on a leadership role can play a significant part in the evolution of the adolescent personality. Opportunities to play authority figures, to dictate right and wrong, and to put forth laws and social agendas are greeted with enthusiasm and serious consideration. Young people involved in every sort of antisocial, destructive, and self-destructive behavior relish playing roles that challenge them to see that justice prevails.

In a group that took place on the same day as a mayoral election, each member was asked to imagine himself or herself as a candidate for mayor. They were to be interviewed about what they would do if elected. As each rose to speak, there were clear changes in posture, attitude, authority, and assurance. In these interviews, group members voiced belief systems, plans, and social commitments. They said they would help the homeless, address the drug problem, and deal with child abuse. There would be proper education, more protection on the streets, and abortion rights—all issues relevant to their daily lives.

In response to a bout of disruptive behavior that was interfering with the work at hand, the artistic team asked the group members to write their own constitution, collectively defining the rules (laws) of the group. A document was authored that included rules prohibiting interruption of others and putting others down, a rule that banned gum chewing, and a rule that required listening. The group members wrote it on a large piece of paper and hung it in the front of the room. The constitution was frequently referred to, usually by group members keeping tabs on their peers. Eventually the rules became more and more internalized.

In both these examples, group members began to make conscious the seeds of their own value systems and ideologies, their commitment to society, and their growing need to "count in the lives of others," as one member put it. They developed an increased understanding of what it meant to function well together.

Another dramatic illustration of adolescents grappling with the development of their own value system happened when a number of groups were dealing with the issue of racism. Each group decided to create a scene about an outsider.

Pedro, a boy from Puerto Rico, has moved into an all-black neighborhood. The newcomer is challenged by a black gang that is out to get him. In every class, soon after the scene begins, a member of the student "audience" rises and yells, "Shoot 'em!" In all six classes there is no option suggested other than "shoot 'em" (meaning Pedro). "That's how it is, miss," the students tell the leader.

The leader asks each class what they think *should* happen. One class suggests that a girlfriend of Pedro's come and shoot members of the black gang.

"How many?" the leader inquires.

"Until there are just a few left. That's how it is, miss," the students repeat.

Disturbed by the unanimous acceptance of this ending, the leader returns next day with another idea: Each class must come up with a *character* for Pedro—a personality and a history. In this way perhaps they will learn *who* it is the gang is threatening—and shooting.

Each class focuses on what Pedro's dream is—to be a teacher, a musician, a politician, or whatever—and discusses what might get in the way of his fulfilling this dream, such as drugs, illiteracy or bad grades in school, his girlfriend's pregnancy, racism, and abuse. Each class gives Pedro a different dream and different obstacles.

Then they repeat the beginning of the scene with the racial confrontation. This time no one in any of the classes wants to kill him. He has become a person, a human being with whom they can identify and toward whom they can feel empathy.

Vital exploration of these issues ensued through discussion and dramatization. Students found themselves, according to one of the group leaders, "expressing ideas, examining beliefs and taking responsibility for those beliefs. They were suddenly not only accepting the world as it is, but reexamining how they want to change it" (J. Rosenfels, CANY group leader, personal communication, December 1992). They discussed the obstacles they faced in their own lives and perhaps for the first time began to consider that there might be ways around the obstacles. There might be a choice as to whether to remain victimized or to confront the problems and find some resolution.

The group leader concluded, "This was a very empowering experience for the group. As I allowed and accepted their worst fears, the issues stopped being a secret and could be publicly explored. The teachers had never seen the students so involved, so inspired to cooperate, and even though there were disagreements, they *wanted* to work them out so the 'play' would succeed" (J. Rosenfels, personal communication, December 1992).

## Empowerment

Becoming empowered rather than accepting the unending misery of victimization is an ongoing theme in the groups. For these young people there is a prevalent feeling of being trapped in a life where change is impossible, in which one must accept the hand that's dealt: "That's how it is, miss." Opening the doors to choices—introducing the very notion of *options* that can be experienced by repeatedly replaying a scene—is extremely liberating.

> Sara, a young female student, plays the role of a depressed girl who is hell-bent on killing herself. She cuts herself off from her friends and family, isolating herself in her room. In one scene, her mother attempts to contact her. Feeling defeated, the mother leaves.
>
> The leader asks Sara what she wants from her mother. "To know that she cares about me," Sara says. The leader turns to the mother, indicating that she might communicate this to her daughter. The mother's response is, "I told her once already." The mother calls her other daughter home from college to see whether she can reach the depressed girl. The sister fares as poorly as the mother. The leader then asks the sisters to reverse roles.
>
> Playing the older sister, Sara finds in herself strength of purpose and becomes animated and determined. By the end of the scene, her affect has completely changed.
>
> The leader asks the sisters to reverse roles again. Sara is asked to pick up the scene where they left off. This time she lets herself be open and responsive, making a genuine connection with her "sister."

Role reversal is a technique commonly used to give each character a perspective on the motivation and emotions of the other. It is also a way of allowing the character, on switching roles, an opportunity to speak to his or her former self.

Sara later revealed that she had a chronic heart problem about which she felt quite hopeless.

## Corrective Family Play

Playing out family dynamics is a popular theme among adolescents. As the source of so much conflict, hurt, deprivation, and lack of self-worth, the family provides the raw material for a substantial number of dramatizations. The initial impulse on the part of these adolescents is to reenact the abuse and misunderstanding so familiar to them. Adolescents commonly take on the role of the harsh, uncaring, punitive parent or the powerless child. Scenes of family conflict typically end with threats, punishments, and ultimatums.

Intervention in these family scenarios is potentially reparative for the participants. Although it is important for the participants, at least initially, to play a scene as they see it, intervention presents an opportunity to rerun the action (several times if necessary) and to introduce other possibilities in the interplay between characters. In this way, scenes are moved in more humane directions, fostering greater connections and more understanding by and among group members.

> A scene is developed in which two students, played by Lisa and Frank, are taking a test. Lisa looks over Frank's shoulder for an answer; Frank gets blamed by the teacher for cheating. The teacher severely reprimands Frank, telling him he must go home and write "Christopher Columbus discovered America" 200 times. Frank returns home and tells his mother what he has to do. His mother is played by Cara, a rather quiet, withholding young girl with a history of abuse. As the mother she becomes furious. She calls Frank a fool and blames him for her having to miss a day of work to go see his teacher at school. She sends the defenseless child to his room without dinner.
>
> The leader praises the scene for its rich authentic quality and for the truth the actors have brought to their characterizations. She supports the expression of anger and frustration by the mother and of helplessness by the child. As a director, the leader suggests to Cara that she might want to try another approach, this time taking on the persona of a more understanding mother, who is open to believing her son's side of the story.
>
> The scene begins again. Cara engages in more dialogue with her "son," though she still hangs on to her punitive attitude.
>
> FRANK.  Mom, I have to write "Christopher Columbus discovered America" 200 times because the teacher thought I was cheating, but it wasn't me.
> MOTHER.  Next time *just don't do it!*

FRANK. I didn't do anything. It wasn't me.

MOTHER. I don't care. You're acting like it's OK, and it's not. Next time it happens I'm going to go to school and whip you in front of the whole class.

The leader then decides to do a scene between Lisa, the girl who did cheat, and *her* father, played by another member of the artistic team.

Lisa admits to her father that she has cheated and says that she feels bad and doesn't know what to do. The actor playing her father models an understanding parent. He tells her, "I understand how you feel. I don't like the fact that you cheated, but I'm proud that you had the courage to be honest with me. People make mistakes. I want you to go back to school and tell the teacher what happened." Lisa tells him that she is afraid, and he reassures her that whatever happens she has his support.

The scene switches back to Frank's home. It is the next morning, and Frank is anxious about his mother's having to accompany him to school. This time Cara relates to him in a more sympathetic way. She apologizes for her temper and tells him not to worry. "Maybe we'll work things out. We'll get the teacher to believe that you didn't cheat."

The miniplay ends in the classroom where Lisa confesses, Frank thanks her, and Frank's mother reassures the teacher, "My son is an honest boy." As his mother is leaving, Frank tells her that he is sorry she had to miss a day of work. "That's OK," she says. "It was important."

The modeling of the actor playing Lisa's father had a dramatic impact on Cara and her characterization. She was able to emulate what she saw the actor do. Thus, she brought a conflict to a constructive resolution. And when the characters experience a healing effect, so, indirectly, do the actors.

## Filling in Maturational Gaps

Drama has the power to create what life has failed to offer. It is possible for lost opportunities to be realized dramatically and for participants to achieve for themselves an otherwise unavailable level of satisfaction.

> In a mixed-age inpatient unit, the group members, about half of whom were adolescents, are asked to think of a time when something in their lives should have been celebrated but wasn't and whom they would have wanted to be with them there. Liana, a young girl from Puerto Rico, says rather sorrowfully that she was not able to celebrate her 15th birthday, her "quinceañera," an extremely important ritual in the lives of Latin American girls. She has never had this rite of passage from girlhood to womanhood because, as she puts it, "I was sick in the hospital." This was a great loss for her.
>
> The group leader has the idea that through dramatization the group might be able to give Liana this rite of passage. The leader asks Liana whether she would like the group to create this event for her. The characteristically melancholy girl breaks into a smile and nods yes. Fortunately, two of the teaching artists are Latin American and know exactly how to help launch this highly ritualized event. Following Liana's lead, they make a list of all the characters and scenes involved in the preparation and enactment of the ceremony. She says she needs a dressmaker to make a dress; handmaidens to help dress her; a procession made up of her friends and their escorts; her mother, father, and godfather; and a band to play music.
>
> The characters are cast and the scene is set. A small group playing the band meet privately in a corner of the room to compose a song for the ceremony. Every person in the group has a role. It is clear that Liana has lived this event in her head many times. She begins by giving a detailed description of her dress to the dressmaker, telling her it should match the shoes, earrings, and hair ornament she plans on wearing. Her chosen handmaidens giggle their way through getting her dressed, wish her luck, and join the procession.
>
> The procession begins with her parents in the lead, the maidens and their escorts following. As they all walk ceremoniously to a designated spot, the band plays the song they have composed just for Liana. The godfather gives his blessings. The father, played by an extraordinarily poetic and sensitive patient, makes a toast recalling Liana's birth, the meaning of her name, his pride in her growth and achievements, his joy in witnessing her passing from girlhood to womanhood, and his eternal love for her.

Liana stands tall and proud, tears running down her face. The room has the feeling of a sacred place. When the ceremony has ended, the group remains still, almost able to see Liana's white dress, the black tuxedos, the candles, and the flowers. For a moment all forget they are in the lounge of an inpatient hospital unit. "I've had my quinceañera," Liana says quietly. It seems to all involved that indeed she has.

## Success and Accomplishment: Creating a Play

For a group that has the luxury of being together for an extended period of time, months of work can culminate in the creation of a play. The process of originating an idea, casting, rehearsing, and performing can be one of the most exciting and arduous endeavors a group can experience. Building a play takes a group into an entirely new realm of collectivity and at the same times puts individual strengths to work for a common purpose.

Everyone in the group has a chance to write, act, and direct. A story line must be developed, characters created, and relationships explored. Scenes must be written and rewritten until they finally fit together in a logical order. Along the way, group members usually become resistant, impatient, and discouraged—all the feelings that in their own lives have led to their inability to follow through a complex task to completion. When a group can tolerate the uncertainty, boredom, and fear accompanying this process, their rewards when the play finally comes together are immeasurable.

The leaders' role in all this is crucial. They must carefully guide the players through a laborious journey. They must show an unflagging belief that, despite periods of chaos and confusion, everything will come together. They have to be keenly aware of all individual and group dynamics at each step so as to intervene and keep the process moving forward.

During the rehearsal of one scene between a teacher and student, Andrea, the girl playing the teacher, becomes more and more frustrated as George, the boy playing the student, persists in yelling in her face, cursing, and refusing to listen to anything she says. At one point, Andrea slaps her hand down on the desk and refuses to go on with the scene.

After a few attempts to redirect and encourage Andrea, one of the leaders enters the scene, taking on the role of another teacher who runs up to Andrea and says, "Do you have a few minutes? I need to talk."

Andrea replies, "Sure."

LEADER. These kids are driving me crazy. I don't know what to do.

ANDREA. What are they doing?

LEADER. They're cursing and shouting, and they won't listen when I speak to them. I know I should be patient and understanding, but sometimes I get so frustrated I lose it. I end up yelling, but that doesn't seem to work. I'm at the end of my rope. Sometimes I feel like crying. I thought that maybe if I spoke to you it might help.

ANDREA. I know what you mean. I go through the same thing myself.

LEADER. What do you do? How do you handle it? You seem so patient and caring all the time.

ANDREA. You just have to be patient, understand that they just can't help it sometimes. When there are problems, I try to talk to them and help them. But I yell sometimes. I get crazy too.

LEADER. Do you ever think of quitting?

ANDREA. Yes, but I won't.

LEADER. I really appreciate your talking to me. It helps to get support. If I'm having a hard time, can I come talk to you again sometime?

ANDREA. Sure.

At this point, the leader motions to George to reenter the scene and says to Andrea, "It seems that someone is here to talk to you. Thanks a lot!" The leader suggests to George that Andrea *really* might be able to help him, so it might be worth his while to listen to what she has to say. George and Andrea replay the scene, this time more successfully.

The leader dealt with Andrea's frustration by entering the scene, mirroring her state of mind, and providing the understanding and support she needed to reenter and behave differently.

This example was part of the rehearsal process for an original play created by a particularly challenging junior high school class, a play that eventually became the highlight of their school year. Before working on this project, individual students had responded to the work with varying degrees of interest and involvement, but it was difficult to establish a cohesive group.

These students had worked most effectively together in a 3-week period during which they developed a lengthy scenario around the struggles of a young teenager. They became so creatively engaged in this work that the leader thought it might be a good idea to do an extended project with them. But when doing a play was suggested, their response was negative: they "hated" the idea. The very thought seemed to evoke a high degree of anxiety. "They broke into subgroups, became more provocative, and began to pick fights" (J. Rosenfels, CANY group leader, personal communication, December 1992).

None of these students had ever been involved in such an endeavor. Why face another failure? Then one day the group wrote a collective poem on the theme, "Being a grown-up means. . . ." Each member contributed a line. When the poem was finished, the leader divided the class into two groups and asked each group to pick one line from the poem and use the line to inspire a family scene. One group created a scene about a problem-laden family unable to work anything out; the other group created a family that was able to talk and settle things.

When the groups came together and presented their contrasting scenes, the leaders suggested these two families and their ways of facing problems could provide a good theme for a play. "OK," said one of the girls in the class, "but I don't want it to have a happy ending. That's a fairy tale. I want it to be about real life."

Gradually, the students developed a scenario without knowing how it would eventually fit together. They worked scene by scene, as if creating individual squares on a quilt that would someday be sewn into a whole. As they explored conflicts and the inner voices and outer relationships of their characters through improvisation, they became deeply interested in the lives of both families. Their relationship to the work began to change dramatically. This was no longer just a class—it had become serious work.

Their improvised scenes were transcribed by their teacher and then returned for rehearsal and revision. Kids who were barely literate or who were simply resistant to reading were now motivated to read their own scenes—their parts in the play. The level of cooperation among classmates began to change as well.

A turning point in the ensemble work occurred one day when one of the leaders was having trouble with her character. She was playing the role of an abusive, alcoholic mother and was experiencing difficulty in making certain choices. She turned to the group. "This isn't working well," she said. "I need your help." First one student and then another stepped in, and soon the entire class was directing the leader. The students offered ideas about her behavior and her inner thoughts. When one suggestion failed, they came up with another. Finally her performance changed. Their directions had paid off, and they had learned firsthand about the real work of an actor.

After this event, the students worked more closely together. They exchanged ideas with one another, listened, and responded, needing less intervention from the artistic leaders. They even rehearsed during the week between classes. "They would be waiting for us when we arrived, getting into character, impatient to start rehearsal. We had never seen them so motivated" (G. Zavala, CANY group leader, personal communication, January 1993).

The performance was a thrilling and exciting event. An audience of family, friends, fellow students, and teachers cheered the actors on. "They really didn't believe until the finish that they would ever perform it," said one of the group leaders. "They had never accomplished anything like that in their lives." The class's teacher reported, "After the finale they all looked at each other and raced out saying, 'We did it! We did it!' punctuating their excitement with 'high fives' all around. When they returned for their final bow, the audience shared their happiness with equal enthusiasm. I couldn't have asked for a better ending to the school year."

## ◆ Conclusion

Young people who are struggling with the formidable task of entering adulthood and who in addition are stigmatized as learning disabled have little hope of realizing their potential. These adolescents, with histories of abuse and neglect and with little chance to express or be recognized for their capabilities and strengths, are in grave danger of living very destructive lives.

CANY engages these troubled adolescents in the dramatic process within a therapeutic environment. In these workshops, play begins to pave the way toward the actualization of who one is and can become. For those with little feeling of self-worth or a shaky sense of identity, theater in this therapeutic context can provide a safe framework in which ego strengths can be developed and healthier interaction with others practiced.

Follow-up studies are needed to determine how much short- and long-term carryover there is to the real world outside the group or the classroom. The degree to which the effects of the work are internalized in the face of life's ongoing demands is a vital question that is yet to be answered. But it is likely, based on the experiences detailed above, that many more students with special needs could be reached and propelled toward richer and more fulfilled lives if CANY's work could be implemented as an essential part of the regular curriculum.

## ◆ References

Erikson JM: Activity, Recovery, Growth: The Communal Role of Planned Activities, New York, WW Norton, 1976

Ormont LR: The Group Therapy Experience: From Theory to Practice, New York, St. Martin's Press, 1992

Rachman AW: Identity group psychotherapy with adolescents: a reformulation, in Adolescent Group Psychotherapy. Edited by Azima FJ Cramer, Richmond LH. Madison, CT, International Universities Press, 1989, pp 30–33

Winnicott DW: Playing and Reality. London, Tavistock, 1971

# CHAPTER 12

# Helping Adolescents Deal With Death on an Inpatient Pediatric Unit

*Penelope Buschman Gemma, M.S., R.N., C.S.*

A dolescent patients with acute and chronic illness in a pediatric hospital may be exposed to the death of a peer. Although individual support from caregivers is essential, the adolescents themselves in one or more group sessions can gain knowledge, explore feelings, share their heightened sense of vulnerability, describe memories, identify coping skills, and lend each other strength. In this chapter, I describe such a group experience focusing on participants, leadership, and process.

On an acute-care unit in a large urban pediatric hospital, there is a fairly constant group of adolescents who are admitted and readmitted. These young people have chronic or life-threatening diseases requiring regular or episodic admissions for treatment of their diseases and the myriad of complications. The illnesses—including cystic fibrosis, asthma, sickle-cell disease, diabetes, cancer, cardiac malfunction, and kidney disease—may involve one or more systems. They may occur with varying degrees of severity and debilitation. In these groupings of adolescents are those with the same disease who may have known each other for many years. Relationships evolve over years of living together in the hospital, where the adolescents develop loyalties, rivalries, and special friendships and interact as sibling members of a family. Indeed, they bring their own family-of-origin roles and functions as they move in and out of this social milieu.

Never are these adolescents more anxious and vulnerable than when a peer dies on the unit. Whether or not the death is anticipated, the adolescents with a life-threatening disease are confronted by their own mortality. They grieve for their peer and for themselves. I have found it helpful to patients and staff to intervene at the time of a death on the unit with one or more group sessions for the surviving adolescent peers, providing permission and opportunity for these young people to talk about the death and the questions and concerns they may have. The group, which is short term, is conducted in a conference room on the unit, and sessions take place close to the actual time of the adolescent's death.

## ◆ Review of the Literature

Groups of adolescents with cancer, which provide the opportunity for interaction with peers and clarification of distorted or incomplete information, have been described in the literature (Baider and De-Nour 1989; Flanagan 1983; Heiney et al. 1988). Brief, problem-focused psychotherapy groups for adolescents also have been described (Heiney and Wells 1988; Raubolt 1985). However, there is little written in the professional literature about short-term support groups for seriously ill adolescents who find themselves serendipitously linked together by illness and their experience of the death of a peer.

## ◆ Inpatient Support Group Experience

In this section, I describe my experience with two group sessions held on an adolescent acute-care unit after the death of Laura, a young patient with cystic fibrosis. The section begins with a brief history of the young woman, highlighting events leading up to her final admission to the hospital, as well as a description of the group participants, the coleaders, and the process.

## History

Laura, a 19-year-old with cystic fibrosis diagnosed at age 18 months, was admitted to the adolescent unit of a large, urban pediatric hospital, where she had spent much of her life.

Laura was the middle child of three children in a Mexican family that had emigrated to the United States just before she was diagnosed with cystic fibrosis. Although Laura's oldest sister was healthy, her younger brother Jose subsequently was diagnosed with cystic fibrosis at the age of 1 year. Their mother was the primary caretaker of both children, as their father was incarcerated and unavailable to the family for most of the children's lives. Mother and children lived in a small apartment in close proximity to the hospital. The children attended school sporadically. As they grew, they became more frequent visitors to the Cystic Fibrosis Clinic and to the pediatric unit.

Laura's illness had worsened, and she responded with anger and dejection. Her pediatrician started her on a trial of antidepressant medication several months before her admission.

Shortly before this admission, Laura, who was involved in a relationship forbidden by mother, exchanged angry words with her mother and left a note saying that she had left home because she found her mother's care too intrusive and overbearing. She promised to contact her mother but did not tell her where she would be staying. Laura went to the home of a peer, a friend with cystic fibrosis whom she knew from previous hospitalizations. This friend, Maria, and her mother welcomed Laura, but they insisted that she contact her family. They invited her to remain with them, and Maria's mother commented that it was like having a second daughter. Her own second daughter had died of cystic fibrosis 8 years before.

At the time of admission, Laura had omitted her nebulizer and postural drainage treatments for many days. Her lungs were congested and she was febrile when she came to the pediatric emergency room requesting admission. She was admitted to the familiar and welcoming adolescent unit. The nursing staff responded warmly to Laura while they initiated her antibiotic treatment. They noted that Laura was talkative and in good spirits despite her medical condition. Laura went to bed early that evening and slept well, interrupted hourly by nurses who checked her respirations and intravenous feedings.

When the nurse went to see Laura at 5:00 A.M., she found her unresponsive with no pulse. A code was called and efforts were made to resuscitate Laura; however, these were to no avail.

Laura's family and pediatrician were called with the sad news. Laura's mother and brother Jose came immediately to the hospital to meet with staff and to grieve for Laura.

Laura's pediatrician, who had known her since she was diagnosed, suggested to the staff and family that her unexpected death might have been the result of a suicidal gesture made after leaving home in anger and despair. This suggestion was shocking to Laura's family, to the nursing and medical staffs, and to the other adolescents on the unit, three of whom had cystic fibrosis. The atmosphere on the unit was bleak. Patients and staff were subdued, struggling with their own feelings of sadness and anger.

At the suggestion of the head nurse, I spoke with all adolescents on the unit, inviting them to participate in a group session during which their feelings and reactions to Laura's death might be discussed. Two young people with anorexia nervosa and asthma who were relative newcomers to the unit decided not to participate. All other adolescents responded with enthusiasm, and a group meeting was scheduled for the following morning.

## Participants

*Maria,* a 17-year-old with cystic fibrosis, was diagnosed at age 2 years. An older sibling had died of the disease 8 years before. Maria's lungs were worsening, and despite fair compliance with her medical treatment, her disease was advancing.

*Louis,* a 16-year-old, had had cystic fibrosis since the age of 3. He had frequented the inpatient unit and known Laura for many years. He had maintained contact with Laura's siblings outside the hospital.

*Tony,* a 16-year-old with cystic fibrosis diagnosed at age 2 years, had been admitted infrequently to the hospital until the age of 15, when his disease began to worsen and his compliance with treatment changed. These events were compounded by a significant family crisis precipitated by the death of his father.

## Leadership

Coleadership for these two sessions was provided by a child psychiatrist who was a consultant to the adolescent service and myself, a clinical specialist in psychiatric mental health nursing. The psychiatric consultant had worked individually with two members of the group during his 6-month assignment to the adolescent unit. He was a valued and trusted member of the unit staff. I had served as a consultant to the nursing staff on the unit for many years and had seen two adolescent members of the group for crisis intervention and short-term psychotherapy during particularly stressful times in their lives. The psychiatric consultant and I had collaborated in other treatment efforts and worked comfortably in our coleadership position with this group.

## First Session

The three group members sat quietly waiting for one of the leaders to begin. They positioned themselves in a tight circle around a conference room table. The predominant mood was anger and sadness. One leader began by saying that we were meeting to talk about Laura's death and the feelings and thoughts that had been stirred up by this unexpected and tragic happening. The group was invited to share feelings, ask questions, and speak candidly, knowing that all that was spoken would remain confidential within the group.

Maria began by talking about her friendship with Laura and the experience of having Laura live with her for 2 days before this last hospitalization. She spoke of Laura's anger with her mother and her need for temporary distance from her family. Laura planned to return to her family in the future. Maria described how her mother had welcomed Laura into their home. Maria stated tearfully and quite emphatically that she did not believe Laura's death had been a suicide for Laura had not been depressed.

Tony added that dying of the disease was bad enough, but the thought of someone with cystic fibrosis taking her life made him angry. He vigorously denied ever having had that thought.

Louis responded with anger at the thought that a person with cystic fibrosis would opt to give in to death rather than fight to live.

Maria asked directly, "Did Laura kill herself? Will you tell us when you know for sure the autopsy results?"

Both leaders responded to the anger in the group, which was heightened by the unknown cause of Laura's death. I suggested that the issue of possible suicide and all the angry feeling engendered by it seemed to take precedence over the sadness of the loss of Laura. There were tears and expressions of sadness. When asked by the coleaders to share special memories of Laura, the group responded with smiles and relief. Maria, Louis, and Tony spent the remainder of the session recalling Laura's leadership in exploits on the unit. There ensued an animated discussion of the pranks and mischief enjoyed by all and led by Laura. There was some rivalry among members as each tried to remember the best and most outlandish story.

The session ended with the recognition of Laura as a ringleader on the unit, a good friend, and a person all would miss. All participants requested a second meeting.

## Second Session

At the time of the session, only Maria and Louis remained on the unit. They had telephoned Laura's younger brother and invited him to join the group. More memories of Laura were shared. The mood in this session was lighter. Maria discussed her intention to be more compliant with treatment, taking her aerosols and doing necessary postural drainage. It was recognized by both participants that Laura had not complied with treatment in a rigorous fashion and that this may have contributed to her untimely death. Maria and Louis discussed their willingness to participate in a new medication trial that required exact compliance and record keeping.

Maria recognized that while their ranks were diminished, the group of adolescents with cystic fibrosis still had each other for support, understanding, and friendship. Tony agreed.

The leaders suggested that additional sessions could be planned if Maria, Tony, and the other adolescents with cystic fibrosis wished. Further meetings were not requested.

## Discussion

The suggestion that Laura might have been suicidal came as a shock to her peers and caregivers. Recognizing a worsening of her disease, her caregivers had not noted changes in Laura's affect. Indeed, Laura was relieved to be hospitalized in a familiar, safe setting.

In my clinical experience, suicide in adolescents with severe, chronic, life-threatening disease is rare. These same adolescents may demonstrate a lack of compliance with prescribed medical regimens. Medications, treatments, and medical appointments may be avoided or omitted altogether. Some adolescents will alter their treatment for periods of time until they become symptomatic. By omitting aerosols, postural drainage, and medications, adolescents with cystic fibrosis deny the disease and challenge those who direct their care. The feeling of invulnerability in chronically ill adolescents is less well founded than it is in a population of healthy young people. Stopping or significantly altering treatment has immediate consequences for these adolescents. The disease course may worsen, requiring hospitalization and more intensive care.

Experimentation with medical compliance generally shifts in the middle and late years of adolescence, when future functioning and plans are linked with the control of the disease. Control depends on the adolescent's assuming more responsibility for care. Although adolescents with cystic fibrosis engage in this medical experimentation, they do not demonstrate overt suicidal behaviors. Rather, their energies are mobilized to fight the disease and to live. Peers support this focus. Not wishing to live as fully as possible is viewed as giving in and, most significantly, as a form of betrayal.

When an adolescent does die of cystic fibrosis, surviving peers seek to find an immediate cause apart from the disease they shared. Complications of another illness, an unexpected response to medication, or extreme lack of compliance may be identified as factors contributing to or hastening the death.

In this informal group format, participants had the opportunity to share with trusted adults the myriad of feelings they had in response to Laura's unexpected death: their fury at her leaving them, their sadness in missing her, their heightened sense of vulnerability, the reworking of their defensive maneuvering, and their renewed determination to be careful and compliant with their treatment, as if they could prevent the worsening of their disease.

In these group sessions, the leaders jointly functioned in a supportive role, offering validation, clarification, and the opportunity for peer reinforcement and support.

## ◆ Conclusion

These short-term group sessions provide an opportunity for the adolescent participants to express their fears, ask questions, and rework their ways of coping, with the support of peers and adult leaders. It is a small but helpful intervention for young people whose lives are threatened by disease and altered by treatment and frequent hospitalization.

## ◆ References

Baider L, DeNour AK: Group therapy with adolescent cancer patients. Journal of Adolescent Health Care 10:35–38, 1989

Flanagan C: Children with cancer in group therapy, in The Child and Death. Edited by Schowalter J, Patterson P, Tallmer M, et al. New York, Columbia University Press, 1983, pp 266–292

Heiney S, Wells L: Successful strategies for organizing and maintaining support groups. Journal of the Association of Pediatric Oncology Nurses 5:32, 1988

Heiney S, Ruffin J, Ettinger RS, et al: The effects of group therapy on adolescents with cancer. Journal of the Association of Pediatric Oncology Nurses 5:20–24, 1988

Raubolt R: Brief problem focused group psychotherapy with adolescents. Am J Orthopsychiatry 53:157–165, 1985

# CHAPTER 13

# Mentally Handicapped Children and Adolescents

*Brendan McCormack, M.B.B.S.,*
*and Valerie Sinason, B.A. Hons, P.G.T.C., M.A.C.P.*

## ◆ Background

Over 300,000 children and adults in the United Kingdom have organically caused mental retardation or learning disability, and over 1 million children and adults in the United Kingdom have mild mental retardation. In the United States, there are between 5 and 6 million mentally and physically handicapped children and adults, an estimated 3% of the population. As in the United Kingdom, poverty was found to have a close connection to mild mental handicap. Draft rejections caused by mental handicap in World War II were 14 times more common in states with low incomes than in those with high incomes, and in some slum areas 10%–30% of schoolchildren were handicapped (Kennedy 1963). Environmentally caused mental handicap is disturbingly common, with an estimated 100,000 children homeless, 11 million children with no direct access to a family doctor, and 500,000 children with malnutrition in the United States (National Commission on Children, Washington, DC, personal communication, April 1990).

Valerie Sinason would like to thank Donald Meltzer & the Clunie Trust and the Tavistock Clinic Mental Handicap Workshop and Research Project.

Given the lack of funding to ameliorate environmental conditions causing mental handicaps, it is not surprising to learn that an extremely small amount of formal treatment is available for those who are emotionally disturbed or mentally ill in addition to their retardation. There is a serious division between mainstream mental health workers with training and experience in individual, group, and family psychodynamic or cognitive therapy and those persons who have the emotional capacity to be with people who are retarded but do not have any training in counseling.

This *cordon sanitaire* has been perpetuated by the widespread denial that severely and profoundly handicapped children, adolescents, and adults have feelings and might experience depression (Dosen and Menolascino 1990), mental illness (Menolascino 1969), sexual abuse (McCormack 1991a; Sinason 1986), developmental crises (Levitas and Gilson 1989), and bereavement (Hollins and Sireling 1989; McCormack 1991b; Hollins et al. 1993), although we are beginning to make some inroads on this misperception. This division extends to clinical literature as well as to mainstream group therapists. The process of mentally handicapped groups and the process of cognitively normal groups are considered to be separate.

There is also a shortage of clinicians for this work. In one regional study in England, Oliver et al. (1987) found that, of 596 self-injuring children and adults in need of treatment, only 12 received any intervention; 11 of these interventions were behavioral and 1 (Sinason 1992) was psychoanalytical.

We also need to bear in mind that although group treatment has a long history with cognitively normal adults (Bion 1959; Foulkes 1946) and adolescents (Azima and Richmond 1989; Phelan 1972), treatment groups for cognitively normal children are still extremely rare, let alone for children with mental retardation.

## Group Activities

Despite the fact that many children and adolescents with learning disability are involved in some sort of group activity, attention to group processes is very patchy. Through experience in our work settings, we consider staff supervision and support or reflection groups to be necessary for these "social" groups to function at their best. A reflection group is a space for reflection that is not for personal therapy, though therapeutic. For example, a teacher in a school for severely and profoundly handicapped children described this moment in her class group:

> Eight-year-old Sarah was having one of her big fits—right in the middle of morning news. John had just managed to tell us his grandmother had died, which he was very sad about, when Sarah took up all the attention, falling onto the floor and wetting herself as well. I told John I was very sorry Sarah had interrupted his news. Her mother had died 3 years ago—a long time now—and she got plenty of attention from us all.

Thinking further about the dynamics of this situation, we could understand that Sarah was giving a bodily communication to the class group of how awful it is to be overwhelmed by something out of control, like having your mother die, being handicapped, or having epilepsy. In fact, the teacher understood that there was a connection between Sarah's mother's death and John's news. However, without support to deal with the painful emotions in the class group, the teacher deprived herself and the group of an opportunity. The context was not a treatment group; it was a class group—a social group. However, it would have been possible to say "John, you can see that Sarah feels very sad for you, too. That may be why she is having a fit right now. Because her mother died too—3 years ago—and maybe she knows what you are feeling like."

Here is another example of group activity in a club for handicapped adolescents. Two volunteers took a group of physically and mentally handicapped young people to a disco. The staff had mixed feelings about this outing, as crowded discos are clearly not easy places for wheelchairs. Inside the disco one young man, Tony, who was severely mentally and physically handicapped with cerebral palsy, went up to an attractive young woman and asked her to dance. "With you?" she asked in shock and then burst into embarrassed giggling with her girlfriends and turned away. Tony stood still for a moment and then banged his head. The dance floor was suddenly quiet. Then, Tony's friends all started rocking and making "handicapped" sounds—sounds representing their emotional pain rather than their organic capacity. The volunteers looked shocked and shouted to Tony, "If you can't manage, we'll just have to take you all home."

In a supervision group afterward, it was possible to consider the humiliation the volunteers felt when a member of "their" group was sexually rejected and then showed them up by making "handicapped" noises when they had hoped to offer a normalizing experience. Only after the volunteers' humiliation was acknowledged was it possible to think of how they had a chance to understand the whole group's humiliation, initially expressed by Tony. On this occasion, they had lost the healing potential for the group by handling the situation as they did.

## Literature

Practitioners working with formal treatment groups of mentally handicapped adolescents rarely make use of the vast body of literature on group therapy with cognitively normal adolescents. Although there are important differences (which we will address), the basic issues remain the same. In highlighting how rare psychotherapy is with this client group, Marian Sigman (1985) pointed out that

> The goals of psychotherapy with retarded individuals are similar to those with nonretarded persons. . . . The process of therapy is similar. In the first stage a relationship is built—sometimes that is the only work of therapy. In the 2nd stage anxiety and aggression are expressed—for some their first opportunity to be negative (Sigman 1985, p. 262).

Sigman added that the central themes in therapy for retarded adolescents have to do with their sense of identity, differentiation, and fear of sexuality—themes that are especially poignant (Hollins and Evered 1990; Hollins and Sinason 1992; Sinason 1992).

## Suitability for Therapy

Before focusing on the specific age groups, we will make some general comments. Many of the published studies concern groups conducted for short periods only (e.g., Pantlin 1987; Meeks 1980) and describe focused and goal-directed groups (Slivkin and Bernstein 1968). Regardless of the kind of treatment, there is no agreement as to what communication skills and degree of intellectual ability constitute suitability and who should be excluded from treatment and on what grounds. Sinason (1986, 1992) and Stokes and Sinason (1992) suggested that "emotional intelligence" is a more significant factor than cognitive abilities. The focus on IQ and disability rating scales can be misleading. Projective tests have been used to show the difference between cognitive and emotional development (Bichard 1990). For example, one adolescent patient who improved dramatically in therapy was profoundly mentally and physically handicapped, had Goldenhar's syndrome, was incontinent and wheelchair based, had no speech, and had blinded herself in one eye (Sinason 1992).

Suitability for therapy is a two-way evaluation. Although adolescents, especially, like being in groups, that does not necessarily mean they will like being in a thinking group. As Meeks (1980) commented, although it is a natural tendency of adolescents to form groups, those groups are not often inclined to study the meaning of behavior. Therefore, suitability for therapy depends on the ability of the patient to tolerate the emotional experience and the ability of the therapist to tolerate and contain the patient. The patient does not need communication skills. (Indeed, if communication skills were necessary, no autistic child or adolescent would ever be treated!) However, communication skills are essential for the therapist. A child psychoanalytic psychotherapy training is particularly helpful, because it strengthens an understanding of nonverbal behavior.

When child or adolescent patients are assessed for group therapy, however, the range of difficulties and the patients' personalities must be carefully considered. Although it can be helpful to have one silent member, a whole group of silent members would not be helpful. One deeply inarticulate, shy member can become the projective home of the group, showing all the fears and wishes in everyone's minds.

Hence, in a largely verbal late-adolescent group convened by Sinason and Julian Lousada (an adult psychotherapist and a principal lecturer in applied social work), we can see the way the whole group can richly benefit from the presence of a silent, more severely handicapped member, Amy.

> BEN.   Are you upset, Amy?
> AMY.   *[Nods yes.]*
> CINDA.   Has your mother died?
> AMY.   *[Shakes head no.]*
> DON.   Did anyone do something sexy that frightened you?
> AMY.   *[Shakes head no.]*
> BEN.   Did you steal something?
> AMY.   *[Shakes head no.]*
> CINDA.   Your social worker has left her job?
> AMY.   *[Shakes head no.]*
> DON.   A boy touched you?
> AMY.   *[Shakes head no.]*
> BEN.   Did you break something?
> AMY.   *[Nods yes and cries.]*

Ben, who has difficulties with theft, followed a theme of breaking and entering; Cinda, who had experienced a series of abandonments, followed the theme of loss; Don expressed his own sexual concerns.

## Secondary Mental Handicaps

Mental disability is associated with problems of intellectual attainment, thinking, and memory. There are many pathways to mental disability, from organic birth defects and brain injury to chromosomal abnormality and psychological trauma. These issues all need to be considered in the course of a group. In addition to a real cognitive deficit and its emotional sequelae, there is also the question of a secondary mental handicap, which is virtually always present (Sinason 1986). By secondary handicap we mean the way "the primary handicap or disability is made worse by defensive exaggerations (secondary handicap)" (Sinason 1992, p. 2). For example, Jeanie, age 8, needed to be taken out of the therapy room to the toilet because she could not open the doors. Even with two hands held together, she lacked the strength and coordination. It was only when the heavy playhouse in the therapy room was pushed over by another child that she showed she had the coordination and strength to accomplish hard physical tasks. Her abnormal left hand was a primary handicap, but she exacerbated her difficulty as a defense against her humiliation at being different. Usually, the degree of secondary handicap only becomes apparent after a period of psychotherapy; therefore, one can never make assumptions about a patient's emotional potential at the start of treatment. By this we mean the internal room in the patient for growth.

However, the cognitive deficit does have implications. Genuine empathy within the group takes slightly longer to build up in a handicapped group compared with a nonhandicapped group; this is also true for therapists of handicapped versus nonhandicapped groups. Julian Lousada commented on a difference faced by therapists of handicapped groups: "I realize that I face a narcissistic injury in not having the freedom to use words in the way I do with a non-handicapped group and that helps me understand what the patients feel like" (personal communication, April 1993).

## ◆ Which Approach Is Best?

The outcome results reported in the literature are not conclusive. Problems with research design, implementation, and evaluation were well reviewed by Pfadt (1991). Some researchers suggest that success was achieved with an unmodified nondirective approach (Yonce and O'Connor 1954); on the other hand, Ringleheim and Polatsek (1957) found no significant results with an analytic nondirective approach. Considering how scarce all treatment resources are for this patient group, there has been surprisingly little rivalry among the different clinicians. Practitioners who might be expected to disagree with each other's approaches cooperate and send referrals to each other.

Because this patient group is more likely to have been deprived of adequate personal attention, being placed in any treatment program offers the chance to make up for emotional deficits. Rudnitzki (1988) saw the group as a "psycho-social prosthesis," and Spinner and Pfeiffer (1986) believed that groups enabled members to compensate for deficits in ego controls. Whatever the kind of adolescent group, however, there is a consensus that increased leadership is needed, as was pointed out nearly 50 years ago by Cotzin (1948). Active leadership has always been needed in child groups because children have even less ability than adolescents to transmute action into symbolic thinking.

## Cotherapy

Most authors suggest that cotherapists are more suitable than single therapists for these groups. That is usually because of the degree of disturbance in the group (Miezio 1967; Piggot 1985). Although it is understood that two therapists symbolically represent a parental couple capable of dealing with the most vulnerable feelings in the group, it is rarely mentioned that two therapists can be a practical necessity in terms of actual violence or fear of violence. Where children have been physically or sexually abused, there is a high likelihood that they will behave violently toward the toys and the furniture in the playroom, their fellow group members, and the therapists.

When patients have epilepsy and other conditions linked to their mental handicap, two therapists provide a safer management team as well. In children's groups, there is often a need for one therapist to escort children to the toilet when they are too young or unable to travel there by themselves. Above all, a couple is optimum for dealing with and containing the grief and anger in the group (McCormack 1991b). Because these patients often have experienced particularly traumatic environments and recurring episodes of abandonment (Friedrich and Boriskin 1976), having two therapists allows them to hate one without feeling that their whole world has been destroyed.

Regardless of the nature of the group, expressions of hostility toward the therapists happen. For example, in an art-therapy group for mentally handicapped adolescents, one girl turned to the older therapist and said, "I can't paint you properly. There isn't enough gray paint." She then laughed. In individual treatment, she was unable to express any hostility—even in humor—toward her therapist. In a psychoanalytically oriented adolescent group convened by Sinason and Isabel Hernandez Halton, a young woman with Down's syndrome was struggling with how to be angry with one of the therapists. After looking most intensely at each in turn, she turned to the Latin American Isabel Halton and asked, "Have you got Down's syndrome? Your voice is funny." Because it was a psychodynamic group, an interpretation was given that she knew very well that Isabel Halton did not have Down's syndrome; rather, the question reflected her observation that Isabel's voice was different, her wish that Down's syndrome was a different language rather than a handicap, and her anger that the therapists were not mentally handicapped. She was then able to agree and laugh with the rest of the group.

## Length of Therapy

When economic resources are scarce, treatment cannot always be offered for the length of time that is considered optimal. Regardless of the type of group, it is crucial that therapists inform their patients at the outset how long the group will be meeting if it is time limited. Six planned months of once-weekly group therapy is far more beneficial than 1 year of group therapy that terminates without warning. Children and adolescents with disabilities are more likely than other patient groups to be moved in and out of different educational and treatment environments with little forethought and acclimatization. Children are more likely than adolescents to be moved to different parts of the country in terms of their foster or adoptive placements. Children with severe handicaps do have a sense of time. The concrete aid of a calendar on which to mark the therapy times helps to develop this sense of time further and allows the children to prepare for endings.

Long-term treatment is necessary when mentally handicapped adolescents receive psychoanalytically orientated group therapy. It takes 1 year to understand and deal with secondary handicaps (Sinason 1990), a second year to deal with the loss and grief at being different that were hidden under the handicapping disguise, and a third year to cope with sexuality issues, dependency needs, and fear of abandonment. There has been a noticeable consensus among psychodynamic practitioners (Bargh 1987; Gravestock and McGauley 1993; Hollins and Evered 1990; McCormack 1991b; Pantlin 1987; Sinason 1992) that a long time needs to be allotted to deal with these key issues. Sinason has shown (1992) how pain at having a disability can be defended against by exaggerating aspects of the disability, thereby creating a disguise.

For children, the issues regarding the length of group psychotherapy are different. The organizer of child psychoanalytic group psychotherapy at the Tavistock Clinic (Susan Reid, personal communication, March 1993) commented that 1 year is an adequate amount of time for group psychotherapy for several reasons. First, on a practical level it ensures a stable period of treatment because parents and caregivers are willing to be escorts for 1 year but might not support treatment if it lasted longer. Second, many children with emotional difficulties are moved to different schools or foster homes, and a longer-term group would cause more disturbance to the children who could not stay. Finally, the speed of developmental change means that 1 year for a child is a far more emotionally significant amount of time than it is for an adult. Although child therapy groups in a full-time residential or treatment setting can last for up to 2 years because there is no travel problem, clinic-based groups, even where they are planned to last 2 years, often have a completely different group of children each year because of moves.

## ◆ Psychoanalytic Group Psychotherapy: Technical and Management Issues

Psychotherapy is not something that is done to someone. It is a reciprocal process, and consent for treatment is essential. Severely handicapped children and adolescents are often not able to express their unwillingness to consent because they are afraid of offending their caregivers. This situation makes it all the more important for the patient's feelings about consent to be carefully explored during the assessment. When a patient is wheelchair based, leaving the room can be hard; such matters have to be discussed thoroughly beforehand. Management of physical difficulties such as incontinence, soiling, epilepsy, and fainting also needs to be discussed with the medical consultant. Confidentiality is an important aspect of therapy; however, child protection issues are paramount. Before therapy starts, child and adolescent patients need to know that if they tell about situations where they have been badly hurt or have hurt others, the therapist will have to alert another member of the team. However, the therapist can preserve the privacy of the patient's language and way of reporting such facts.

The therapist needs to be careful not only of his or her use of language but also of his or her tone of voice. It helps the group when the therapist deals with hostility toward him or her in a facilitating and direct way. For example, when Jim, age 17, kept looking at his watch to see whether it was time for the session to end, Sinason commented, "You really are sick to death of me right now. When is this horrid group going to end?" Jim and the group burst out laughing. After that, it was far easier for them to acknowledge feeling angry with the group or the therapists.

## The Group Process

When clients are functioning at an infantile level (partly due to actual handicaps and partly due to emotional problems), the therapist and group function as an "auxiliary brain" (Hollins et al. 1993); they aid the development of thinking.

In the following dialogue from a 4-year group convened by Sinason and Julian Lousada, it is possible to see how members can take on this auxiliary-brain function and help each other face issues of rivalry.

Wendy suddenly looks devastated.
MARY.   What's the matter, Wendy?
WENDY.   Someone's cross with me.
VALERIE.   Who?
BEN.   Me?
WENDY.   No.
KAREN.   Me?
WENDY.   No.
VALERIE.   Me?
JULIAN.   Me?

WENDY.  No.

MARY.  Me?

WENDY *[shyly and crying]*.  Yes.

MARY.  Me? Cross with you? Why?

WENDY.  What I said.

MARY.  What you said? What could have made me cross? *[Long pause.]* Ah . . . are you worried I will be cross you are being paid for your nursery placement and I don't get any money for mine?

WENDY *[crying loudly]*.  Yes.

MARY.  Of course I'm not. I am pleased for you. *[She hugs Wendy.]*

This dialogue, after 4 years, contrasts vividly with the way the groups speak in the early sessions, where the main way of relating is in dyads with the therapists. Sinason is researching these linguistic changes as part of a research project with Sheila Bichard and Judith Usiskin at the Tavistock Clinic. It takes 12 sessions to develop a linked, juxtaposed series of monologues. The content of these monologues shows why reciprocal emotional contact was so painful.

ALEX.  I had a dog that starved and was put down.

BONNIE.  I had a pet that went blind.

CHARLES.  My mother has got cancer.

DARLA.  When I was little, I had to go to Great Normal Street Hospital [her poignant interpretation of Great Ormond Street Hospital].

EDWARD.  I had a puppy that was put down.

Apart from the content of the group material, the process closely follows the process of other groups, whether one uses the chart of group stages in Yalom et al. (1967) or the one in Garland et al. (1965). Each stage is longer, however, because of the patients' real cognitive deficits and their difficulty in processing thought. A nonhandicapped adolescent group might show rivalry over who is the most attractive; however, a mentally handicapped adolescent group discusses who is the most or least handicapped.

The processes in children's groups of moving from infantile dyads with the therapist to empathy with others in the group are very similar to the processes in adolescent groups, except that some of the children's cooperative empathic behavior shows itself in play.

In a group for severely mentally handicapped children, many of whom had been sexually abused, the nature of the communication changed between 10 months and 22 months, as can be seen in the case example below. The group was set in a playroom that has a playhouse, dressing-up clothes, drawing equipment, baby carriages, and a range of puzzles and toys. The extent of sexual abuse in this group is very worrying (Sinason 1988, 1989, 1993).

### Case Example 1: At 10 Months

Tom rushes to the giant teddy bear and simulates anal penetration—punching the teddy in the head and bending him over the sink. His face is pale, and he looks about to have an epileptic fit. Jill sits drawing a picture of a beautiful princess. She looks at Tom for a moment but says nothing. The beautiful princess is given a particularly low-cut dress. Tracy-Ann sits next to Jill and grins as she watches Tom. She picks up a baby doll and suggestively splits its legs apart and looks at me aggressively. I comment that everyone is showing the group that difficult, hurtful sexy thoughts are on their minds, but no one wants to talk to anyone else about them.

### Case Example 2: At 22 Months

Tom rushes to the giant teddy bear and simulates anal penetration. "Go on. Fuck the teddy," shouts Jill. "No," says Barry. "You don't have to. Just because she says." Tracy-Ann looks up from her drawing. "Why are you doing that again, Tom? Did your dad do something to you again?" "Fuck off," shouts Tom, throwing the teddy away and returning to the table where the rest of the group is. "Coward! Pimp!" shouts Jill. "You are too frightened to fuck the teddy." I comment that everyone was either trying to make one person do the horrid sexy thing or helping them not to.

At this stage, the children were still too damaged to offer total empathy as a group. However, the benefit of the group was that hopeful feelings of ending abusive behavior could be located in one person and sadistic wishes to perpetuate the abuse could be located in another. In individual therapy, the children would not have had the same freedom to share their unbearable experiences.

## ◆ Conclusion

Children and adults with mild, severe, and profound mental or multiple handicaps and emotional disturbance can do well in groups. Although our focus here has been psychoanalytically orientated groups, the lessons learned from them can be applied to other settings, including supervision of primary care workers.

The group processes described in this chapter are familiar to any mainstream therapist. What, then, is holding back mainstream therapists from working with mentally handicapped children and adolescents? There is the fear of being stupid and not understanding what is being said if a patient has a severe speech defect. However, over and beyond such moments are the fear of getting close to the handicap itself and the guilt at not being handicapped in the same way. These two feelings impede treatment of the parents of our patient group as well as our patients themselves. Richard Ruth (1990) commented that traditional psychoanalytic thinking tends to view "developmentally disabled persons as largely lacking in meaningful inner lives and therefore the capacity to benefit from psychotherapy" (p. 168). However, on the basis of the literature we cite in this chapter, it looks as if that view is beginning to change.

## ◆ References

Azima FJ Cramer, Richmond LH (eds): Adolescent Group Psychotherapy. Madison, CT, International Universities Press, 1989

Bargh J: Play Back the Thinking Memories. Pamphlet. London, National Children's Bureau, 1987

Bichard S: Psychological assessment of change. Paper presented at meeting of the Royal Society of Medicine, London, March 9, 1990

Bion W: Experiences in Groups. New York, Basic Books, 1959

Cotzin M: Group psychotherapy with mentally deficient problem boys. American Journal of Mental Deficiency 53:268–283, 1948

Dosen A, Menolascino FJ: Depression in Mentally Retarded Children and Adults. Amsterdam, The Netherlands, Logon Publications, 1990

Foulkes SH: On group analysis. Int J Psychoanal 27:46–51, 1946

Friedrich WN, Boriskin JA: The role of the child in abuse. Am J Orthopsychiatry 46:580–590, 1976

Garland JA, Jones HE, Kolodny R: Explorations in Group Work. Boston, MA, Boston University, 1965

Gravestock S, McGauley G: Talk given at Tavistock Clinic Mental Handicap Workshop, London, England, January 6, 1993

Hollins S, Evered C: Group process and content: the challenge of mental handicap. Group Analysis 23:55–67, 1990

Hollins S, Sinason V: Jenny Speaks Out and Bob Tells All. London, Sovereign Series, 1992

Hollins S, Sireling L: The Last Taboo (video on death and mental handicap). London, England, St Georges Hospital Medical School, 1989

Hollins S, Sinason V, Thompson S: Individual and group psychotherapy, in New Directions in Mental Handicap. Edited by Bouras N. Cambridge, England, Cambridge University Press, 1993

Kennedy JF: Message from the President of the United States relative to mental illness and mental retardation. 88th Congress, 1st session, Document No 58. Washington, DC, U.S. Government Printing Office, 1963

Levitas A, Gilson S: Psychodynamic psychotherapy with mildly and moderately retarded patients, in Mental Retardation and Mental Illness: Assessment, Treatment and Service for the Dually Diagnosed. Edited by Fletcher R, Menolascino F. Lexington, MA, Lexington Books, 1989, pp 71–109

McCormack B: Sexual abuse and learning disabilities. BMJ 303:143–144, 1991a

McCormack B: Thinking, discourse and the denial of history: psychodynamic aspects of mental handicap. Irish Journal of Psychological Medicine 8:59–64, 1991b

Meeks JF: The Fragile Alliance. Melbourne, FL, Robert E. Krieger, 1980

Miezio S: Group therapy with mentally retarded adolescents in institutional settings. Int J Group Psychother 17:321–327, 1967

Menolascino FJ: Emotional disturbances in mentally retarded children. Am J Psychiatry 126:168–176, 1969

Oliver C, Murphy GH, Corbett JA: Self injurious behaviour in people with mental handicap: a total population study. Journal of Mental Deficiency Research 31:147–162, 1987

Pantlin AW: Group analytical psychotherapy with mentally handicapped patients. Group Analysis 18:44–53, 1987

Pfadt A: Group psychotherapy with mentally retarded adults: issues related to design, implementation, and evaluation. Research in Developmental Disabilities 12:261–285, 1991

Phelan J: Adolescents Grow in Groups. Edited by Berkovitz I. London, Butterworths, 1972

Piggot C: Discussion on the paper by A. W. Pantlin. Group Analysis 20: 51–53, 1987

Ringleheim D, Polatsek I: Group psychotherapy with a mentally deficient group, a preliminary study. American Journal of Mental Deficiency 60:144–151, 1957

Rudnitzki G: Group therapy with disabled young people: effects of modified group analytic techniques. Group Analysis 21 (27):169–180, 1988

Ruth R: Some trends in psychoanalysis and their relevance for treating people with mental retardation, in Treatment of Mental Illness and Behavioural Disorders in the Mentally Retarded: Proceedings of the International Congress, May 3 and 4, 1990. Edited by Dosen A, Van Gennep A, Zwanniken GJ. Amsterdam, Logon Publications, 1990, pp 167–177

Sigman M: Individual and group psychotherapy with mentally retarded adolescents, in Children With Emotional Disorders and Developmental Disabilities: Assessment and Treatment. Edited by Sigman M. New York, Grune & Stratton, 1985, pp 259–276

Sinason V: Secondary mental handicap and its relationship to trauma. Psychoanalytic Psychotherapy 2:131–154, 1986

Sinason V: Smiling, swallowing, sickening and stupefying: the effect of abuse on the child. Psychoanalytic Psychotherapy 3:97–111, 1988

Sinason V: Uncovering and responding to sexual abuse in handicapped patients in psychotherapeutic settings, in "Thinking the Unthinkable": Papers on Sexual Abuse and People with Learning Difficulties. Edited by Brown H, Craft A. London, Family Planning Association, 1989

Sinason V: Individual psychoanalytic psychotherapy with severely and profoundly mentally handicapped patients, in Treatment of Mental Illness and Behavioural Disorders in the Mentally Retarded: Proceedings of the International Congress, May 3 and 4, 1990. Edited by Dosen A, Van Gennep A, Zwanniken GJ. Amsterdam, Logon Publications, 1990, pp 71–81

Sinason V: Mental Handicap and the Human Condition: New Approaches from the Tavistock. London, Free Association Books, 1992

Sinason V: Disability and abuse in Baillieres clinical paediatrics, in Child Abuse. Edited by Hobbs C, Wynne J. London, Bailliere Tyndall, 1993, pp 69–87

Slivkin SE, Bernstein NR: Goal-directed group psychotherapy for retarded adolescents. Am J Psychother 22:35–45, 1968

Spinner D, Pfeiffer G: Group psychotherapy with ego impaired children: the significance of peer group culture in the evaluation of a holding environment Int J Group Psychother 36:427–446, 1986

Stokes J, Sinason V: Secondary mental handicap as a defence, in Psychotherapy and Mental Handicap. Edited by Waitman A, Conboy-Hill S. London, Sage, 1992, pp 46–59

Yalom ID, Houts PS, Newell G, et al: Preparation of patients for group therapy. Arch Gen Psychiatry 17:416–427, 1967

Yonce K, O'Connor N: Measurable effects of group psychotherapy with defective delinquents. J Mental Sci 100:944–952, 1954

CHAPTER 14

# Adolescents Who Abuse Substances

*David W. Brook, M.D.*

Group psychotherapy has a central role to play in the treatment of adolescents who abuse substances. The appropriate use of a variety of group techniques can address issues of adolescent development such as separation from the family, psychosexual development and pubertal growth, and closer relationships with peers of both sexes, as well as those psychosocial issues of particular relevance in adolescent substance abuse.

Drug abuse by adolescents is particularly harmful because both the use of substances of abuse and the psychopharmacological effects of such substances interfere with the normal developmental tasks of adolescence. Growth and development are delayed or go astray in pathological directions. Psychosexual development, separation and the establishment of independence, peer relationships, and vocational and education goals are all adversely affected by adolescent substance abuse. It is important to keep these developmental issues in focus during the group treatment of adolescents who abuse substances.

With these issues in mind, it is clear that group psychotherapists treating adolescents who abuse substances must have knowledge of a

This chapter is based in part on work done in the Department of Psychiatry and Behavioral Sciences at New York Medical College, Valhalla, New York.

number of related disciplines: group and individual psychotherapy, child and adolescent development, and substance abuse etiology, prevention, and treatment. A broad knowledge of psychopathology and a biopsychosocial perspective are also essential for such a group therapist.

In this chapter, I explore the rationale for the use of group techniques in this population. First, there is a brief literature review. The next section of the chapter consists of a discussion of the biopsychosocial developmental bases of adolescent substance abuse, focusing particularly on the role of groups in the course of adolescence. Then comes a brief exposition of the various types of adolescent substance abuse, including comorbidity and the difficult issues involved in polysubstance abuse and dual diagnosis. A brief discussion of patient selection comes next. The fifth section comprises an exploration of the various techniques of treatment, focusing on the central role of group treatments and the relationship of such treatments to the developmental basis of adolescent substance abuse. An illustrated case example is included. The sixth section contains a discussion of the curative factors at work in adolescent group psychotherapy. Last, there is a brief discussion of the role of group techniques in the prevention of adolescent substance abuse and adolescent acquired immunodeficiency syndrome (AIDS).

## ◆ Literature Review

Although groups have been widely used in the treatment of adolescents who abuse substances, their use has not often been the object of scientific study, as evidenced by the relative paucity of articles in the professional literature. Group psychotherapy for the treatment of persons in general who abuse substances has been studied and written about extensively (Cooper 1987; Galanter et al. 1991; Kanas 1982; Vanicelli 1982, 1984; Yalom et al. 1978).

Group psychotherapy with adolescents has been used for treatment and for prevention of substance abuse. Coleman (1978) examined the use of sibling group therapy with 10- to 13-year-olds with older siblings who abused substances, but results were inconclusive.

Wunderlich et al. (1974) developed a program of short-term group psychotherapy for drug-abusing adolescents who were referred by juvenile court and found less recidivism in participants. Rachman and Raubolt (1985) focused on the role of the leader in adolescent groups, emphasizing the leader's giving the group active direction. Birmingham (1986) discussed the outpatient treatment of adolescents who abuse substances. Vanicelli et al. (1984) discussed aspects of the therapeutic contract.

Bratter (1989) made the point that because there have been no attempts to quantify the theory and techniques for group work with adolescents who abuse substances, few group therapists know how to cope with these difficult-to-treat patients and there have been no efforts to systematize innovative treatment approaches. Theoretical frameworks, using appropriate techniques, can yield data that can be quantified in some way. One can then apply appropriate statistical analysis to test such data. By and large, this has not yet been done in the field. However, despite the lack of outcome studies and descriptions of long-term group treatment efforts, certain points are made in the literature about these adolescent patients. According to Levin (1987), the aim of treatment is to substitute the ties of relationships for those of addiction. Group psychotherapy for adolescents offers peer support and peer confrontation, lessening transferences that may interfere with the dyadic treatment of adolescents (Anderson 1982; Trapold 1990).

Drug abuse commonly begins in early adolescence. The Monitoring the Future survey has been conducted annually since 1975 among 16,000 seniors from 130 high schools nationwide and since 1991 among nationally representative surveys of eighth and tenth graders (more than 15,000 students per grade per year). These surveys revealed that although drug use among most adolescents had been declining through the 1980s, abuse continued at a high level; moreover, the early 1990s showed significant increases, particularly among eighth- and tenth-grade students. As recently as 1989 more than half of high school seniors had tried an illicit drug, and this figure was at 43% in 1993. More than a quarter of the class of 1993 had tried a drug other than marijuana, and alcohol and cigarette smoking continued at a high level (alcohol 87%, cigarette use 62%) (Johnston et al. 1994).

The three most commonly used drugs in adolescence (besides cigarettes) are alcohol marijuana, and inhalants (Johnston et al. 1994). Marijuana acts as a gateway drug (Kandel 1982), and its use is a necessary but no sufficient condition for the future use of other illicit drugs. It was found that 26% of marijuana users also used other illicit drugs, compared to 1% of nonusers of drugs and 4% of users of legal drugs (Kandel 1982). Marijuana is the most commonly used illicit drug, and inhalants are in second place. (Among eighth graders, inhalants rank highest.)

A small but significant number of users of illicit substances begin in the sixth grade or earlier. For example, among eighth graders in 1993, 4% reported using marijuana in sixth grade or earlier, and 11% reported having used inhalants.

Despite the geographic spread of the use of crack (smokable cocaine), crack and cocaine use declined in the late 1980s and stabilized in the early 1990s.

## ◆ Developmental Bases of Adolescent Drug Abuse

Substance abuse may be regarded as the result of the interaction of an inherited genetic predisposition (genotype) with certain environmental stimuli that bring the predisposition to overt phenotypic expression. There is good, if incomplete, evidence for this *risk-diathesis model* of drug abuse. Twin and adoption studies, as well as family biological studies of the children of alcoholic persons in particular, have shown the likelihood of a genetic predisposition. Probably, there are a number of types of genetic predisposition to drug abuse, as suggested by the typology of alcoholism proposed by Cloninger et al. (1981). Current studies suggest that an inherited disorder of neurotransmitter functioning or metabolism may be at the root of the genetic predisposition. This disorder may involve the neurotransmitters dopamine or serotonin, or both.

As in adults, adolescents develop three types of substance use disorders. These are substance abuse, substance dependence, and the organic brain syndromes caused by the various substances of abuse.

DSM-IV (American Psychiatric Association 1994) lists 10 classes of substances of abuse and gives definitions of the substances and of their associated disorders. The main differences between adult and adolescent substance use disorders rest on the shorter length of time adolescents have been using substances. A shorter duration of use usually means that adolescents show fewer (if any) psychosocial sequelae of chronic use and fewer of the more severe pathophysiological effects of abuse or addiction and that they are less likely to develop organic brain syndromes secondary to substance use (Kaminer 1991).

The environmental stimuli that may serve as the precipitating risk factors for drug abuse include many psychological variables. These stimuli may cause adolescents to begin and maintain drug use and may bring about the progression from drug use to drug abuse. Such psychosocial stimuli may be divided into a number of domains (Brook et al. 1992a), including personality, peer, family, and environmental contexts.

It should be noted that drug abuse is commonly found in association with other kinds of problem behaviors such as delinquency, precocious sexuality, school failure and dropout, and other comorbid psychiatric disorders. The most common psychiatric disorders found in adolescents who abuse substances are affective disorders, conduct disorders, and anxiety disorders (Kaminer 1991). It should be noted that the relationship between substance abuse and psychiatric disorders in adolescence is common (perhaps seen in 75% of all cases of substance abuse) and complex. Whether there is a common genetic or psychosocial vulnerability to both kinds of disorders (Brook and Cohen 1992) or whether one kind of disorder precedes and predisposes to or influences the other kind remains a controversial area of current investigation.

To treat substance abuse disorders successfully, it is important to institute the appropriate treatment for any coexisting comorbid disorder. This can be done in a day program or on an inpatient unit with a specially designed mentally ill chemical abusers (MICA) program. It is very difficult to treat dually diagnosed adolescents with severe degrees of psychiatric disturbance on an outpatient basis alone. In addition to having problems related to the nature of the symptoms and the degree of illness, many of these adolescents require the use of various psychopharmacological approaches or other interventions that are best started on a day program or inpatient unit. Group psychotherapy can play a very important role in such MICA units. Once a dually diagnosed adolescent patient is stabilized, referral for longer-term outpatient group psychotherapy may be indicated.

One explanation of the relationship between substance abuse and psychiatric disorders is the self-medication hypothesis (Khantzian 1985). According to this hypothesis, persons abuse substances with specific pharmacological characteristics to medicate disturbed ego states and states of affective dysregulation. The specific substance used depends on the type of intrapsychic disturbance. For instance, a highly anxious person might use alcohol or a sedative-hypnotic drug to relieve anxiety; a depressed person might use a stimulant such as amphetamine or cocaine. This hypothesis, while potentially useful in enhancing our understanding and the effectiveness of treatment interventions, needs experimental confirmation. It may be that in genetically predisposed people, self-medication may play a role in the development of substance abuse in conjunction with the influence of other risk factors.

Particularly of note is the strong relationship found between substance abuse and adolescent suicide. Rich et al. (1986) reported findings from the San Diego Suicide Study that substance abuse and suicide were strongly related in 70% of suicides completed under the age of 30 years. It is well known that suicide attempts often follow intoxication (Brent et al. 1987). Perhaps the adolescent most at risk for suicide is a white male who is intoxicated, has access to firearms, and is not receiving professional treatment (Kaminer 1991). Of course, all suicide threats or gestures must be taken seriously and dealt with by appropriate measures, often including hospitalization. Knowledge of the patient's risk factors for suicide helps in determining how to deal with a suicide threat. There are also strong correlations between adolescent substance abuse and parental substance use and between adolescent substance abuse and physical and sexual abuse of adolescents of both sexes. Indeed, especially in dually diagnosed adolescents, physical and sexual abuse may be the rule. An attempt should always be made—at an appropriate time and with tact and care—to elicit a history or other evidence of such abuse.

# ◆ Psychosocial Risk and Protective Factors

The psychosocial risk factors for adolescent substance use and abuse have been thoroughly explored by Brook et al. (1990). An impaired child-parent mutual attachment relationship in a child with a genetic predisposition to drug abuse results in a high level of childhood aggression and further impairment of the family interactions. The child does not internalize parental controls well and identifies poorly with the parents. These problems lead to difficulties with peers and in school, resulting in isolation, depression, poor social skills, poor problem-solving skills, temper tantrums, and early delinquency.

In addition, the continuation of an impaired adolescent-parent relationship results in rebelliousness, sensation seeking, risk-taking, and further deviant behavior. Such an adolescent is likely to be impulsive and depressed, have difficulties in school, and associate with drug-using peers. Drug abuse, delinquency, and precocious sexual behavior further interfere with the adolescent's development and the normal psychosocial tasks of adolescence. With continued impairment of the relationship between the parents and the adolescent, the influence of the drug-using peer group becomes magnified, resulting in further drug use and abuse.

The interactions between parents and child work mutually and reciprocally, with feedback effects acting as influences in both directions. Parents influence the child through parental personality and parental child-rearing practices, and the child's characteristics affect the parent-child relationship (Brook and Brook 1990). These developmental mechanisms affect the adolescent's personality, which in turn affects the parent-adolescent relationship. An example of this mutual reciprocal interaction is the finding that childhood aggression predicts less mutuality in the parent-adolescent relationship, which is related to adolescent unconventionality and more adolescent drug use (Brook et al. 1992a).

The interactions of risk factors and protective factors for adolescent drug use are complex and have both direct and indirect effects. For instance, the parental trait of conventionality, a protective factor against adolescent drug abuse, is related to a more positive parent-child mutual attachment relationship (protective) and the internalization of parental values, which are connected with greater adolescent conventionality (protective). Greater adolescent conventionality is related to less peer drug use and low or no adolescent drug use. The effects of protective factors such as parental conventionality, parents and peers who do not use drugs, a positive parent-child attachment relationship, and so forth can mitigate the noxious effects of harmful risk factors and environmental stimuli during growth and development. For instance, a firm attachment to one parent can counteract the effect of the risk factor of marital discord on adolescent drug use. The influence of sibling drug use (a risk factor) is lessened by associating with peers who do not use drugs (a protective factor). Other risk and protective factors also interact similarly to influence the end result of more or less adolescent drug use (Brook and Brook 1990).

It should be kept in mind that the two strong predictors of adolescent drug use are aggression in childhood and associating with drug-using peers in adolescence (Brook et al. 1992b). Parental substance use and abuse, whether legal or illicit, are also significant risk factors, as is parental psychopathology. As a part of the treatment of adolescents who abuse substances, every attempt also should be made to treat parents and family members.

Another important characteristic of adolescent development must be considered in the treatment of adolescents who abuse substances. During the course of adolescence, adolescents become less attached to parents and family and more attached to peers, both individual peers and peer groups. This process is accentuated and occurs earlier or in a disturbed way in the case of adolescents who abuse substances. This characteristic of adolescent development has significance for treatment; it is usually easier to treat younger adolescents who are still attached to their families than older adolescents who have already formed strong attachments to substance-abusing peers and peer networks. This difference may not apply to adolescents in an enmeshed family (Kaufman 1985), in which a role reversal often occurs. According to Kaufman, an enmeshed family is one in which family members are intensely overinvolved; they have an increased sense of belonging that requires them to give up much autonomy. It may be equally difficult to treat younger and older adolescents in such families, because in both cases, autonomy is similarly impaired.

Groups play a significant role in childhood and adolescent development. The early nuclear or extended family group—including the mother-child dyad, early childhood peer groups, school groups (in which children and adolescents spend most of their waking hours), the family group of later childhood and adolescence, and the various peer groups of adolescence—all play crucial roles in normal growth and development, as well as in the development of adolescent substance abuse. The developmental importance of groups, both in the family and with peers at play and in school, points to the importance of using groups and group approaches in the treatment of adolescent substance abuse.

## ◆ Selection of Patients

Patient selection criteria for groups of adolescents who abuse substances are based on the general patient selection criteria for group psychotherapy (Brook 1980). In addition, some selection criteria are based on the nature of adolescence and on the issues involved in adolescent substance abuse. According to Scheidlinger (1985), adolescents in crisis, adolescents with fragile egos, psychotic adolescents, sociopathic adolescents, and paranoid adolescents do not belong in a group. Although not documented at present, it is likely that adolescents who associate less with drug-using peers and who value academic achievement more will do better in group therapy. The absence of overt self-destructive behavior, the presence of a relatively good sense of self-esteem, and the presence of a positive mutual relationship with parents or a parental surrogate are also likely to indicate a good prognosis. A history of delinquency or early childhood aggression probably indicates a relatively poorer prognosis.

Adolescents whose substance abuse does not result in severe disability may be suitable for outpatient groups, as may adolescents with a relatively intact support system, those with a history of rehabilitation treatment with only a brief relapse, and those who binge as opposed to using substances every day (Phillips 1989).

Adolescents with a history of more severe disability, dual diagnosis, or a severely impaired and dysfunctional family are more likely to benefit from group psychotherapy in a structured day program, a therapeutic environment, or an inpatient setting. A more restrictive inpatient setting is also indicated for physically dependent patients, patients who have failed at outpatient treatment, and intravenous drug abusers (Kaminer 1991).

Those factors found to be related to patient selection and completion of treatment in adolescents included being middle-class, not using opiates, an older age at first use, a concurrent educational program, and the absence of polydrug abuse (Rush 1979). The presence of a comorbid psychiatric diagnosis was related to poor treatment outcome in adults, but there are as yet no good outcome studies of the treatment of dually diagnosed adolescents (Kaminer 1991).

## ◆ Treatment Techniques

Because of the development of adolescent substance abuse in family and group settings, family therapy and group psychotherapy are of particular importance in the treatment of substance use disorders (Ball and Meck 1979). Henderson and Anderson (1989) and Scheidlinger (1985) recommend outpatient group psychotherapy as the treatment of choice for substance-abusing adolescents.

The goals of group therapy for adolescents who abuse substances are complex. They include teaching patients the value of themselves and other people and helping patients to learn to relate to other people in a responsible and mutually helpful way (Shaw 1992). Group psychotherapy can help adolescents to contain and redirect rebellious feelings in socially acceptable and positive ways. It can allow adolescents who have previously had few successes to experience interpersonal success, with enhanced self-esteem as the result (Birmingham 1986). The therapist must keep in mind the necessity of helping the patient establish control over the substance abuse, or the addiction if it is present. Most therapists agree that the goal of abstinence for the adolescent is of primary importance for successful therapy (Vanicelli 1992). Involving the family members or surrogate families in the treatment process is also crucial. Indeed, some therapists will not treat adolescents who abuse substances unless at least some family members are included in the treatment in some way. Family therapy and multiple family group therapy are often used for this purpose.

Several types of groups are appropriate for use in the treatment of adolescents who abuse substances. Often an adolescent may be treated in a number of different groups concurrently. Such groups can include male and female groups, a substance abuse education group, a 12-step group, a relapse prevention group, a vocational group, a group for learning problem-solving skills, a leisure education group, a medication group, a health group, an outside family group, an activity group, and so forth. Recently, several centers have begun to hold groups for the early treatment and prevention of the physical abuse of women by men, something for which both men and women who abuse substances are particularly at risk. Such groups can have memberships made up of men only, women only, or both sexes together. Although many authors suggest that substance abuse groups be made up of substance abusers only, more data need to be gathered and evaluated to understand this issue more fully.

In the past, many group psychotherapeutic approaches to the treatment of persons who abuse substances have been based on interpersonal and psychodynamic interpretive techniques (Ends and Page 1957; Khantzian 1985). These techniques, which are based on support and the interpretation of certain unconscious conflicts, can be useful. However, for adolescents in particular, behavioral techniques based more on interventions focusing on the here and now in the group may be more efficacious (Galanter et al. 1991).

For example, persons who abuse drugs may be responding more to conditioned responses set off by specific cues, rather than attempting to handle emotional conflict through drug-using behavior. Certainly, a group therapist treating drug-abusing adolescents must know about both kinds of issues and must be able to use a blend of treatment approaches. A number of authors suggest the use of structured guidelines, including behavioral contracts prohibiting substance use (Birmingham 1986). Corey and Corey (1987) also point to the importance of structure and limit setting and even suggest themes for group discussion with role-playing to emphasize focusing on feelings.

Specific techniques for use with adolescents who abuse substances include the provision of a supportive group environment. Even confrontational group programs such as Daytop provide support for members to be able to express themselves freely. Because impulsivity and acting-out are characteristic of both adolescents and persons who abuse substances, the group therapist must be prepared to deal with these issues with consistent, reasoned limit setting. Often in a day program setting or an inpatient setting, behavioral rewards or deprivations may be used with good results. Adolescents who abuse substances also have difficulty tolerating anxiety and may direct primitive transferences toward the therapist. These feelings may be diffused in the group among the other group members (Kanas 1982). Peer pressure and peer support are also powerful forces for behavioral change in groups and may be particularly useful in decreasing denial (Galanter et al. 1991).

Certain psychopharmacological approaches may be useful in the treatment of adolescents who abuse substances, perhaps in conjunction with group psychotherapy. The use of medications for the treatment of adolescents who abuse substances needs further study and evaluation. Certainly, medication treatments such as methadone maintenance, naltrexone, and disulfiram may have a place in the treatment of selected adolescents.

Patients seen in groups should also be seen in individual sessions to assess the presence of continuing symptoms and to explore issues that a patient is unable to bring up in the group setting. Preparation of patients for group and introduction of the therapeutic contract are also best accomplished in early individual sessions, usually before the patient joins the group. Individual sessions are also useful for assessing the patient's ability to benefit from group therapy. As noted above, psychotic or intellectually impaired patients often do not do well in a group setting and so are relatively contraindicated for group treatment (Brook 1980).

Groups for adolescents who abuse substances may be time limited or long-term, depending on the treatment setting, the goals of treatment, and financial and managed care issues. Groups for learning problem-solving skills, for example, may be time limited and use a step-by-step approach (Galanter et al. 1991). Such steps include the following:

- Recognition of the problem
- Definition of the problem
- Formulation of several possible alternative solutions
- Selection of the best alternative solution after examination of the pros and cons of each alternative

Such time-limited groups can increase members' ability to plan ahead, although their relationship to long-term abstinence is unclear.

As noted, educational and other kinds of groups can provide opportunities for behavioral change through patient interaction and active participation. Such groups can operate on a surface level but can also be used to explore issues of self-esteem, affective expression, and problem-solving skills.

For longer-term outpatient groups, an interactional approach, as developed by Yalom et al. (1978) and Vanicelli (1982), can be useful. Such an approach emphasizes self-disclosure and the expression of feelings in a safe, nonjudgmental setting. Patients are encouraged to attend Alcoholics Anonymous (AA), and abstinence is a primary goal of treatment. Limit setting and confrontation of denial are more effective when done by other group members. It can be difficult to find an appropriate AA group for an adolescent, and the therapist's active help in this regard is useful. Adolescents can benefit from inclusion in adult AA groups, but there are often many difficulties in terms of age-appropriate goals and developmental tasks, the increased vulnerability of some adolescents to the influences of certain psychopathic adults, and the lack of adolescent peer support.

Groups for adolescents who abuse substances must strike a balance between being focused on the group and group issues and being focused on the individual group member. A complex and shifting interplay develops between the group's issues and the individual member's issues. This interplay may be facilitated by the use of a group-centered approach, which refers to the focus of the leader and the group on issues of the group as a whole, the interactions between its members, and the meaning of each issue and interaction for each member. This interplay requires sensitivity and skill on the part of the group therapist. There is also an interplay between the interactional processes occurring in the group and behavioral and supportive issues. For instance, a hostile interchange in the group may be used to illustrate and explore the behavioral skill of anger control. Balancing these processes and using interpretation to explore group and individual interpersonal and unconscious processes to promote insight and self-understanding also require sensitivity and skill (Rutan and Stone 1993). The most useful and lasting changes occur in the here and now of the group process, and the leader must have the knowledge and ability to keep the group members focused on the interactions in the group, despite the presence of ongoing denial, acting out, and other forms of resistance.

The example cited below illustrates a number of the issues discussed in this chapter. It is taken from one session of a community meeting held on a daily basis in a day MICA program for dually diagnosed adolescents. The adolescents present were from 15 to 18 years old, with nine boys and seven girls present.

### Case Example

A staff member opened the session by announcing the names of the eight level III patients who were eligible to go on the next field trip and asked that they bring in consent forms signed by their parents.

Nick then discussed how his father, back in the home after a period of incarceration, was trying to push him around and dominate him by setting overstrict and unreasonable rules for his conduct. He had managed to achieve a working relationship with his mother that involved mutual compromises, and his father's reentry into the home was disturbing the delicate balance. He had slept at a friend's house for two nights the past week to avoid angry confrontations with his father.

Ray said that he was also angry with what went on in his family as his parents frequently quarreled loudly, particularly when his father was drinking. He also often felt that he had to sleep at a friend's house to escape the turmoil at home. Nancy Ann spoke about her conflicts with her brother, who beat her and tied her up. She felt that her parents were unable to protect her, and related the story of her brother's recent investigation by Child Protective Services (New York State has a mandatory child abuse reporting law). She felt afraid he would beat her up more because she told her therapist about him and it resulted in a Child Protective Services investigation.

One of the staff members asked if the patients felt safe in talking about themselves in therapy. Susan said that she did, because she trusted the staff and her therapist; she also said that all these issues were bound to come out in the open sooner or later anyway. Ramona brought up her angry feelings at a male teacher, whom she felt was too strict with her. A number of the other patients said that they felt angry at this particular teacher because he had been absent for a week because of illness, leaving them to be taught by a substitute teacher who didn't really know them and whom they felt they couldn't really trust. A staff member said that people often felt angry when they felt abandoned.

Peter described a fight he had gotten into over the prior weekend, stating that he felt so angry he could have killed the other person. A staff member asked if there were other ways people could deal with crises or troubling feelings without fighting or using drugs or drinking. Lavinia said that she always tried to talk things over with friends when she felt troubled or upset. Steve discussed how badly he felt when he learned two of his friends were killed in an auto accident involving drunken driving. A number of the other patients said they saw the article in the paper about this accident and that they felt bad for Steve. Arthur said he tried not to get in a car with friends who had been drinking, but many patients said that although that was a good idea, it wasn't always possible to know if someone had been using substances. A staff member announced that 10 of the patients had to report for urine screens, and the group meeting ended on that note.

Although this example illustrates several points discussed earlier, there are a few especially salient issues. The adolescents' concern with intrafamilial conflicts and their difficulties in handling angry feelings are clearly seen. Examining the adverse sequelae of substance abuse is done in the context of group support. Interpersonal conflicts and dependence on staff in the program setting are frequently discussed. Examination of alternative, non-self-destructive ways of dealing with life stresses is an ongoing process. The example also illustrates one of the uses of a system of rewards and punishments (deprivations) and mentions the use of random urine testing.

# ◆ Curative Factors

A number of curative factors have been noted to be particularly important in the treatment of adolescents who abuse substances. According to Butler and Fuhriman (1983), self-understanding, catharsis, and interpersonal learning were valued in outpatient therapy groups. Corder et al. (1981) found that adolescents identified similar factors as being helpful in groups. Of course, the role of the leader must be emphasized because he or she creates the appropriate group atmosphere for limiting setting, support, growth, and abstinence (De Blassie and Sallee 1982).

The group's limit-setting ability can help the adolescent internalize the ability to set limits and can aid in the further development of an internal locus of control. Group members point out self-destructive behaviors and suggest alternative ways of handling disturbing affects and of responding to disturbing behavioral cues. A peer-counseling function comes into play, which also provides peer support.

Through supportive confrontation, group members become aware of dysfunctional responses and behaviors and learn to evaluate difficult situations more realistically and appropriately. Group members are helped to confront denial and accept responsibility for their actions. Through the affective interchange occurring in the group, group members learn to trust and help one another. Adolescents who come to be concerned with each others' lives may form extragroup relationships, which have the potential for aiding or hindering further growth. Such relationships can be supportive and should not necessarily be regarded as antitherapeutic. It is important for adolescents to discuss their extragroup contacts in the group, because this discussion fosters self-examination and decreases potentially destructive clique formation. Through the establishment of mutual trust, the group may help the adolescent members develop autonomy and responsibility and may act as a transitional object or substitute family (Scheidlinger 1985), facilitating emotional growth.

Adolescents who abuse substances tend to come from disturbed families (Galanter et al. 1991). Therefore, recent research into the psychosocial familial etiology of adolescent substance abuse may further our understanding of possible curative factors that play a role in group therapy with these adolescent patients. Other psychosocial domains have also been found to be of importance in the development of adolescent substance abuse. Recent studies of risk and protective factors for adolescent substance use (Brook et al. 1990) reveal a complex set of psychosocial risk factors acting in the peer, personality, family, school, and environmental domains. Certain factors are particularly important: the nature of the parent-adolescent mutual attachment relationship, the adolescent's association with substance-abusing peers, the presence of early aggression, and the presence of certain personality attributes such as unconventionality, risk taking, sensation seeking, delinquency, and precocious sexual behavior. Group approaches directed at altering these risk factors or increasing the presence of protective factors (e.g., associating with peers who value academic achievement) may serve as powerful curative influences. Although these findings are too new to have found widespread clinical applications, the use of adolescent group therapy to change the nature and intensity of such risk factors promises to provide a more direct therapeutic approach to the psychosocial causes of adolescent substance abuse.

For example, the use of multiple family groups may be an innovative approach to changing the nature of the parent-adolescent bond, an area of difficulty often seen in the families of adolescents who abuse substances. A group that explores the pros and cons of risk taking may provide the adolescent with alternative ways of dealing with destructive impulses and difficult feelings. This research-based approach is new, but initial exploration of its uses indicates a positive and direct way to bring curative factors to bear on the core problems of adolescents who abuse substances.

## ◆ Group Techniques in the Prevention of Adolescent Substance Abuse and AIDS

Education in elementary school can play an important role in the prevention of adolescent substance abuse and AIDS. Classes and group discussions that present children with factual information are necessary starting points for preventing later morbidity. However, classroom education alone—even that which focuses on teaching protective personality traits such as responsibility—has only limited value. Probably more effective are group efforts (Corey and Corey 1987) that focus children's attention on the interactions between people that lead to initiation into drug abuse and on risk taking that might lead to further morbidity—for example, violent behavior and its effects or the development of infectious diseases, such as AIDS or sexually transmitted diseases. Focus groups and peer counseling groups can be particularly useful for this purpose. These groups can be led or guided by trained teachers or guidance counselors who have received special training in the use of group techniques. These group leaders also must understand the psychosocial risk and protective factors that lead to substance abuse in genetically predisposed individuals.

Efforts at helping adolescents at risk to understand how such psychosocial factors affect their own lives and the lives of their family members are particularly useful. Family therapy, including multiple family groups, can also help expose the noxious role that psychosocial risk factors play in interactions in the family. Such treatment can result in changed familial and peer interactions, leading to decreased substance abuse. A complete discussion of the role of such psychosocial risk and protective factors in adolescent substance abuse was published previously (Brook et al. 1990).

For adolescents already getting treatment for substance abuse, relapse prevention efforts have particular value in helping avoid further morbidity, disability, and risk-taking behavior. Relapse prevention groups explore ways in which adolescents can alter their behaviors and handle affective and interpersonal stresses without resorting to substance abuse or other risk-taking behavior. Such groups can also explore those predisposing personality, family, and peer factors that make individuals vulnerable to relapse. Groups can also help participants develop both general and specific coping skills, using a cognitive-behavioral approach (Marlatt and Gordon 1985).

Substance-abusing adolescents very often engage in precocious and risky sexual behavior and risky drug behavior. Therefore, it is important to educate these adolescents about AIDS and to teach them ways to prevent infection with the human immunodeficiency virus (HIV). Adolescent girls, in particular, are at risk for infection because of engaging in prostitution to get money for drugs or directly exchanging sex for drugs. Group techniques are useful to help adolescents focus on the avoidance of inappropriate, risky sexual behavior (Frost 1992; Grant 1988).

# ◆ References

American Psychiatric Association: Diagnostic and Statistical Manual of Mental Disorders, 3rd Edition, Revised. Washington, DC, American Psychiatric Association, 1987

Anderson SC: Group therapy with alcoholic clients: a review. Advances in Alcohol and Substance Abuse 2:23–40, 1982

Ball JD, Meck DS: Implications of developmental theories for counseling adolescents in groups. Adolescence 14:529–534, 1979

Birmingham M: An out-patient treatment programme for adolescent substance abusers. J Adolesc 9:123–133, 1986

Bratter TE: Group psychotherapy with alcohol and drug addicted adolescents: special clinical concerns and challenges, in Adolescent Group Psychotherapy. Edited by Azima FJ Cramer, Richmond LH. New York, International Universities Press, 1989, pp 163–169

Brent DA, Perper JA, Allman C: Alcohol, firearms, and suicide among youth. JAMA 257:3369–3372, 1987

Brook DW: Selection of patients for group psychotherapy. Issues in Ego Psychology 3:32–36, 1980

Brook DW, Brook J: The etiology and consequences of adolescent drug use, in Prevention and Treatment of Drug and Alcohol Abuse. Edited by Watson RR. Clifton, NJ, Humana Press, 1990, pp 339–362

Brook JS, Cohen P: A developmental perspective on drug use and delinquency, in Advances in Criminological Theory, Vol 3. Crime Facts, Fictions, and Theory. Edited by McCord J. New Brunswick, NJ, Transaction Publishers, 1992, pp 231–251

Brook JS, Brook DW, Gordon AS, et al: The psychological etiology of adolescent drug use: a family interactional approach. Genet Soc Gen Psychol Monogr 11:111–267, 1990

Brook JS, Whiteman M, Cohen P, et al: Childhood precursors of adolescent drug use: a longitudinal analysis. Genet Soc Gen Psychol Monogr 118:197–213, 1992a

Brook JS, Hamburg BA, Balka EB, et al: Sequences of drug involvement in African-American and Puerto Rican adolescents. Psychol Rep 71: 179–182, 1992b

Butler T, Fuhriman A: Curative factors in group therapy: a review of the recent literature. Small Group Behavior 14:131–142, 1983

Cloninger CR, Bohman M, Sigvardsson S: Inheritance of alcohol abuse. Arch Gen Psychiatry 38:861–871, 1981

Coleman JC: Current contradictions in adolescent theory. Journal of Youth and Adolescence 7:1–11, 1978

Cooper DE: The role of group psychotherapy in the treatment of substance abusers. Am J Psychotherapy 41:55–67, 1987

Corder BF, Whiteside L, Haizlip T: A study of curative factors in group psychotherapy with adolescents. Int J Group Psychother 31:345–354, 1981

Corey MS, Corey G: Groups: Process and Practice, 3rd Edition. Pacific Grove, CA, Brooks/Cole, 1987

De Blassie RR, Sallee N: Counseling with the young adolescent. Journal of Early Adolescence 2:25–30, 1982

Ends EJ, Page CW: A study of three types of group psychotherapy with hospitalized inebriates. Quarterly Journal of Studies on Alcohol 18: 263–277, 1957

Frost JC: Group psychotherapy with HIV-positive and AIDS patients, in Group Therapy in Clinical Practice. Edited by Alonso A, Swiller HI. Washington, DC, American Psychiatric Press, 1993, pp 255–270

Galanter M, Castaneda R, Franco H: Group therapy and self-help groups, in Clinical Textbook of Addictive Disorders. Edited by Frances RJ, Miller SI. New York, Guilford, 1991, pp 43–451

Grant D: Support groups for youth with the AIDS virus. Int J Group Psychother 38:237–251, 1988

Henderson DC, Anderson SC: Adolescents and chemical dependency. Social Work in Health Care 14:87–105, 1989

Johnston LD, O'Malley PM, Bachman JG: National survey results on drug use from the Monitoring of the Future Study, 1975–1993, Vol. 1: Secondary school students (U.S. DHHS [NIH] Publication No 94-3809); Vol. 2: College students and young adults (U.S. DHHS [NIH] Publication No 94-3810). Rockville, MD, National Institute on Drug Abuse, 1994

Kaminer Y: Adolescent substance abuse, in Clinical Textbook of Addictive Disorders. Edited by Frances RJ, Miller SI. New York, Guilford, 1991, pp 320–346

Kanas N: Alcoholism and group psychotherapy, in Encyclopedic Handbook of Alcoholism. Edited by Kaufman E, Pattison EM. New York, Gardner, 1992, pp 1011–1021

Kandel DB: Epidemiological and psychosocial perspectives on adolescent drug use. Journal of the American Academy of Child Psychiatry 20: 328–347, 1982

Kaufman E: Substance Abuse and Family Therapy. Orlando, FL, Grune & Stratton, 1985

Khantzian EJ: The self-medication hypothesis of addictive disorders: focus on heroin and cocaine dependence. Am J Psychiatry 142:1259–1264, 1985

Levin JD: Treatment of Alcoholism and Other Addictions: A Self-Psychology Approach. Northvale, NJ, Aronson, 1987

Marlatt GA, Gordon JR (eds): Relapse Prevention: Maintenance Strategies in the Treatment of Addictive Behaviors. New York, Guilford, 1985

Phillips KL: Chemical dependence treatment review guidelines. Gen Hosp Psychiatry 11:282–287, 1989

Rachman AW, Raubolt RR: The clinical practice of group psycho-therapy with adolescent substance abusers: strategies for clinical intervention, in Alcoholism and Substance Abuse: Strategies for Clinical Intervention. Edited by Bratter TE, Forrest G. New York, Free Press, 1985, pp 338–364

Rich CL, Young D, Fowler RC: San Diego Suicide Study, I: young vs. old subjects. Arch Gen Psychiatry 43:577–582, 1986

Rush TV: Predicting treatment outcome for juvenile and young adult clients in the Pennsylvania substance abuse system, in Youth Drug Abuse. Edited by Berschner GM, Friedman AS. Lexington, MA, Lexington Books, 1979, pp 629–656

Rutan JS, Stone WN: Psychodynamic Group Psychotherapy, 2nd Edition. New York, Guilford, 1993

Scheidlinger S: Group treatment of adolescents: an overview. Am J Orthopsychiatry 55:102–111, 1985

Shaw S: Group psychotherapy with adolescents, in Adolescent Substance Abuse. Edited by Lawson GW, Lawson AW. Gaithersburg, MD, Aspen, 1992, pp 121–130

Trapold, M: Adolescent chemical dependency, in Family Therapy and Beyond: A Multisystemic Approach to Treating the Behavior Problems of Children and Adolescents. Edited by Henggeler SW, Bordwin CM. Pacific Grove, CA, Brooks/Cole, 1990, pp 246–277

Vanicelli M: Group psychotherapy with alcoholics: special techniques. J Stud Alcohol 43:17–37, 1982

Vanicelli M: Removing the Roadblocks: Group Psychotherapy With Substance Abusers and Family Members. New York, Guilford, 1992

Vanicelli M, Canning D, Griefen M: Group therapy with alcoholics: a group case study. Int J Group Psychother 34:127–147, 1984

Wunderlich RA, Lozes J, Lewis J: Recidivism rates of group therapy participants and other adolescents processed by juvenile court. Psychotherapy: Theory, Research and Practice 11:243–245, 1974

Yalom ID, Bloch S, Bond G, et al: Alcoholics in interactional group therapy. Arch Gen. Psychiatry 35:419–425, 1978

# CHAPTER 15

# A Five-Phase Model for Adolescents Who Abuse Substances

*Henry I. Spitz, M.D., and*
*Susan T. Spitz, A.C.S.W.*

Psychotherapists from diverse clinical backgrounds and theoretical orientations have searched for innovative and intelligent approaches to troublesome but commonly encountered treatment problems. Working with adolescents is a challenge in itself. When psychologically symptomatic teenagers also have a presenting complaint of substance abuse, the clinician's task becomes even more complex. In addition, when adolescents are psychologically symptomatic, a set of family dynamics almost invariably must be factored into a comprehensive treatment plan.

As a consequence, treatment of adolescents who abuse substances raises issues that involve individual, group, family, self-help, and psychopharmacological interventions. The primary focuses of this chapter are the theoretical and clinical issues that face the group therapist who works with adolescents and how group psychotherapy can play a critical role in the rehabilitation, growth, and development of this patient population.

## ◆ Scope of the Problem

Current estimates (Dusenbury et al. 1992) suggest that three million adolescents in the United States are considered problem drinkers and that 400,000 teenagers need active substance abuse treatment. Although cigarettes and alcohol are the most popular substances of abuse, there is still abuse of other drugs, most notably cocaine (particularly "crack"), marijuana, heroin, and hallucinogenic substances.

Because adolescence is such an emotionally intense and often stormy and confusing stage of life, it is often difficult to distinguish between "normal" experimentation with mind- and mood-altering substances and behavior that indicates more serious psychological disturbance.

Negative prognostic factors for developing addictive patterns and for having increased difficulty in gaining and maintaining long-term abstinence have been studied. Adolescents who begin using potentially addicting substances before age 15 years are at highest risk for developing intractable patterns of addiction (Robins and Pryzbek 1985). Familial factors such as parental history of substance abuse, emotional rejection, and deprivation are also correlated with a greater tendency for teenagers to become excessively involved with substance use.

Semlitz and Gold (1986) reemphasized that peer group influences are perhaps the most important interpersonal or social factors affecting the introduction to drug experimentation and potential substance abuse in adolescents. Much of the rationale for the use of a group format in working with adolescents rests on the recognition of the peer vector as a credible and potent force for influencing adolescents' attitudes and behavior.

Other general risk factors include poverty, low self-esteem, affective disorders, and possible biological factors such as a genetic predisposition to drug or alcohol abuse. These elements are thought to be significant in the genesis and maintenance of adolescent addictions.

## ◆ Overview of Groups for Adolescents Who Abuse Substances

The types of groups and the context within which they are conducted are varied indeed. Groups take place on inpatient psychiatric services, in residential treatment centers, and most commonly in an outpatient setting. The composition of the group is usually designed to accomplish some specific treatment goals, and the apparently homogeneous nature of these groups can be misleading. Although it is true that most groups are homogeneously composed of adolescents, they are heterogeneous for many other factors within the same group. Often members of the same group abuse different drugs and may be at different points in the recovery process. Similarly, there are obvious differences among types of groups: a multiple family group, an adolescent self-help group, and a therapeutic community meeting all are aimed at helping the adolescent, but they do so from different vantage points and place emphasis on different therapeutic factors.

Broadly speaking, the two primary types of groups for adults who abuse substances are the psychotherapy group and the self-help group, which is some form of the 12-step program. Numerically, more adults participate in self-help groups. This is not the case with adolescents for several reasons. Emotional immaturity and developmental lags due to excessive involvement with drugs make it much harder, if not impossible, to have self-governed and consistently led peer groups with defined rules, goals, and appropriate limits. Professional group leadership helps provide a structure within which a therapeutic group experience can transpire.

Regardless of the group leader's theoretical orientation or leadership style, there is a clear consensus among clinicians who work with persons who abuse substances that the top priority in treatment is to get the addiction under control. Without an attempt at accomplishing this goal, therapeutic intervention of any kind is deemed useless.

The sections that follow focus on the outpatient psychotherapy group. We try to highlight the specific issues faced by group leaders and members when constructing and conducting a model that addresses the specific needs and problems presented by the addicted adolescent patient.

## ◆ Phase 1: Evaluation and Orientation

Many critical and often neglected phases that determine the eventual success or failure of a new group take place long before the first session. The pregroup phase encompasses the screening, evaluation, diagnosis, and preparation of prospective group members before group entry.

For the adolescent, the pregroup phase should include an assessment of motivation for therapy. Is the teenager here of his or her own volition or as the result of a family intervention or court-mandated treatment? A core element of this phase is a thorough diagnostic evaluation, including neuropsychological or other testing, to make an accurate individual diagnosis. It is essential to take a specific drug history as a routine part of the intake process. Issues of dual diagnosis often emerge and must be factored into a treatment plan that takes into account both the severity of any psychopathology and the extent and type of drug abuse.

A central element of any pregroup phase is the education and orientation of new members. This element takes on added meaning when working with adolescents. It is wise to take several individual sessions, if necessary, to ensure that the new member understands the nature of the group and how it will be useful. A typical orientation has a large educational component and includes the following:

- The general purpose and size of the group
- The role and activity level of the leader
- Where the group will be held and the physical arrangement of the room itself
- The time period of each session and whether the group is short term or open-ended
- Rules about regular attendance
- Some discussion of whether new members will be joining over the course of the group
- Whether urine testing for drugs is part of the group design
- Confidentiality
- The policy regarding contact among members outside of formal sessions
- Whether anyone will be observing or taping the group sessions
- Some discussion of how other simultaneous therapies will be coordinated
- Plans for inpatient hospitalization if it becomes necessary

The therapist should leave a good deal of time for the adolescent to ask questions. This question period yields valuable data regarding myths, misconceptions, and fears that might interfere with the adolescent's ability to participate in the group.

A successfully conducted first phase results in a carefully selected and well-prepared group with realistic expectations about the experience that lies ahead. Two other distinct advantages of careful pregroup preparation are a reduction in the dropout rate (Piper 1982) and a sense of early postures, roles, or resistances certain group members are likely to exhibit. An added benefit of spending adequate time in preparing adolescents for groups is that it begins the process of forming a positive therapeutic alliance.

## ◆ Phase 2: Entry Into the Group

Once an adolescent has achieved some semblance of emotional equilibrium and is not actively using drugs, he or she is ready to enter the group. The tasks for the leader in the earliest stages of the group center around getting the group launched, setting a therapeutic climate of trust and mutual respect, and providing a stable structure most conducive to the creation of therapeutic group norms.

These goals are attained by active group leadership starting in the first session. The group leader may chose to begin the initial session with a review of some of the elements discussed individually with members during their orientation phase. A set of ground rules or an early treatment contract is a typical clinical translation of this principle of review.

A representative example of this process occurs when the leader goes over the group guidelines at the start of the first session. Drug treatment groups for adolescents begin with each member agreeing to abide by a set of firm but fair rules that includes a number of themes. The group is told that its purpose is for members to help support and assist each other in abstaining from all mind- and mood-altering substances. Second, members must make an agreement to be absolutely honest about any drug use and never to come to group under the influence of any drug.

Furthermore, regular attendance is required, and a policy concerning how many absences are acceptable (less than one per each 2-month period) is instituted. Random urine testing for drugs is also a component of the initial group design, as is the request that group members refrain from social contact outside the regular sessions. Group leaders openly state that it may be necessary to communicate with other people involved in the adolescents' therapy or with the families, or both.

Special emphasis is given to the importance of confidentiality in the group. A clear distinction must be made between a transfer of learning, a therapeutic event that helps teenagers use the information from group sessions constructively in life outside the group, and ordinary gossip, which is a true breach of confidentiality. Serious breaches of confidentiality are presented to members as one of the nonnegotiable grounds for dismissal from the group.

Anyone who has worked with adolescents who abuse drugs knows that it will be difficult for them to consistently comply with the set of limits imposed by the group leader. The occasional use of a drug is best handled as an experience from which an adolescent can learn about the antecedents and cues that motivated this particular lapse in a pattern of sobriety. Obviously, a regular pattern of "slips" is destructive for the group and the individual, and such members usually require more intensive treatment, such as inpatient hospitalization.

To be a positive role model for the members, the group leader must make this initial position statement. In so doing, he or she sets the stage for group members to have a set of standards and expectations placed on them that forms the backdrop for the drama that will unfold as the group progresses.

## ◆ Phase 3: Establishing a Working Group Climate

Yalom (1985) underscored the value of creating an atmosphere of cohesion early in the life of the group. He also wisely noted that cohesion, while necessary and desirable, is not always synonymous with a sense of comfort, nor is it always easy to establish. The adolescent substance abuse group is an example of a group in which establishing cohesion can be a monumental struggle.

Bratter (1989) vividly described establishing cohesion:

> Without exception, the first few sessions will be characterized by massive mistrust and alienation. A countertherapeutic climate will prevail until the leader decides to confront deliberate deceit and demand honesty. Addicted and alienated adolescents are both dishonest and manipulative. These adolescents trust no one because they fear being hurt. (pp. 168–169)

Some of the suggestions of Riester (1993) concerning adolescent groups in general are particularly helpful for the leader charged with the task of maintaining group stability and developing some sense of group cohesiveness in groups composed of adolescents with drug abuse problems. Riester emphasized matching group structure to "the developmental level of the patients in the group" (p. 223). This matching helps facilitate the use of homogeneous factors in the group to develop a sense of peer similarities and eventual peer support, leading to group cohesion. Riester's emphasis on matching group structure in a way that is "congruent with the developmental level of the patients in the group" helps facilitate the use of homogeneous factors in the group to develop a sense of peer similarities and eventual peer support, leading to group cohesion.

Similarly, Riester issued the caveat that "the unwanteds will press the therapist to reject the group and thereby confirm their negative self-image while recreating a familiar emotional encounter with authority figures" (p. 228). Therefore, group leaders must be understanding about many early resistances to group in general and, as a corollary, to cohesion itself. The varied forms this resistance may take in adolescent substance abuse groups include relentless testing of the leader; requests for therapist self-disclosure, especially surrounding the issue of the leader's own personal experiences with drugs; a variety of verbal and nonverbal acting-out behaviors; and being provocative in an effort to sabotage the leader and the group.

Because the group process is dynamic over time, the leader can expect retreats from a cohesive state even after it has been established.

The drug-addicted adolescent's tendency to regress, to be wary of parental figures, and to be interpersonally insecure with peers all contribute to a fluctuating sense of group solidarity.

# ◆ Phase 4: The Middle or Working Stage of the Group

Although group cohesion is necessary, it is not sufficient unto itself. According to the original concept of Yalom (1985), cohesion is a necessary precondition for change rather than the sole goal of a therapeutic group experience. Perhaps more to the point with adolescents is the issue of the leader's ability to take charge of the group experience and exercise control over the sequencing of group interventions. Using this model, the leader would initially aim for cohesion to pave the way for the next major therapeutic thrust—the management of confrontation.

Cohesion, or peer support, can be viewed as a cushion or buffer against the potential impact on group members of confrontation by the therapist. Confrontation of members by the leader is a hallmark of the middle or working stage of adolescent substance abuse groups. Much has been written about the appropriate use of confrontation when working with adolescents. The group therapist has to be clear on the goal, form, and timing of a group or individual confrontation. A rule of thumb for confrontation in substance abuse groups with adults (Spitz 1987) is that before a leader confronts a member he or she should be sure that the confrontation is conscious, voluntary, and designed to achieve a specific result, usually in the here and now.

Careful attention to the use of confrontation helps safeguard against other occupational hazards frequently present when working with teenagers who abuse drugs. Countertransferential anger or rage masquerading as "authenticity" or some other euphemism for the therapist's inappropriate use of confrontation not only confuses adolescents but contributes to the perpetuation of many damaging experiences they have already been subjected to in their families.

Rachman and Raubolt (1985) addressed the subject of confrontation in adolescent substance abuse groups in an in-depth and thoughtful manner. These authors described a confrontational style called the "caring confrontation." This consists of the therapist being simultaneously "tough and tender" by "direct confrontation of the substance abuser in an empathic atmosphere of genuine concern, compassion and caring" (p. 368). Excessive use of negative confrontation—as in the form of a caricature of an old group meeting at Synanon (a therapeutic community of drug abusers only)—leads to "an increase in tension, anger, hostility, and resentment, to the exclusion of positive feelings, empathy, concern, or caring" (p. 367).

The middle stage of adolescent drug abuse groups is the longest of the stages of group development. During this stage, goals other than achieving a drug-free existence are in evidence. When an adolescent drug abuse group is well along in a working phase, some recognizable themes should emerge. Examples of these themes are age-related concerns, including family problems, peer relationships, issues related to power and the abuse of power, competition, concerns about aspects of identity and sexuality, and school or work difficulties. Drug-related topics such as acquiring self-monitoring techniques, developing problem-solving skills, managing painful emotional states (most notably, anger, depression, and anxiety) without resorting to drug use as self-medication, and developing a drug-free social network are also prominent at this period in the group.

## ◆ Phase 5: Transition out of the Group

The two major tasks of the final phase of the group are separating from the group and solidifying a plan for relapse prevention. Members who are ready to leave the group are encouraged to review their experience. This review consolidates their own accomplishments and, by a process of peer identification, instills a sense of realistic hopefulness in the remaining group members. Group feelings can be intense during this phase; teenagers who remain in the group may feel envious or demoralized. The leader can genuinely counter the negative effects of a member's departure by using the departure to deal with unresolved issues of loss and separation and by reminding group members how they have played a key role in helping one of their peers attain a level of success. This may be the first opportunity many drug-abusing adolescents have ever had to experience their positive interpersonal impact on someone and to gain an understanding of the benefits of sharing, collaborating, and altruism.

Concrete plans for aftercare and extramural contact with group members are also regularly discussed at this juncture. On occasion, a party or ritual of some sort to mark the end of someone's group membership may be used as a catalyst for mobilizing feelings in the remaining group members that will become the subject matter for future sessions.

## ◆ Additional Treatment Issues

As is the case with all specialized groups, traditional technique must be reassessed in light of its value for the group in question. Certain clinical choices have particular significance when the group is composed of adolescents with drug issues. In conceptualizing and constructing the group, some leadership decisions come up for review. With adolescents, the choice of whether to work alone or in cotherapy is emblematic of the types of considerations facing group leaders.

The case favoring cotherapy with male and female group leaders rests largely on providing a substitute parental pair, which will undoubtedly stimulate emergence of family issues in the group. Those who advocate cotherapy for adolescents who abuse substances believe that the greater opportunities for role modeling a collaborative relationship between adults, handling differences respectfully, sharing the work load, and monitoring potential countertransferential pitfalls far outweigh the usual objections raised about excessive expenditure of staff time and cost inefficiency.

Proponents of the male-female leadership team state that the presence of such a team can lower the dropout rate in adolescent substance abuse groups. Mintz (1963) suggested that when a group member has anxiety in relationship to a parent of one sex, he or she is likely to flee from group if there is only one therapist and that therapist is the same sex as the parent. However, if there are male and female therapists, the member can lean on the less feared therapist, whose active and supportive role thereby enables the member to stay in group during times of high anxiety instead of dropping out.

The question of family involvement in treatment planning takes on special significance when working with addicted adolescents. How to recruit and incorporate the family of the addicted adolescent is always a clinical priority. Family therapists, especially those who approach families from a general systems point of view, take the position that adolescent drug abuse is a symptom of family dysfunction and that most, if not all, families in which there is an addicted adolescent should be seen in family therapy. At times, the group experience occurs simultaneously with the family therapy and aims primarily at peer issues and themes other than familial ones.

There is, however, a large interest in group therapy circles in the use of the multiple family group as another effective modality; it includes both the identified patient in each family and his or her family. Tucker and Maxmen (1975) first delineated the great potential advantages inherent in the multiple family group model.

The advantages listed by Tucker and Maxmen included deisolation, socialization, support, imparting information, catharsis, problem solving, promoting therapeutic competence in family members, instilling a sense of hopefulness, patient support, interfamily learning, and facilitation of group therapy. Multiple family therapy also is a rich source of data.

Kaufman (1985) echoed this enthusiasm and applied multiple family group therapy to the treatment of alcoholic and drug-abusing patients, citing the advantage such groups offer for "the integration of other family members who have a role in perpetuating the substance abusing system as well as the power to change the system" (p. 174). These groups always contain a large psychoeducational component; thus, they provide a nonthreatening way of teaching families with a chemically dependent member about the relationship between family factors and drug abuse. The groups allow identification of codependency; enabling behaviors; excessive use of denial defenses; dysfunctional family patterns of enmeshment, rigidity, scapegoating, coercion, and guilt induction; and the detouring of parental-marital tensions by focusing on an addicted child. Alternative, more adaptive behavioral solutions are sought in the group as families and therapists pool their resources and experiences.

Another benefit derived from multiple family groups is the ability to "fill in" single-parent families with sorely needed support elements generated by these groups, which can be large (15–20 members). Cross-family learning, in which one member or one family sees itself mirrored in the actions of another, is a powerful experiential learning process that regularly transpires in the multiple family group.

Family groups also serve as a reservoir of information and advice for their membership. Those who could benefit from a 12-step program are encouraged to join Alcoholics Anonymous, Al-Anon, Nar-Anon, and the fellowship programs created specifically for adolescents and young adults.

Because multiple family groups are big, there are at least two leaders. Sometimes a small team will lead a particularly large or network-like multiple family group. Each staff member on the team must clearly understand his or her designated role and function in the group to minimize confusion among the members and also to avoid the tendency for staff members to get into competitive or overlapping roles. When role definitions among staff members are clear, troublesome issues common to substance-abusing families, like interpersonal and intergenerational boundary blurring, are helped considerably.

Like homogeneous adolescent drug abuse groups, multiple family groups try to strike a balance between strong supportiveness and appropriate confrontation of members—not only by leaders but also by the members themselves. Theme-oriented meetings are another popular format for the multiple family group. This format serves the dual purpose of 1) facilitating group members' participation and 2) helping families whose equilibrium has been affected by addiction to strengthen healthy identifications through group interaction around shared life experiences—that is, the group leaders can model clear and open communication in their relationships as a model for family members to use in their own discussions at home.

## ◆ Is Group Therapy the Treatment of Choice for Addicted Adolescents?

The enthusiasm for group therapy shown by many workers in the field raises the question of why groups are believed to be essential, if not the definitive therapeutic approach for chemically dependent adolescents. Raubolt and Bratter (1974) presented a compelling argument for group therapy as "the treatment of choice for adolescent drug abusers." Their argument is based on six factors:

> (1) Peer group relationships, so central to adolescent development, are mirrored in group experiences. (2) Adolescents often accept peer groups as therapy experiences in preference to being seen alone or with their families. (3) The social elements present in groups blend with age-related social concerns shared by adolescents. (4) Groups provide clinicians with "therapeutic leverage" necessary to promote change, set limits, help test reality, and confront problematic behavior. (5) Groups assist greatly in the consolidation of adolescent ego identity through the evolution of individual and group identifications made through relationships that originate in the group. (6) Groups provide a place where experimentation is encouraged, thereby permitting constructive use of fantasy, the expression of emotion, creativity, and the development of alternatives to self-defeating, drug-taking behavior. (p. 56)

Perhaps the salient point is not that group therapy is superior to other therapies. Rather, the key question is what collaborative role group therapy can play in the comprehensive approach to the notoriously complex clinical dilemma of adolescent substance abuse. The broad applicability of group therapy and its ability to facilitate combinations of different techniques and therapeutic points of view make group an ideal template for the creation of eclectic and innovative treatment models for chemically dependent adolescents and their families.

## ◆ Summary

Whether the venue in which an adolescent substance abuse group meets is an inpatient ward, a halfway house, or an outpatient setting, the group therapist must be active and sincere about his/her interest in helping adolescent drug abusers. He or she must carefully select adolescents who can tolerate and benefit from group pressure and confrontation in a supportive group milieu. Teenagers who have coexisting major psychiatric illness are usually inappropriate candidates for the groups that emphasize high degrees of confrontation and pressure.

Not only the treatment potential but also the preventive benefits of group membership have been explored. Educative approaches involving either just adolescents or adolescents and their "significant others" are proliferating as part of preventive drug abuse programs.

More formal research is needed to clarify the advantageous and deleterious elements in the composition, leadership style, and inherent properties of groups themselves. However, there is much to suggest that group therapy will continue to enjoy a position of prominence in the field of substance abuse in general and that is has superb qualities that specifically relate to the problems presented by adolescents at risk for addiction.

# ◆ References

Bratter TE: Group psychotherapy with alcohol and drug addicted adolescents: special clinical concerns and challenges, in Adolescent Group Psychotherapy. Edited by Azima FJ Cramer, Richmond LH. Madison, CT, International Universities Press, 1989, pp 163–189

Dusenbury L, Khuri E, Millman RB: Adolescent substance abuse: a sociodevelopmental perspective, in Substance Abuse: A Comprehensive Textbook, 2nd Edition. Edited by Lowinson JH, Ruiz P, Millman RB. Baltimore, MD, Williams & Wilkins, 1992, pp 832–842

Kaufman E: Multiple family therapy and couples groups, in Substance Abuse and Family Therapy. Orlando, FL, Grune & Stratton, 1985, pp 173–192

Mintz E: Special value of co-therapy in group psychotherapy. Int J Group Psychother 15:127–132, 1963

Piper WE, Debanne EG, Bienvenu JP: A study of group pre-training for group psychotherapy. Int J Group Psychother 32:309–325, 1982

Rachman AW, Raubolt RR: The clinical practice of group psychotherapy with adolescent substance abusers, in Alcoholism and Substance Abuse: Strategies for Clinical Intervention. Edited by Bratter TE, Forrest CG. New York, The Free Press, 1985, pp 349–375

Raubolt RR, Bratter TE: Games addicts play: implications for group treatment. Corrective Social Psychiatry 20:3–10,1974

Riester AE: Creating the adolescent group psychotherapy experience, in Group Therapy in Clinical Practice. Edited by Alonso A, Swiller HI. Washington, DC, American Psychiatric Press, 1993, pp 219–236

Robins LN, Pryzbek TR: Age of onset of drug use as a factor in drug and other disorders, in Etiology of Drug Use: Implications for Prevention (NIDA Research Monograph No 56). Edited by Jones CL, Battjes RJ. Washington, DC, U.S. Government Printing Office, 1985, pp 85–135

Semlitz L, Gold MS: Adolescent drug abuse: diagnosis, treatment and prevention. Psychiatr Clin North Am 9:455–473, 1986

Spitz HI: Cocaine abuse: therapeutic group approaches, in Cocaine Abuse: New Directions in Treatment and Research Edited by Spitz HI, Rosecan JS. New York, Brunner/Mazel, 1987, pp 156–201

Tucker GJ, Maxmen JS: Multiple family group therapy in a psychiatric hospital. Journal of Psychoanalysis in Groups 27:34–43, 1975

Yalom ID: The Theory and Practice of Group Psychotherapy, 3rd Edition. New York, Basic Books, 1985

# CHAPTER 16

# Adolescents Who Have Eating Disorders

*Ellyn Shander, M.D., and*
*Sheila A. Orbanic, R.N., M.S.*

W ith burgeoning health care costs, mandated utilization review, and increasing pressure on financial resources available for health care, the treatment provider has a compelling obligation to consider the efficient allocation of resources. Considerations include the modality of the prescribed treatment and the likely benefits. Clinicians are required to seek out and use the most cost-effective therapy. Minimally effective care at significant cost is neither in the patient's best interest nor in the best interest of third-party providers. It has been our experience that group psychotherapy is an essential, efficient, and cost-effective intervention for the treatment of patients with eating disorders.

Active, goal-oriented group therapy stimulates feelings and responses in the individual, precipitating introspection and involvement seldom attained under other conditions. Participants in group are able to get a sense of other patients' life experiences. Shared experience sets the stage for future endeavors undertaken in individual and group therapy. As therapy progresses, relationships strengthen, and a common purpose and relatedness unfold within the group.

Mutual empathy emerges as a result of group members sharing experiences, strengthening the foundation of group work. The individuals learn to be self-reflective, gain insight, receive and offer criticisms, articulate feelings, and reinforce healthy coping skills.

Many patients with eating disorders use *intellectualization* as a defense mechanism to avoid experiencing core feelings. In group, we urge participants to speak from their gut and heart, not from their heads. This expression of raw emotion establishes a therapeutic arena where patients can practice tolerating uncomfortable feelings without fleeing. Group therapy also requires that each member listen and give feedback to her peers, thereby building communication skills while reinforcing group cohesion.[1] This process is difficult for patients with narcissistic personality traits, but encouraging active group participation can still be helpful.

This chapter not only synopsizes the commonalities among patients with eating disorders—their symptoms, personalities, communication styles, and family dynamics—but also provides an outline of specific group therapy techniques. We have found that these techniques and exercises effect positive behavioral change and challenge the numerous cognitive distortions harbored by most patients with eating disorders.

Specific criteria for eating disorder diagnoses can be found in DSM-IV (American Psychiatric Association 1994). In addition to anorexia nervosa and bulimia nervosa, DSM-IV (American Psychiatric Association 1994) contains research criteria for diagnosis of compulsive overeating (binge-eating disorder). A review of the diagnostic criteria in DSM-IV is useful in the context of this chapter.

## ◆ Part 1: The Person Behind the Criteria . . . The Feelings Behind the Behaviors

Emotions shape our actions, perceptions, and mind-set, creating our human experience. Healthy relationships are enhanced by putting

---

[1] The terms *she, her, and herself* are used in this chapter because our typical group member was female.

feelings into words. Children learn to express feelings through experiencing and interacting with their environment and by imitating family members who demonstrate and encourage the healthy expression of emotions. Ideally, children acquire the social skills and judgment necessary to cope with life stressors.

Adolescents with eating disorders, however, have significant difficulty in spontaneously recognizing and freely expressing a full range of emotions. They have not learned to express, have not been encouraged to express, or lack the self-esteem to express their feelings. Patients worry that their feelings will be uncontrollable, so feelings are denied.

It is not uncommon to hear a group member say, "I don't feel anything" or "I never think about how I feel. I'm dead inside." A group member who does express her own feelings frequently experiences guilt and accuses herself of being selfish. Guilt feelings can create and perpetuate the self-destructive cycles of starving, bingeing, and purging, which the teenager feels powerless to stop. Group therapy becomes a powerful ally in an arduous battle between the adolescent's normal developmental journey toward self-actualization and the destructive forces of enmeshed relationships, perceived helplessness, and perpetual childhood.

Adolescents with eating disorders, like most teenagers, are flooded with hormonal and developmental changes, as well as societal and peer pressures. They are emotionally unequipped to handle the onslaught of feelings and developmental changes and grow increasingly frightened. As their sense of helplessness grows, they desperately search for some control and stability in their lives. Unable to verbalize their internal fears, they learn to control an external entity—food.

To summarize, patients with eating disorders, whether they are bingers, restrictors, purgers, laxative abusers, or compulsive overeaters, use eating behaviors to *neutralize* overwhelming feelings. These troubled adolescents feel powerless in their lives and believe that what they say is valueless. As their weight drops or increases, they feel a false sense of power and control. Soon, the cycle of starving and bingeing takes hold and monopolizes teenagers' time and thoughts. In this manner, they no longer face societal or peer pressure and are too preoccupied with their eating behaviors to think about how they feel.

Often, an adolescent with an eating disorder is the distress signal for a dysfunctional family system. Such a family often discourages individuality by disrespecting personal boundaries and discounting the adolescent's opinions and feelings. Love is not experienced as unconditional, but rather as something that is earned through top grades or remarkable athletic performances. Many of these parents convey the importance of physical appearance and maintaining "the perfect image."

The anorexic adolescent and, often, her family present a re-stricted, rigid affect, rarely displaying genuine, spontaneous emotion. The teenager's restricted affect parallels her self-imposed starvation. The untreated anorexic patient emphatically defends her own happi-ness, denying the existence of personal or familial stressors. Ironically, her emaciated physique betrays her artificial happiness and broadcasts her unspoken, emotional turmoil.

In contrast, bulimic individuals and their families are typically more volatile and affect laden. Bulimic patients frequently report feeling frustrated and angry, but verbalizing these feelings is followed by remorse and guilt. Bulimic adolescents use concealed, frenzied binges and exhaustive vomiting to dampen and restrict their turbulent affects.

An eating disorder can stem from a variety of physically and emo-tionally painful experiences. Issues involving alcoholism, unresolved grief, molestation, incest, physical abuse, or emotional abuse often lie below a thin layer of "emotional ice." In group, we see plastic smiles and mechanical statements camouflaging desires for self-validation, individu-ality, mutual respect, and unconditional love. As group members share similar family experiences, group becomes a powerful place to feel safe.

## ◆ Part 2: Techniques of Group Therapy

A creative and active style is necessary in leading an eating-disorders group. Passive leadership or a nonconfronting style allows individual and group distortions in thinking and behaviors to go unchallenged. A provocative therapeutic approach is necessary to prevent inappropriate behaviors from remaining hidden and unarticulated or, worse, validated by silence.

We use varied techniques to effect change in the following problem areas: cognitive distortions, affect intolerance, inability to problem solve, poor communication skills, and deficits in self-sufficiency.

## Cognitive Distortions

Patients frequently display cognitive distortions in group therapy that provide important substance for the therapeutic process. The group leader should point out such distortions and encourage the group to participate in examining these behaviors. This process allows the group to reflect on their own thought distortions. The process of improving self-awareness and mastery is thereby advanced.

Some cognitive distortions are presented below:

**Overgeneralization.** Patients with eating disorders tend to negatively overgeneralize their potential. They live in fear of taking risks. Failure would prove to them that they are losers and confirm their perception of a never-ending pattern of defeat.

*Example:* Such a patient might say, "I'll never be able to go to college because I'm so stupid."

*Intervention 1:* Ask each group member to discuss one event in her life when she took a risk and was proud of her actions. This exercise helps group members to see that they can be powerful and take risks successfully, even if the event was actually a small incident.

*Intervention 2:* Encourage discussion of things people have done previously that made them feel good about themselves. Press everyone to come up with her own personal scenario, and assist those with very negative opinions about themselves to participate positively.

**Labeling.** Patients with eating disorders usually label *who* they are based on *what* they weigh. They often believe others judge them using the same distorted thinking, based on their physical appearance.

*Examples:* Patients might make statements such as "There's no way I can go to school today, I'm so fat! Everyone will notice me" and "I weighed myself this morning! I feel great—I lost one-half pound!"

*Intervention:* Encourage discussions as to the absurdity of tying one's self-esteem to a number on the scale. Explain that when people use an arbitrary number such as weight to inflate self-esteem, it places them at risk for the *flag phenomenon:* When the wind blows, the flag looks great, but when there's no wind, it droops—flat and deflated.

Obviously, self-esteem that depends on weight, appearances, and outside opinions is very vulnerable. When other group members present similar behavior patterns, it is easier for a patient to understand this concept.

**Blaming.** Patients with eating disorders minimize and ignore their internal affect and discomfort while magnifying their difficulties with eating. All that is left looming in front of their eyes are huge plates of food they cannot eat, or food that beckons them to self-destruction. By displacing their feelings and anxieties onto their plates, they avoid real issues.

*Example:* Patients might say, "All my problems come from food."

*Intervention:* "It's not the food, it's the feelings!" This theme phrase is repeated any time food or food-related behaviors are mentioned during group. The phrase is also repeated as a reinforcement of the group rule: *We do not talk about food, we talk about feelings!* This repetition is done with the intention of continuously refocusing the group on the underlying feelings that fuel the food-related symptoms.

## Affect Intolerance

Alexithymia is the inability to identify emotions—a hallmark of patients with untreated eating disorders.

*Examples:* "I'm numb," "I have no feelings," and "I feel confused."

*Intervention:* Group therapy teaches patients how to identify their emotions and offers them skills to practice tolerating these new affective states. We couple a concrete visualization with the visceral experience of feelings. We ask group members to visualize a bell ringing whenever they notice that they are feeling sad, glad, happy, angry, and so forth. Then, we encourage them to report these emotional experiences in group.

Often, patients will confuse states of mind with true affective states.

For example, "I feel confused" reflects a state of mind, whereas "I feel fat" reflects a state of physical-biological being. When someone makes an "I feel" statement that is not an affective statement, it behooves the group leader and the other group members to point it out. Having identified various affects, we teach different options that can be used to respond to inner feeling states:

1. If the affect is very strong, the patient can decide to put it on a back burner and not respond to it immediately. We remind the patients that this is not an example of "stuffing" feelings, but containing the feelings until the patient chooses to deal with the feelings in a safe place, such as in individual therapy, with a friend, or in another group.

2. It is prudent to have a list of activities that group members can use for self-soothing or distraction. For example, loneliness can be assuaged by seeking out a friend, playing a tape, writing in a journal, or simply going out for a walk. We call these options *survival skills*. (See Table 16–1 for a list of survival skills.)

   In some groups, it can be useful to make a "survival bag"—a homemade fabric bag filled with written ideas of things to do when affective flooding occurs. Alternatively, each group member could be asked to fill a pocket-sized memo book with survival-skill suggestions. These items can function as concrete reminders to delay or thwart the use of eating-disorder behaviors to dilute affect.

3. "Move a muscle—change a mood" has its origins in Alcoholics Anonymous and refers to the power people can exercise over their own internal affective states by physically changing their situations. This concept is stressed in group.

4. Doing nothing but experiencing the affect and "riding the wave" is another alternative to dealing with some affective states. One can imagine that feelings are like waves—they get to the shore and are time limited. We ask patients to visualize being a surfer and riding their feeling waves, anticipating that their feelings will end on the shore.

In summary, group members need to learn to identify and tolerate affective states to offset the temptation to use automatic eating behaviors to neutralize feelings. The objective is to give group members a variety of new tools to deal effectively with their affect.

Often, a group member will say, "But I don't know what to do with my urge to binge [or urge to starve, take laxatives, vomit] when I'm upset." We recommend that despite any internal turmoil, "even when there are earthquakes, tornadoes, or volcanoes going off in your feeling place, you have to remain sober!" Of course, sobriety for each group member is abstaining from any eating-disorder behavior and following her meal plan.

**Table 16–1.**   Survival skills

- Remove yourself from the noxious environment.
- Use the phone to call someone. Verbalize those feelings!
- Visit a friend.
- Make a plan that you can put into action when things get intense:
    Take a bath.
    Do your nails.
    Take a walk.
    Go to the library.
    See a movie alone or with a friend.
    Do a puzzle.
- Ride out the "feeling wave." Keep in mind that the feelings will end.
- Express your feelings through another medium—for example, artwork, journal writing, or singing along to a favorite album.
- Go shopping within your budgetary limits.
- Exercise or dance—unless overexercising is a problem.
- Choose a confidant you can trust—someone who is a good listener (for example, a therapist).
- Don't berate yourself when you slip. Start fresh! Start over!
- Be good to yourself. Be your own best friend. Use positive self-talk.
- Meditate in a special place (e.g., nature).
- Look at something beautiful, peaceful, serene—or fun and exciting.
- Ask for a hug from a person—or get one from a stuffed animal.

## Inability to Problem Solve

Patients with eating disorders often have difficulties finding solutions to fairly routine dilemmas normally encountered in daily living. These difficulties stem from their tendency to exhibit concrete thinking, often stubborn and inflexible character styles, and a high incidence of learning disabilities. The cumulative outcome is a low frustration tolerance.

When these teenage patients approach situations that may require complex planning and decision processes, their anxiety increases as their self-esteem decreases. Adolescents with eating disorders have difficulty making college schedules, planning daily routines or activities, and—most apparently—deciding whether to meet their own needs or those of someone else. Many of these patients have had to make decisions and take risks within high-achieving families with critical parental figures.

*Example:* A typical statement is "I don't know what to do! I think I want to study art history, but I know my parents think I should study business. Who cares? I'll never graduate anyway. . . ."

*Intervention:* We use the group to model problem solving in a supportive atmosphere. As group members come to expect the group to be a place to troubleshoot their problems, they tend to spontaneously bring in personal life dilemmas. To facilitate this process, structured exercises with cards containing difficult life situations can also be passed out.

Here are examples of such a structured exercise: "Your friends ask you out for dinner; you want to be included in the group, but you're already counting calories in your mind and cannot bear to eat in front of them. What do you do?" Or: "Your stepmother invites you to her birthday party the day before your history exam. You don't want to go because of your anxiety about the exam, but your dad will be furious if you decline. What do you do?"

Often, if one group member has difficulty articulating a pattern of constructive actions, the group will be asked to brainstorm ideas. Group members are reminded that trying to achieve perfect solutions is unrealistic, but developing effective problem-solving techniques is achievable.

## Poor Communication Skills

Typically, patients with eating disorders have inadequate communication skills. They are rarely direct and fear rejection and revenge (Riebel 1989). These young women often are convinced that people should be able to read their minds. They have perfected the ability to anticipate the needs of emotionally erratic parents as a survival skill. Often these patients are overpolite, indirect, and unable to make their needs known. Built-up frustration and anger are then turned inward or are neutralized by an eating-disorder frenzy. The most common reason for a slip is an uncommunicated need or wish related to a significant person in these patients' lives. Left unresolved, this need or wish leaves the patients feeling victimized and helpless.

*Example:* A patient might say, "I'm in the hospital because I don't want to eat, I guess. The rest of the family is fine. Well, maybe my mom is overprotective. But I could never tell her . . . I'd hurt her feelings."

*Intervention:* A very powerful intervention in group is to ask if anyone has any "instant replays" she would like to present in group. The group member who volunteers presents a vignette of a situation that she wishes could have been handled differently. She explains the characters in detail, and the roles are assigned to other group members. It is useful for the presenting patient to play the adversary, mean parent, or selfish friend. Meanwhile, the other players model the affect they feel the situation merits. The group leader can direct the scenario as little or as much as he or she feels is justified to enhance the learning experience. After each dramatization, the group critiques the performance and describes the assertive techniques that were implemented.

The final part of the exercise involves the presenting patient playing herself and using the newly acquired assertiveness techniques to confront the adversary in her scenario. Our goal is to foster the insight and self-esteem that enable patients to use the skills and confidence gained during group in home, school, or work situations.

### Assertiveness Techniques

**Broken record.** The broken-record technique refers to repeating the same phrases in a conversation despite escalating emotion during the course of the discussion. For example, "You're not listening to me. I understand that you want me to go to Uncle Bob's for Thanksgiving, but I don't feel comfortable there and I'm not going." The patient is told to repeat the same phrase three or four times to the person she is talking to, without getting louder and more excited. She may then choose to remove herself from the encounter altogether with a statement such as "You're not able to hear me right now, so I'm going for a walk."

**The formula.** Patients are taught to rely on "the formula" whenever they feel perplexed by stressful situations and can't put their feelings into words. It is a reliable technique that can be used not only in group but also in real-life scenarios. The formula is as follows: "I feel [blank] when you do [blank], so please don't do that!" For example, "I feel worthless when you pick on my friends, so please don't do that!"

## Deficits in Self-Sufficiency

Patients with eating disorders are notoriously poor at self-soothing and self-monitoring skills in stressful situations. Lack of these skills is precisely what has led them to self-soothe with primitive bingeing or restriction of food.

*Example:* A patient who lacks these skills might say, "My friends aren't home, my parents are arguing and I've got a math test tomorrow. I can't deal with this! I'm not eating dinner tonight . . . maybe I can at least lose another pound!"

*Intervention:* We teach "good mommy skills." Ask the patients to imagine what a good mommy would do or say in various situations when soothing a small child. In their role as a good mommy, patients are asked to take their inner child for a walk as they repeat self-soothing phrases like "You deserve to treat yourself well because you're a good person, and I like you" and "Everyone makes mistakes—you can try again!" This skill is termed *self-talk* and is especially useful when patients are overgeneralizing negative life experiences or characteristics. (See Table 16–2 for other self-talk phrases.)

Another tool that enhances self-inquiry is a prepared, written form given out to the group. It lists questions that are to be answered at the end of the day to check for daily self-sufficiency. Below are some examples:

1. Did I stuff my feelings today during a situation when I could have been more assertive? What was the scenario when I did that? What happened? What could I have done differently? (The scenario could also be used as an instant replay in the next group.)
2. Did I follow my meal plan today? Was I good to myself and did I give myself the fuel I need to live healthily?
3. Did I act like a victim today? How will I avoid this behavior tomorrow?

This self-awareness is crucial for the development of the self-soothing and self-regulation that this patient population so desperately needs.

In summary, patients with eating disorders are plagued with cognitive distortions, affect intolerance, and difficulties with problem solving. They frequently lack adequate communication skills and are deficient in ego strengths. Group therapy is an influential and effective therapeutic vehicle for changing behavior in these young women. This process accelerates individual behavioral changes. The goal is to

**Table 16–2.**   Positive self-talk messages

- I'm not going to vomit [starve, binge]. I'm going to face my feelings!
- I'm worth it! I deserve to be healthy!
- I deserve to take care of myself!
- I come first. I'm not going to put others before me!
- Hang in there kid, it's going to be OK!
- I'm allowed to eat. I need energy to deal with my feelings!
- I give myself permission to eat, even if my "sick side" doesn't want to.
- If I can do it tomorrow, I will do it today!
- Even if I feel awful now, I must stick to my meal plan and eat three meals!
- I can do it no matter what anyone else says. I will conquer this!
- I have to eat to live! There's always hope and things can get better!

turn a previously ego-syntonic symptom into a foreign pattern, which over time becomes awkward and uncomfortable. These patients can change their eating behaviors as they begin to talk about and tolerate very painful feelings.

This type of group requires an active and evocative group leader who readily challenges patterns of dysfunction (Hornyak 1989) and takes an active role in reshaping responses to difficult life situations. It can be a moving, rewarding, exhilarating, and exhausting experience for both the patients and the therapist!

## ◆ Conclusion

When evaluating patients with eating disorders, the therapist must

1. Identify what the symptom is "solving" for the patient.
2. Convince the patient of the validity of the therapist's observations by presenting hypotheses in an active and empathic manner.
3. Help build alternative ego skills to help patients develop affect tolerance until they can self-regulate their feelings.
4. Use principles from Alcoholics Anonymous to promote the idea that every slip (i.e., binge, purge, starvation, laxative or diuretic abuse) is an attempt to neutralize feelings. Patients must figure out what precipitated the slip so they can be empowered to commit themselves to sobriety again.
5. Work on behavioral changes while constantly connecting patients to their underlying emotional needs.
6. Try to keep the situation in perspective. These patients often frustrate therapists because the rate of behavioral change is slow. Remember, if you are addressing their underlying life problems, most patients will recover. It simply takes time, creativity, and patience.

# ◆ References

American Psychiatric Association: Diagnostic and Statistical Manual of Mental Disorders, 3rd Edition, Revised. Washington, DC, American Psychiatric Association, 1987

American Psychiatric Association: Diagnostic and Statistical Manual of Mental Disorders, 4th Edition. Washington, DC, American Psychiatric Association, 1994

Hornyak L: Experiential Therapies for Eating Disorders. New York, Guilford, 1989

Riebel LK: Communication skills for eating-disordered clients. Psychotherapy 26:69–74, 1989

# CHAPTER 17

# Suicidal Adolescents

## Don R. Heacock, M.D.

Although there has been a threefold increase in adolescent suicide in the past 20 years, and despite the fact that suicide is the third leading cause of death in adolescents, group psychotherapy for suicidal adolescents remains underused and is seldom written up in the literature. Berman and Jobes (1991), Pfeffer (1986) and Sudak et al. (1984), leading researchers and authors in the area of suicide in children and adolescents, devoted less than one page in their books to the use of groups with suicidal children and adolescents. Other authors have given even less space to this type of therapy. The reasons for this underrepresentation in the literature are complex, but they probably have much to do with the fact that group therapy itself has generally been considered a secondary or adjunctive therapy compared with individual and other therapies. Also, many therapists working in this area have the erroneous impression that group therapy with suicidal adolescents can cause contagion or spread of suicidal behavior. These myths, added to the usual difficulty in treating adolescents, probably account for the underuse of group therapy with suicidal adolescents.

In contrast, Ross and Motto (1984) and Scheidlinger and Aronson (1992) are strong advocates of group therapy for suicidal adolescents. Scheidlinger believes that group therapy is the treatment of choice for these patients because they are intensely peer oriented.

Scheidlinger and Aronson (1992) also suggested that one should play down the suicidal and even therapeutic aspects of the group with the adolescents themselves and instead should emphasize that they are attending a "rap" group for general discussions. Although this suggestion makes good sense with adolescents, we at the Lincoln Medical and Mental Health Center have found that a very powerful icebreaker and supportive factor is to tell each patient that the others in the group have also made suicide attempts. This immediately establishes a bond among the patients and promotes the concept of universalization—so important in group psychotherapy.

Ross and Motto (1984) sounded the caveat that in treating these patients a good backup hospital or emergency room is important. I wholeheartedly endorse this assertion—particularly with high-risk suicidal adolescents.

We have successfully used group therapy with suicidal adolescents in the Child/Adolescent Outpatient Psychiatric Service of the Lincoln Medical and Mental Health Center, a large municipal hospital in the South Bronx (with a mainly Hispanic and black inner-city catchment area population). The Langley Porter and San Mateo programs in California have also effectively used group therapy with suicidal adolescents.

# ◆ Types of Therapy

## Outpatient Versus Inpatient Groups

Outpatient group psychotherapy with suicidal adolescents has some uses and goals that are different from those of inpatient group psychotherapy. This chapter's central focus is outpatient groups, but inpatient group therapy with suicidal adolescents is also very important. As part of the regular treatment regimen of suicidal adolescents in a hospital setting, group therapy adds much to the healing process. Ward rules and regulations, concerns about confinement, separation from friends and family, and living in close proximity to other more seriously ill patients make inpatient treatment more difficult for the patient. On the other hand, the fact that one has a captive audience allows better group attendance and easier accessibility to patients and family. Inpatient groups have the same internal dynamics as outpatient groups, with the considerations just mentioned. Key differences between inpatient and outpatient adolescent groups were described by Heacock (1980).

## Group Therapy in the School Setting

A very promising approach that lies somewhere between inpatient and outpatient group therapy is group therapy at school. I have had experience in a local high school where groups have been effective. Groups of adolescents with varying degrees of suicidal and homicidal ideation responded well to therapy done during the school day. The captive-audience concept ensured the contact with patients, yet the stigma (for the adolescents) of hospitalization was avoided. Problems of logistics and absenteeism were minimized also. Rewards in the form of academic credits, food (pizza), and even cash were added inducements to maintain interest in treatment.

## Individual Therapy Concomitant
## With Group Therapy

All adolescents who have made serious suicide attempts should be offered group psychotherapy, despite the observation that less than one-third of suicidal adolescent patients referred for therapy will follow-up.

Outpatient group therapy can be offered to all, but some simultaneous individual therapy is necessary. At the Lincoln Medical and Mental Health Center Adolescent Group Program, patients are given an appointment for individual therapy with one of the group cotherapists once every 4 weeks. Individual therapy is needed monthly because there are often things that the adolescent will not discuss in the group. Every effort, however, should be made to get the adolescent to discuss all problems in the group.

# ◆ Suitability for Group Therapy

## Screening of Patient

A self-screening technique is used at Lincoln Medical and Mental Health Center in the sense that patients who miss two or more sessions and then fail to respond to follow-up letters or even to Mobile Crisis Team visits are referred for follow-up to Special Services for Children. Patients who specifically request individual therapy and who cannot be persuaded to try group are offered only individual therapy.

## Indications and Contraindications for Group Therapy of Suicidal Adolescents

If the patient has a social hunger (a desire to be a part of a community of peers), this is a strong indicator for group therapy. The patient also must be able to relinquish some of his or her own needs temporarily to benefit from group therapy—needs such as the desire to talk about themselves and their own problems whenever they wish.

The majority of suicidal adolescents fall into this category, but a few do not. Contraindications to group therapy for this adolescent population are extreme depression, severe impulsivity, destructive acting out, and ostentatious homosexuality. Severely addicted or overtly psychotic teens also do not do well in groups. The markedly different aspect of their pathology compared with that of the group as a whole makes treatment difficult. Slavson (1950) said that patients must be grouped on the basis of similarity of syndromes rather than similarity of symptoms. Even though suicidality is a powerful common symptom, *severely* paranoid or psychotic suicide patients are better treated in individual therapy.

We did not find the cluster effect—the contagious quality of suicidal behavior in susceptible adolescents (see Shaffer and Gould 1987)—to be a significant factor in our high-risk suicidal adolescent patients. Scheidlinger and Aronson (1992) also found that actual suicide attempts by members while in a therapy group did not present unmanageable problems to the therapist when discussed rationally in therapy sessions.

## Use of Assessment Instruments

Many useful assessment instruments are available now in the field. At the Lincoln Medical and Mental Health Center, Child/Adolescent Outpatient Psychiatric Service, we use the "Evaluation of Imminent Danger for Suicide" instrument, developed at the Division of Child Psychiatry, Columbia University, by Rotheram-Borus and Bradley (1990). Results of this test can indicate whether an adolescent is in "potential imminent danger." In the Lincoln Medical and Mental Health Center Child/Adolescent Outpatient Psychiatric Service, we use this assessment instrument every 6 months. We also rely on the clinical judgment of the cotherapists to determine whether suicidal patients are improving or worsening. Each suicidal adolescent is followed closely with the help of this instrument. The patient's specific answers to questions are particularly helpful in following the progression or resolution of problems. When there are indications of very high or increasing risk, hospitalization has to be considered.

Shaffer, one of the leading researchers in the field of adolescent suicide, stressed (Shaffer and Gould 1987) the importance of a clear definition of the patient population, sensitive measures for change, and good operation techniques in research. The instrument mentioned above and many others now in use are an important beginning in doing research in the area of adolescent group therapy.

## ◆ Phases of the Group

Most adolescent therapy groups go through three phases: a beginning, a middle, and an end phase. The beginning phase starts at the first meeting after the screening sessions. In the first session, the leader(s) put the patients at ease and explain the nature of the group and the group rules and regulations. Adolescents are initially shy, mistrustful, and not talkative. They look to the leader(s)—not to each other—at first. The leader(s) must explain that the patients should say what comes to mind, but it is especially important for them to talk about troubles, worries, problems, and particularly feelings such as anger, depression, and mistrust. The patients are asked to put impulses into words, not into actions. They should also be punctual and keep confidential whatever is discussed in the group. Associating outside the group is discouraged because it dilutes the push to talk about problems in the group itself and therefore can contribute to acting out.

The middle phase occurs when patients discuss their suicidal feelings, loss and grief, and family problems. Common themes for discussion are drugs, sex, parents, school, coping devices, and specific individual problems. With support by the therapist or cotherapist, the adolescents begin to look at and talk to each other—not to the therapists. They then feel free to attack the therapists or even each other verbally.

The last phase involves movement toward termination. This phase is especially hard for suicidal adolescents, who have issues of termination and separation at the core of their conflict. Time must be left for adequate discussion of these important issues, and provision must be made for supportive contact and help if a relapse occurs after the group therapy stops.

## ◆ Long-Term Versus Short-Term Groups

Suicidal adolescents often may respond to short-term therapy. Patients from lower socioeconomic groups also do well in short-term therapy.

Suicidal patients generally struggle mightily against their own and their families' denial of their suicidal intent. This denial probably occurs because of the sense of shame, failure, and incompetence that the family often feels at the idea of having a suicidal child. Adolescents are generally also negatively oriented to any form of psychotherapy. "I'm not crazy!" they say, and "What will my friends think of me?" Although patients have stayed for varying periods of time in group therapy, those who stay longest generally improve the most.

## ◆ Adjunctive Factors That Contribute to Successful Clinic-Based Group Therapy

### Use of the Mobile Crisis Team

At the Lincoln Medical and Mental Health Center, Child/Adolescent Outpatient Psychiatric Service, patients who remain at high risk for suicide (as determined by the clinical judgment of both cotherapists, parental assessment, and the "Evaluation of Suicide Risk Among Adolescents" instrument) are told that continued group therapy is essential. The hospital's Mobile Crisis Team is used to help maintain contact and to see that these patients come to therapy and take their medication if medication is ordered. The Mobile Crisis Team has given us another approach and an added dimension in our therapy with high-risk adolescents. Because of these patients' passivity and poor motivation due to the deadening effects of life in the inner city, we have found that close cooperation with an active and dynamic Mobile Crisis Team is essential for successful outpatient group therapy of suicidal adolescents. Individuals who are part of this team must be aggressive and positively oriented. A more detailed report on the use of the Mobile Crisis Team in outpatient therapy with children and adolescents is forthcoming.

## Parental Involvement

Parental involvement and participation are key factors in this form of therapy. Those adolescents who benefit most are those whose parents support the therapy. The parent(s) are seen in family sessions before starting therapy—preferably on the hospital unit or ward, if that is possible. Family therapy (initially and once every 3 months) has been found to be very helpful; however, frequently only one interested parent or family member will attend.

As in almost all child and adolescent work, a good relationship with the parent(s) and other family members helps therapy with the adolescent. However, building a good relationship is easier said than done in many cases, and herein lies the art and skill of the child and adolescent therapist. A poor relationship with a parent can mean the end of therapy with the adolescent. At the very least, the parent must be kept from sabotaging therapy.

## Medication

Another therapeutic adjunct to successful group therapy with suicidal adolescent patients is medication. Antidepressants such as desipramine, fluoxetine, and sertraline can be very helpful. Lithium carbonate, thioridazine, haloperidol, and hydroxyzine can make the difference between success and failure in therapy with adolescents.

## Cotherapy

One male and one female cotherapist, both experienced in work with suicidal adolescents, are the ideal leadership team for this type of therapy. They are the best choice for several reasons: 1) a family atmosphere is re-created, 2) the adult therapists act as role models for the patients, and 3) the patients see how mature adults discuss and settle differences while maintaining mutual respect and a continued working relationship. Cotherapists are also good because each can check the other's blind spots. If one is absent, the other is there to take the group. Additionally, the patients' hostility and anxiety are directed toward both therapists, rather than toward just one. Recording and numerous other group chores can also be shared. An important caveat, however, is that the working relationship in the group should be clear to both therapists. Is one therapist first between equals, or are they essentially both leaders with the same authority? This should be frankly and openly discussed, clarified, and worked through before cotherapists work together.

At Lincoln Medical and Mental Health Center, residents in adult psychiatry rotating through the Child/Adolescent Division are sometimes also allowed to be cotherapists. As they develop more ease and competence with this technique, their role changes from that of participant-observer to that of actively involved therapist. They learn much from the experience and also can contribute much. Residents are given orientation lectures and literature on adolescent group therapy and adolescent suicide before entering the group.

## ◆ Characteristics of the Best Patient Population and Grouping

### Gender Issues (The Coed Group)

Adolescent girls attempt suicide four to five times more often than adolescent boys. Consequently, many more girls than boys are available for this therapy. Boys complete suicide four to five times more often than girls; however, obviously and tragically, group therapy is feasible only with a living patient. It is still our feeling at the Lincoln Medical and Mental Health Center, Child/Adolescent Outpatient Psychiatric Service, that a mix of girls and boys would be better than all boys or all girls. Yet it is not easy to find boys for this type of therapy in a hospital clinic setting.

## Other Factors Relating to the Mix of Patients

A mix of factors other than the common one of suicidality is desirable for this type of group therapy. A range of diagnoses, ethnic groups, and educational and vocational interests can add to the therapy. However, the caveat as stated by Slavson (1950) above must be kept in mind: that the best mix is one where patients have a similarity of syndromes, or a similarity of their core dynamics.

## ◆ Description of the High-Risk Suicidal Adolescent Therapy Group at Lincoln Medical and Mental Health Center

Since September 1990, a high-risk suicidal adolescent outpatient group has existed in the Lincoln Medical and Mental Health Center, Child/Adolescent Outpatient Psychiatric Service. The principles described above are based largely on that group experience. The group consists of approximately eight girls and boys, mostly Hispanic, with some African American members. Most adolescents were referred for this weekly therapy group after a period of days on the pediatric ward, usually after an overdose of pills. Their suicide attempts were generally serious ones. Diagnoses were typically schizophrenia, conduct disorder, major depressive episode, and dysthymia. About one-third of the patients were given antidepressant medication, usually fluoxetine or desipramine. One was put on lithium. (The patient receiving lithium had a psychotic relapse, was hospitalized for 6 months, and then returned to the group—where she did well as long as she continued to take fluoxetine as prescribed [20–40 mg/day].)

At some time early in the patients' group experience, they are asked to share their suicide attempts in detail with the group members. So far, all have been willing to do this.

Since the start of the group, there have been no completed suicides, but two patients made another suicide attempt and were rehospitalized. When patients fail to come to two appointments, the Mobile Crisis Team gets sent to the home. This has had interesting ramifications. The patients called the Mobile Crisis Team worker "the truant officer." They railed against him, but the staff sensed that the patients felt more secure knowing that they would not be allowed to drop out with impunity—and that they were important enough to get followed up.

Some case examples from the program follow.

### Case Example 1

Three girls, Maria, Gina, and Maryetta, were hospitalized at the same time after suicide attempts. They had been acquainted on the outside via school contacts. While playing with a Ouija board game, one (a schizophrenic adolescent) got a message through the board to kill herself. She made a serious attempt, and later the others got the same "message" through the Ouija board; they also made attempts, were admitted to the hospital, and then were referred for group therapy. To date, one patient is out of therapy, one (the original schizophrenic girl) is still in the group, and one is in individual therapy.

### Case Example 2

Another patient, Lucia, who has a severe conduct disorder, tells stories of violence, death, and mayhem in her neighborhood at almost every session. She is a 16-year-old Hispanic girl who fits the image of the "gun moll" (or Bonnie, of the movie *Bonnie and Clyde*). She has sold crack and has used it herself at times, but denies using it now. She comes regularly to the sessions despite her severe sociopathic background. She appeared depressed for almost a year but improved when put on desipramine and later fluoxetine. She tearfully described the death of four boyfriends in drug-related gang shootouts. The group urged her to get out of her South Bronx neighborhood before she herself was killed, but she said she would never leave because "I love the street life." Three months before this writing, she began living with a 45-year-old man who appears to care for her. He bought her beautiful clothes, and she lived with him in his apartment in New Jersey. It appeared that she had given up on young boys her age because, she says, "they all get killed."

## Case Example 3

Another patient, Marita, a 17-year-old Hispanic girl, lives with her 10-year-old brother and her drug-selling mother in a housing project apartment. She described in the group how her mother had become enmeshed in the process of selling drugs (crack) to pay off loan sharks. She tells of her fear that other drug pushers will burst into her apartment one day to kill her mother because of some real or fancied conflict over the drugs the mother is selling. The group has tried to get this patient to take her little brother and move to a relative's house, report the mother to the police, or talk the mother into moving elsewhere and giving up the drugs. The patient is unable to act on any group suggestions and remains paralyzed in this frightening situation day after day.

## Case Example 4

Finally, there is Melia, an obese 18-year-old Hispanic girl, who rarely misses a session and has been coming for 2 years. She was accused of lesbianism by other group members because she constantly touched them as she talked. With the therapist's support, she told of her lesbian feelings and her suicide attempt, which occurred because her uncle raped her. As she told of her feelings in the group sessions, she stopped touching the other members, who all now accept her as a group member. She is still unable to lose weight but has graduated from high school and is now a freshman at New York University. She is doing well there and serves as an educational role model for the other group members, who all have various degrees of academic difficulty.

# ◆ The Future for Group Psychotherapy With Suicidal Adolescents

Because a large number of adolescents attempt suicide but a small number actually complete suicide, future group therapy with suicidal adolescent patients might well focus on 1) school-based preventive groups (including groups in junior high school) and 2) groups for high-risk adolescents whose suicidal behavior brings them to hospital emergency rooms. Among teenagers, serious suicidal behavior increases when they reach high school age, generally at age 15 years. Introducing group therapy with a focus on suicide before this time—for example, to junior high school students right in the schools themselves—would reach a great number of adolescents who would eventually be at high risk for suicide. Like others, we feel that the group focus should not be just on suicide but on mental health in general. However, the faculty and other staff who refer students to these mental health discussion groups held in their junior high and high schools need to have a keen sensitivity to suicide-related issues.

Finally, group therapy as described in this chapter should be available in all adolescent therapy clinics. These high-risk patients should be identified in the emergency rooms and or after admission to the wards of hospitals. Aggressive recruitment methods and meticulous follow-up, including use of the Mobile Crisis Teams, should be used to reduce the initial no-show rate after referral. Limited diagnostic and therapeutic family contact, individual sessions, and medication should be part of the basic group therapy approach.

Group psychotherapy with suicidal adolescents is an underused modality of treatment, yet some authorities believe it is the treatment of choice for these patients. Adolescents are naturals for therapy groups because of their intense peer orientation. These adolescent therapy groups can be time limited (6 months) or longer term (1–2 years), depending on the needs of the patient. Groups can also be open or closed. We at Lincoln Medical and Mental Health Center, Child/Adolescent Outpatient Psychiatric Service, favor the open-ended group, with patients' therapy individualized as to length of treatment. In short, it is hoped that this chapter makes it clear that group therapy for suicidal adolescents is alive and well.

# ◆ References

Berman AL, Jobes DA: The treatment of the suicidal adolescent, in Adolescent Suicide—Assessment and Intervention. Washington, DC, American Psychological Association, 1991, pp 181–182

Heacock DR: Therapeutic groups with hospitalized adolescents, in A Psychodynamic Approach to Adolescent Psychiatry: The Mt. Sinai Experience. Edited by Heacock DR. New York, Marcel Dekker, pp 291–304

Pfeffer CR: Adjunctive treatment modalities for suicidal children, in The Suicidal Child. New York, Guilford, 1986, pp 264–265

Ross CP, Motto JA: Group psychotherapy with suicidal adolescents, in Suicide in the Young. Edited by Sudak HS, Ford AB, Rushforth NB. Boston, MA, John Wright, 1984, pp 420–421

Rotheram-Borus MJ, Bradley J: Evaluation of Imminent Danger for Suicide. Tulsa, OK, National Resource Center for Youth Services, 1990

Scheidlinger S, Aronson H: Group psychotherapy with suicidal adolescents. Paper presented at the annual meeting of the American Psychiatric Association, Washington, DC, May 1992

Shaffer D, Gould M: A study of completed and attempted suicide in adolescents (Progress Report, Grant No MH 38198). Rockville, MD, National Institute of Mental Health, 1987

Slavson SR: Selection and grouping of patients, in Analytic Group Psychotherapy. New York, Columbia University Press, 1950, pp 240–242

Sudak HS, Ford AB, Rushforth NB: Suicide in the Young. Edited by Sudak HS, Ford AB, Rushforth NB. Boston, MA, John Wright, 1984

Trautman PD, Shaffer D: Treatment of child and adolescent suicide attempters, in Suicide in the Young. Edited by Sudak HS, Ford AB, Rushforth NB. Boston, MA, John Wright, 1984, p 313

# SECTION IV

# Groups in Broader Societal Context

CHAPTER 18

# Teen Line: A Listening Post for Troubled Youth

*Elaine Leader, Ph.D.*

Most adolescents who have some kind of personal problem rely primarily on their friends for help (Carr 1981; Prediger et al. 1974). Friendships are generally characterized by mutuality or a willingness to be helpers to each other. According to Carr (1981), many adolescents have the ability to be attentive and supportive, are sensitive to others, and can express thoughts and ideas in ways that do not threaten the esteem of others. They are, however, frequently drawn into giving advice. Nonetheless, research has demonstrated that the skills involved in effective helping can be learned by a variety of laypersons, including paraprofessionals (Carkuff 1969), high school students (Carr and Saunders 1979), and junior high and even elementary-age students (Bowman and Myrick 1980).

## ◆ The Growth of Peer Counseling

The past 20 years have seen an enormous increase in the proliferation of peer counseling programs. Most have arisen to address the need for mental health care, a need that far outweighs the services that the mental health profession can provide (Reguir et al. 1978). The combination of a rising need for counseling services, cutbacks in mental health funding, and shortages of professionals has resulted in parapro-fessionals being trained to meet this need. At the same time, self-help groups have mushroomed to address shared or common concerns, using support and catharsis as problem-solving interventions (Carr 1981). Similarly, school systems, swamped with demands for counsel-ing services that professionals are unable to meet, are rapidly develop-ing peer counseling programs. For example, the Peer Assistance Network of Texas reported that the number of school districts in the state with peer programs grew from 15 in 1987 to nearly 300 in 1992.

What constitutes peer counseling? According to D'Andrea and Salovey (1983, p. 3), peer counseling is both a method and a philoso-phy. Its goal is to promote personal growth and development through a helping relationship. Peer counselors help counselees clarify thoughts and feelings and explore various options and solutions, but they do not give advice. They are listeners, clarifiers, and information providers. They use active listening and problem-solving skills, along with knowledge about human growth and mental health, to counsel people who are peers—peers in age, status, and knowledge.

## ◆ Why Teen Line?

Telephone counseling has become a widely established means for providing crisis intervention since the development of the early sui-cide prevention services in the United States (Litman et al. 1965) and the Samaritan Movement in Britain (Central Office of Information 1978). These early community-based suicide prevention services, with their highly acclaimed hot lines, were followed by the establishment of college-based peer counseling services, some of which include both telephone and in-person programs (Hinrichsen and Zwibelman 1981). However, it was not until the 1980s that telephone counseling services targeted specifically for teenagers appeared. Even today, services staffed by teenagers are relatively rare. In an annotated and indexed bibliography of peer counseling publications (Carr 1992), only 3 of 750 entries from 1980 through 1992 describe teen-to-teen telephone counseling services, indicating the paucity of such services compared with school-based peer programs.

## ◆ What Is Teen Line?

A 17-year-old boy calls, saying he is depressed a lot. His brother died a year ago. The caller explains he has problems meeting people and making friends. He is currently hanging out with his cousins, who are in a gang.

A 14-year-old girl from Northern California calls, complaining that all her friends are drinking and doing drugs. She got in a fight with a certain friend because of that friend's drinking. She doesn't agree with her friends doing drugs and drinking, but she doesn't know how to handle it.

These are just two examples of the 1,400 calls that are handled at Teen Line every month. (All examples of calls in this chapter were taken from actual call sheets.) Teen Line is a hot line staffed by trained teenage volunteers who provide teenage callers a place where an empathic peer will listen to them and, when necessary, give additional help through referrals.

Teen Line is accessible through its toll-free number to any teenager in California. Most callers are between the ages of 13 and 19 years old, although preteen callers and those in their 20s are not unusual. Of the 1,400 monthly calls, 70% originate from Los Angeles County, 24% from other California counties, and 6% from other parts of the United States. The average call lasts 20 minutes. Based on Teen Line in-house surveys, an estimated 38% of callers are Hispanic, 36% are Caucasian, 14% are Asian, and 6% are African American, reflecting the multicultural nature of the local community.

Teen Line volunteers come from a variety of school, socioeconomic, and ethnic backgrounds. Teenagers from minority groups are actively recruited to apply as volunteer listeners through specific outreach to minority churches, youth groups, and predominantly minority-populated schools.

Teen Line developed as a service program of The Center for the Study of Young People in Groups, a nonprofit corporation affiliated with the Department of Psychiatry at Cedars-Sinai Medical Center in Los Angeles. It is funded by individual donations, corporate gifts, and foundation grants. In-kind support is given by Cedars-Sinai.

Since 1981, Teen Line has been open every night from 6:00 to 10:00 P.M. It is staffed by more than 60 adolescent volunteers between the ages of 14 and 18 years, each serving as a listener for one evening a week for a minimum of 1 year. Each teen participates in 60 hours of training and a minimum of 12 sessions of observing before working on the Teen Line. On each shift is an adult mental health professional referred to as an RA (resource associate), who has also participated in training and is involved on a volunteer basis. More than 25 adult volunteers currently are participating.

# ◆ What Are the Problems?

The Los Angeles riots of 1992 are testament to the many problems faced by youth today. Alienated young people found expression for their disillusionment and frustration through participation in rioting, setting fires, and looting businesses. A cursory glance at the newspaper or watching the news on television serves as a constant reminder of the many problems confronted by youth, particularly in Los Angeles County.

## Increase in Gang Participation

> A 13-year-old boy calls. He is tagging with a gang and wants to get out. He has been tagging for 4 years.
> A 15-year-old calls who wants to leave the gang but is afraid of the consequences.

A source from the Los Angeles Police Department reports that an estimated 56,800 Los Angeles youths are involved in gangs. In his almost 10 years' experience in working with gang youth, he found that while the average age of a gang member is 22 years old, the decision by young persons to be in a gang comes much earlier, in many cases as young as 9 or 10 years old. Puberty seems to be the time at which many youths, particularly boys, become actively involved in gangs—so by the time they are anywhere from 13 to 16 years old, they are already firmly ensconced in the gang life-style.

Another alarming trend is the gang participation of "taggers," who are usually a younger group starting around age 11 years. Until recently, taggers have primarily been known for painting graffiti and did not involve themselves in violent gang activities. However, now it is feared that they are using their experience as taggers as a foundation for later gang participation, or that in some cases they are being forcefully recruited by resident gangs.

## Increase in Use of Weapons by Youth

A 15-year-old girl calls. She tried to commit suicide on Saturday. A gang member is threatening her brother, and her brother has been shot at several times. She used to be in a gang herself and wants to go back.

A 14-year-old girl joined a gang 3 weeks ago because she wanted a family, but now they want her to do a drive-by and shoot someone so she can be "one of them." She wants to leave but is afraid she'll get beaten up.

Weapons seizures increased 29% in Los Angeles from September 1988 to June 1990 ("Childhood: Fearing for Your Life" 1991). The same survey also found that 1,076 weapons-related incidents occurred in Los Angeles in 1987, compared with 469 in 1985.

At Washington Preparatory High School in Los Angeles, when three randomly selected classes were polled ("Childhood: Fearing for Your Life" 1991), it was revealed that

■ One-third of the students said they had either been shot, shot at, or caught in gang gunfire.
■ All of the more than 100 students interviewed said that they were constantly in fear of being shot.

## Increase in Youth Arrests

A 17-year-old boy called who is in a reformatory school for rape. He has been there for 2 weeks and has to stay till he's 21.

A 16-year-old girl calls who was date raped. She's terrified she might be pregnant or get AIDS (acquired immunodeficiency syndrome). She's scared about reporting the rape and having the guy arrested.

A 12-year-old called because he can't control his stealing. He says he steals anything he can. He's never been caught and wants help before it gets serious.

Table 18–1 displays arrest rates for juveniles (ages 10–17 years) in Los Angeles County for 1990. It is clear that many youths need preventive and intervention measures to aid them in making the right choice about involvement in crime, including both the individuals committing the offenses and those being victimized by the crimes.

## Increase in Youth AIDS

A 16-year-old boy called with questions regarding forms of protection against AIDS.

A 17-year-old girl wanted information about having an AIDS test. She'd had sex and hadn't used protection.

AIDS has been among the top five causes of death for adults in California (California Department of Health Services 1991). It is becoming a growing concern among teen populations. Nationwide, the Centers for Disease Control and Prevention reported 789 full-blown

**Table 18–1.** Juvenile arrests reported for Los Angeles County, 1990

| Offense | Juveniles arrested |
| --- | --- |
| Motor vehicle theft | 7,406 |
| Burglary | 7,164 |
| Assault | 4,796 |
| Robbery | 4,591 |
| Drug law violations | 3,675 |
| Theft | 3,256 |
| Homicide | 407 |
| Forcible rape | 202 |

*Source.* California Department of Justice 1991.

cases of AIDS in youths 13–19 years old as of December 1991. As of March 11, 1992 (unpublished data), Children's Hospital in Los Angeles reported 33 cases of AIDS in youths 13–19 years old. This may seem like a small number, but when it is compared with the 1989 figure of 3 youths in the same age group, it represents an alarming increase.

However, statistics do not tell the whole story because youths infected with the human immunodeficiency virus (HIV) are not included—only those youths with full-blown symptomatology are actually counted.

It should also be noted that the Centers for Disease Control and Prevention (1991) estimates that for every reported case of AIDS, there are anywhere from 2 to 10 unreported cases. In addition, given that it can take as long as 10 years for an HIV-infected person to develop symptoms of AIDS, the fact that AIDS was the second leading cause of death among 25- to 34-year-olds in California is of particular concern because it is likely that many of these people were infected in their teen years (California Department of Health Services 1991).

## Increase in Teen Pregnancies

> A 15-year-old called who thinks she might be pregnant. She and her boyfriend had sex a month ago. They used a condom, but she's late getting her period so she's worried.
>
> A tearful 13-year-old calls who thinks she is pregnant and doesn't know what to do. She's scared to tell her parents.

Los Angeles County leads the state of California in other less than notable ways. Table 18–2 indicates the county's high birth rates to teens. The 521 births to mothers under age 15 years account for 40% of the total births in that category in California.

## Increase in Teen Suicide

> A 15-year-old girl called who has tried to commit suicide several times, ever since she was 4 years old. She doesn't really want to die.

She just wants all her problems to work out, but she can't see a way for that to happen.

A 14-year-old girl called who has been thinking about killing herself. She was molested by her mother's boyfriend when she was 7 years old but hasn't told anyone.

A national study of 11,631 high school students in grades 9 through 12 conducted by the Centers for Disease Control and Prevention (1991) reveals that in the 12-month period studied, 1) 3.6 million youths nationwide considered suicide, 2) 2.1 million youths devised a plan for suicide, and 3) 1 million youths made a suicide attempt. Of the 1 million youths nationwide who attempted suicide, 276,000 sustained injuries that required medical treatment ("Study Shows" 1991).

The Los Angeles County Inter-Agency Council on Child Abuse and Neglect (1990) reported 43 adolescent suicides in 1989, which is a 26% increase over the previous year's total of 34.

## Increase in Risks for Los Angeles Youth

A 16-year-old boy calls whose alcoholic father has deserted the family. There isn't enough money, and he's scared they'll end up homeless and on the street or in a shelter.

An 18-year-old girl called who had run away from home with

**Table 18–2.** Los Angeles County births to teenage fathers and mothers, 1989

| Age, yrs | Births to teenage fathers | Births to teenage mothers |
| --- | --- | --- |
| Under 13 | 3 | NA |
| 13 | 7 | NA |
| 14 | 20 | 521[a] |
| 15 | 129 | 1,226 |
| 16 | 497 | 2,559 |
| 17 | 1,084 | 4,088 |

*Note.* There were 16,186 births with no age stated for the teenage fathers. NA = not applicable.
[a]Number of births to mothers younger than age 15 years.
*Source.* California Department of Health Services 1991.

her boyfriend because of physical and verbal abuse. Now her boyfriend has walked out, she can't go home, and she can't support herself on her part-time job.

In a recent study conducted by the Center for Study of Social Policy, it was found that California teens are especially vulnerable to crime and poverty and to the resultant stresses ("Poverty, Violence" 1992). Between 1988 and 1989, it was found that among California teens

- There was a 15% increase in the violent death rate.
- There was a 4% increase in juvenile incarcerations.
- There was a 6% increase in teen pregnancy.
- Thirty-three percent of California youths (1.5 million youths) live below the poverty line.

It is obvious that these appalling figures indicate that a large number of Los Angeles youths are at risk. Sadly, the problems of these adolescents continue to outpace the availability of traditional help. For some youths, the first step in reaching out for help is a call to Teen Line. For others, a friend recognizes a need and serves as a bridge to get help for the friend by calling the hot line.

## ◆ Teen Line Call Statistics

Between 1981 and 1992, the hot line serviced over 127,000 calls. In 1991 and 1992 alone, over 33,000 calls were answered. In a sample month, the six most common reasons for calling were

1. Dating relationships (161 calls)
2. Parental concerns in the family (69 calls)
3. Relationships with friends (52 calls)
4. Sex information and concern (40 calls)
5. Suicide (20 calls)
6. Sex-related relationships (20 calls)

Figure 18–1 shows data compiled from call sheets dated March 15, 1992, through April 15, 1992. Data similar to those shown in

Figure 18–1 were found in other surveys of calls, indicating that this month is representative (D. Alter-Starr, M. Arvelo, and N. Geshke, unpublished master's research, University of California—Los Angeles School of Social Welfare, May 1992). Other issues discussed in calls include alcohol, drugs, gang activity, pregnancy, depression, loneliness, running away, physical abuse, sexual abuse, general family concerns, and self-esteem, to name a few.

## ◆ Teen Line Outreach

Teen Line serves an important function within the community through its extensive outreach program conducted by the staff. For the September 1990–August 1991 school year, presentations were made to 47 schools and youth groups, with a total attendance of 7,848 young people. Additionally, the Teen Line video was shown to 6,663 youths through the cooperation of school faculty members, other organizations, and health fairs. Teen Line cards (with the hot-line number on

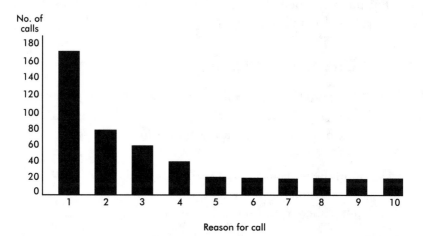

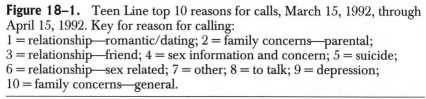

**Figure 18–1.**  Teen Line top 10 reasons for calls, March 15, 1992, through April 15, 1992. Key for reason for calling:
1 = relationship—romantic/dating; 2 = family concerns—parental;
3 = relationship—friend; 4 = sex information and concern; 5 = suicide;
6 = relationship—sex related; 7 = other; 8 = to talk; 9 = depression;
10 = family concerns—general.

it) were given to 92,550 students in the Los Angeles Unified School District (LAUSD) schools alone. A well-received safe-sex brochure produced by Teen Line was distributed to 51,240 students, also at LAUSD schools.

These results were achieved by one part-time Teen Line outreach staff person and two unpaid outreach interns, accompanied by Teen Line listeners. The effectiveness of this outreach program is attested to by the following figures: teen callers learn about the hot line from Teen Line posters, fliers, and cards (29%), friends and word of mouth (43%), magazines (9%), television and radio (8%), relatives (4%), and school newspapers (1%).

## ◆ Teen Volunteer Benefits

Although the mission of the agency is to provide teen callers with a safe, nonjudgmental, and positive peer listening service that guarantees anonymity, there is a very positive side benefit for the volunteer teen listeners. The expectations and time commitment involved for the teen volunteers are quite comprehensive and taxing, yet Teen Line has been able to involve over 60 volunteer youths annually and, to date, has trained over 500 teens.

Why do these teens do it? Perhaps because they learn firsthand how important and rewarding it is to help others and to give back to their own community. Too few opportunities are available to adolescents for exercising a sense of social commitment. Teen Line offers such an opportunity; contributing makes a difference—not only to society but also to the volunteers themselves (S. Zalusky, "Social responsibility and empathy in adolescent volunteers," unpublished dissertation, California School of Professional Psychology, Los Angeles, February 1988, p. 188).

In their study of 22 subjects who had participated as peer counselors in a 12-month high school peer counseling training program, Hahn and Le Capitaine (1990) found a substantial impact on the personal development of peer counselors. Likewise, in a study comparing Teen Line volunteers with a matched nonvolunteer peer group, Zalusky (unpublished dissertation, 1988) found that the volunteers' level of social concern and empathy was significantly higher than that of their nonvolunteer peers. She pointed out the need for programs to address the adolescents' wish for individual growth as well as their wish to be helpful. At Teen Line, both wishes are accommodated in the design of the intensive training program, wherein teen volunteers begin the process of learning the invaluable lesson of how much is gained by giving to others.

## ◆ The Training Program

A paradox inherent in the training program lies in the need to train the teen volunteers in effective communication skills while recognizing that the teens have a communication style and demeanor that are immediately comprehended and accepted by their peers. The success of the training has been contingent on maintaining a balance between respecting the expertise that is inherent in the teens who enter the program and teaching them new methods of response. A full description of the training program is contained in an unpublished manual (E. Leader, T. D. Lipton, and P. Wisne, "The Why and How of Teen Line," June 1983).

### Screening Procedures

There are many criteria for determining whether teen applicants are suitable. The primary one is that the teen applicant must have experienced and competently dealt with problems and conflicts in the past. The ability to develop strategies for solving personal problems and the willingness to consult others when needed are crucial to the life experience of an effective hot-line listener.

The personality variables examined during the screening procedure are emotional maturity, intellectual development, ability to understand others, tolerance of differing value systems, and willingness and capacity to commit time and energy. These criteria are evaluated during four stages in the screening procedure: 1) a listener questionnaire, 2) an individual interview with a clinician, 3) a task-oriented group interview, and 4) a parent-teen orientation meeting.

**Listener questionnaire.** The five-page completed questionnaires are evaluated along several dimensions:

1. Level of self-disclosure and its appropriateness to context
2. Coherence in the expression of ideas
3. Awareness of limitations
4. Appearance of written response (orderly versus disorderly)
5. Content as it expresses intellectual and emotional development

**Individual interview.** An interview schedule and the teen applicant's questionnaire provide guidelines for the 30- to 40-minute individual interview. Although the interview is not a formal mental status review, one of the purposes is to pick up any severe psychopathology that would rule out the applicant's acceptability as a Teen Line volunteer.

Questions on the interview schedule are designed to ascertain the degree of openness, maturity, and commitment of the prospective volunteer, as well as to explore the capacity for empathy. Problem-solving processes and the ability to acknowledge one's own strengths and weaknesses are other aspects examined. In exploring the motivation of the applicant and the degree of separation and individuation from family ties, the interviewer is able to determine the teen's degree of readiness to participate in the program.

**Task-oriented group interview.** The group interview is specifically designed to reduce performance anxiety and strives to promote a supportive atmosphere so that an open, in-depth discussion of the most challenging aspects of hot-line work may take place. It is structured to promote discussion and introspection—a format used throughout the training program.

The group interviewers evaluate how each applicant functions within the structure. Is there an openness in admitting limits of competence? Is there a willingness to expand these limits? Is the applicant tolerant of opposing viewpoints? Does the applicant dominate the group process or withdraw from it? How profound is the applicant's insight into his or her own personality? Does the applicant understand the struggles of others, particularly those struggles that are different from his or her own?

**Parent-teen orientation meeting.** The purpose of the parent-teen orientation meeting is to introduce new applicants and their parents to the staff and to explain what the program requires of the volunteers. After a videotape about Teen Line is shown, an explanation of the philosophy of the program, the serious nature of the commitment, and an overview of the training are given. There is also an open forum for questions answered by a panel of teen listeners. The meeting concludes with a tour of the facility and the Teen Line telephone room.

## Training Program Objectives

The training program has three objectives:

1. To promote the development and/or enhancement of those behaviors, attitudes, feelings, and thought patterns that are exemplified in an effective hot-line listener
2. To respect, support, and enhance the expressed individuality of each of the trainees
3. To impart a general body of knowledge concerning the psychological aspects of adolescence

The training program seeks to help the adolescent organize and augment prior learning and to put it into a coherent framework. Great emphasis is placed on the encouragement and reinforcement of the unfolding individuality of each teen.

A vital component of the training is the learning of active listening skills. The elements that define effective listening are numerous, complex, and interdependent. The initial assessment of a call requires the listener to use attributes such as quick thinking combined with good judgment to determine whether the call is a crisis or a noncrisis situation. If it is a crisis, the effective listener assesses the seriousness of the crisis and chooses a plan of action appropriate to the situation.

Qualities required of the teen listener include concentration, empathy, independence, observation, self-knowledge, and adaptability.

The training program becomes a living laboratory in which old behavior patterns and attributes are reinforced and strengthened and new ones are introduced and experienced. Although certain patterns of thought and behavior are essential to effective hot-line work, the way in which each individual exhibits these patterns is unique.

## Training Program Format

The training program format consists of 13 weeks of intensive instruction with two 2-hour meetings each week. One session per week is devoted to development of listening skills; the other focuses on a topic concerning the psychology of adolescents. Three or more observations of evening shifts are also expected during the formal training period. At completion of formal training, volunteers participate in monthly supervision groups and in-service staff meetings. The structure is multifaceted and based on the observations that

- Adolescents need to be actively engaged in the learning process.
- Adolescents desire situations that allow them to demonstrate their sense of responsibility, knowledge, maturity, judgment, and expertise.
- Adolescents yearn to be appreciated for their individuality and creative expression.
- Adolescents seek purposeful and meaningful activity both as an end in itself and as a source of recognition.

The sessions are structured to elicit the above situations. Sessions are held in a circular seating arrangement that promotes reciprocity and exchange of information rather than a separation between educator and student. When the trainer does give a didactic presentation, this presentation is interspersed with the contributions of the teens and takes the form of giving new information, as well as providing an overview and summary. Questions are posed, and time is allotted for introspection and response. Finally, the trainer facilitates experimentation within the session through experiential exercises that serve to illustrate the basic concepts being discussed.

In summary, the training session format comprises five essential elements that may or may not occur in the following order: 1) question, 2) introspection, 3) discussion, 4) didactic presentation, and 5) experimentation.

These five elements represent a diversity of experience: internal and external expression, active and receptive participation, cognitive and experiential learning, supportive and challenging instruction, and group and individual focus. This model, in its comprehensiveness, promotes an intense and engaging learning experience. It is used in all training activities.

## Group Process in the Training Group

As in all group experiences, the development of group cohesion and identity is important in the Teen Line training program.

In the initial training sessions, icebreaking, naming, listening, and mirroring exercises are used to generate group cohesion and identity. Interpersonal relating in the form of questions about each other's school and activities is used by the trainer to encourage group process and the development of group bonding. Group rules and regulations, particularly with regard to prompt attendance at all sessions, provide firm boundaries within which the group members can have a creative learning experience and begin to develop a group identity.

Because of their interpersonal sensitivity and high level of maturity, many of the teens who are accepted in the program have felt different from their peers and some have even felt isolated. They are often concerned with those less fortunate than themselves who have been recipients of scorn and ill treatment. A few of them have personally suffered the pain of being ostracized from a peer group for reasons based on insecurity and jealousy.

Like an adolescent therapy group, the goal of a Teen Line training group is to provide a climate in which all members can feel accepted by peers. The trainer pays particular attention to the development of specific roles within the training group. For example, by attending to the group process he or she can forestall a quiet trainee from becoming an isolate. Likewise, a training group member who monopolizes the conversation and has difficulty allowing others to contribute can become disruptive to group process and group learning.

Occasionally, a training group member may be so disruptive to group learning that the group member is asked to leave the program. The teen is counseled by the trainer and guided toward a volunteer activity more suited to his or her developmental and idiosyncratic needs. When a teen is asked to leave the group, the trainer helps the group to process this event in the same manner as a therapy group would process the loss of a group member. Most times, there is a sense of relief and a rededication to the group learning task by the remaining training group members.

# ◆ Conclusion

Peer programs such as Teen Line provide a meaningful role for young people—something that society seldom does. The skills learned in peer counseling involve cognitive, intrapsychic mechanisms and behaviors for dealing with both environmental situations and inner emotional states. These skills are acquired at Teen Line through its intensive training experience and as a result of the responsibilities inherent in staffing a hot line.

For the many adolescents who contact Teen Line, talking with an empathic, caring, and nonjudgmental peer helper is, at the very least, an opportunity to clarify concerns and explore options. For 10%–15% of the callers, Teen Line provides specific referral for more definitive evaluation and treatment at appropriate community organizations. And, for an undetermined but very significant number of adolescents, contacting Teen Line can be lifesaving.

# ◆ References

Bowman R, Myrick R: "I'm a junior counselor, having lots of fun." The School Counselor 28:31–39, 1980

California Department of Health Services: Vital Statistics of California 1989. Sacramento, CA: California Department of Health Services, 1991

California Department of Justice: Criminal Justice Profile 1990. Sacramento, CA, California Department of Justice, Division of Law Enforcement, Bureau of Criminal Statistics, 1991, p 55

Carkuff R: Helping and Human Relations: A Primer for Lay and Professional Helpers, New York, Holt, Rinehart & Winston, 1969

Carr RA: Peer Counseling: An Indexed and Annotated Bibliography. Victoria, BC, Canada, Peer Resources, 1992

Carr RA: Theory and practice of peer counseling. Paper presented at the annual meeting of the National Consultation on Vocational Counseling, Ottawa, January 1981

Carr R, Saunders G: The Peer Counsellor Starter Kit. Victoria, BC, Canada, Department of Psychological Foundations in Education, University of Victoria, 1979

Centers for Disease Control and Prevention: Attempted suicide among high school students—United States, 1990. MMWR 40(37):633–635, 1991

Central Office of Information: Britain, 1978: An Official Handbook. London, Central Office of Information, 1978

Childhood: fearing for your life. Los Angeles Times, May 13, 1991, section A, p 1

D'Andrea VJ, Salovey P: Peer Counseling: Skills and Perspectives. Palo Alto, CA, Science and Behavior Books, 1983

Hahn JA, Le Capitaine JE: The impact of peer counseling upon the emotional development, ego development, and self-concepts of peer counselors. College Student Journal 24:410–420, 1990

Hinrichsen JJ, Zwibelman BB: Differences between telephone and in-person peer counseling. Journal of College Student Personnel 22:315–319, 1981

Litman RE, Farberow NL, Schneidman ES, et al: Suicide prevention telephone service. JAMA 192:107–111, 1965

Los Angeles County Inter-Agency Council on Child Abuse and Neglect (ICAN): Child death and child abuse/neglect in Los Angeles County, 1989. El Monte, CA: Los Angeles County Inter-Agency Council on Child Abuse and Neglect, 1990

Poverty, violence haunt state's youth. Los Angeles Times, March 23, 1992, section A, p 3

Prediger D, Roth J, Noeth R: Career development of youth: a nationwide study. Personnel and Guidance Journal 53:97–104, 1974

Reguir DH, Goldberg ED, Taub CA: The de facto mental health services. Arch Gen Psychiatry, 6:191–198, 1978

Study shows a million teen suicide attempts. Los Angeles Times, September 20, 1991, section A, p 1

# CHAPTER 19

# Culture and Ethnicity

*Alberto Serrano, M.D., and*
*Susan Hou, M.D.*

## ◆ A Frame of Reference

The significance of culture and ethnicity in mental health was discussed in the early literature, mostly by sociologists and anthropologists. More recently, we have seen a growing interest in providing mental health services relevant to different ethnic groups. However, relatively few articles in the group psychotherapy literature cover this topic. There are even fewer publications on the use of groups for children and adolescents that address cultural and ethnic issues.

Psychotherapy training programs have often underplayed the role and significance of culture and ethnicity. Furthermore, there have been few suitable role models for teaching and supervision. Scheidlinger (1968) recommended training in cultural sensitivity for therapists using group approaches in community mental health settings. Bloombaum et al. (1968) also discussed the risk of cultural stereotyping among psychotherapists.

Serrano and Ruiz (1991) noted that a culturally sensitive therapist must become aware of and work through his or her own fears and biases about patients of different racial and ethnic extraction. Cultural and language factors often make it difficult for patients and therapists of different backgrounds to establish an effective therapeutic alliance. If future therapists are to become sensitive to the relevance of this dimension, training curricula should include reading and supervised experiences in cultural issues.

The concept of the melting pot prevalent in the United States for much of this century has been more recently replaced by a growing acceptance of cultural diversity. A new interest in specialized training in this area has emerged. Clinicians have become more aware of how ethnicity and culture "define ways in which people perceive their relationship to nature, people and institutions" (Dawkins et al. 1980, p. 384). Dawkins et al. underline that those "worldviews constitute our psychological orientation in life and can determine how we think, behave, make decisions and define events" (p. 384). As clinicians, we need to avoid oversimplifications: ethnic groups are not homogeneous, and cultural stereotyping should be prevented.

English (1983) classifies these worldviews into four major categories. First is the *bicultural/multicultural worldview,* which "draws upon multiple sources of cultural and socialization experiences" (p. 18). This view is bicultural, with traditional values of the background culture and those of the mainstream society seeming to coexist without apparent dominance or replacement. A person with such a worldview is able to use old and new cultural traditions without "melting" them. Second is the *acculturated/assimilated worldview.* Acculturation involves the acquisition of beliefs, attitudes, and behaviors of a social group of which one is not a national member and refers to taking on "values, norms and role expectations of the dominant group" (p. 19). Assimilation is an end state in which primary group ties develop with the dominant group. Third, a *native oriented/traditional worldview* emphasizes holding onto symbols, norms, behaviors, values, and beliefs of one's background ethnic-cultural traditions while remaining relatively isolated or impermeable to mainstream influences. Finally, a *transitional-marginal worldview* refers to "individuals who are suspended between their original ethnic identity and the mainstream culture" (p. 19). These persons typically lack a strong identification with their cultural roots and have limited adaptive capacity or no commitment to joining the mainstream culture.

We should recognize that these four categories often overlap. In our clinical observations, we find frequent individual variations depending on different life cycles or in the context of critical life events.

The number of publications that address the subject of group therapy for children and adolescents of various cultures is limited. These few articles can be found scattered in social work, psychology, psychiatric, and educational journals, demonstrating that the treatment of children in groups encompasses the expertise of multiple professionals and underscoring the need for wider dissemination of these experiences.

The literature reviewed reflects a broad spectrum of clinical applications, mostly by nonpsychiatric therapists. A good number of the reports are about the use of school-based groups with a psychoeducational emphasis. The following are common goals frequently described in the literature:

- To improve school performance—behaviorally and academically
- To enhance adaptation to a second culture
- To improve language skills
- To create a support system
- To address racial tensions in school

Despite the apparent heterogeneity of these reports, it is possible to recognize the following common issues: 1) isolation, 2) language, and 3) countertransference.

## ◆ Isolation

It is typical for children and adolescents from a different ethnic background to experience themselves as isolated from the dominant cultural group. The unfamiliar ways can make these youths feel inadequate, inferior, stigmatized, and even persecuted. Man (1992) report on the benefits of group psychotherapy with children of Asian origin, which they found more effective and less threatening than individual counseling. Peer group support offered a structure where racial issues could be openly discussed, with a resulting reduction of the members' sense of isolation. Lothstein (1985) also noted that groups for latency-age black children decreased their sense of alienation and were less stigmatizing than individual therapy. Hardy-Fanta and Montant (1982) described a group therapy model with Hispanic female adolescents that they found to be effective in reducing these teenagers' sense of isolation. Bilides (1991), Lopez (1991), and Markward (1979) also reported on the use of ethnically homogeneous groups with children and adolescents isolated within the mainstream culture. The group experience is associated with increased self-esteem and decreased acting out.

## ◆ Language

Those who remain in the land of their birthplace often take the facility with which they speak the predominant language for granted. The literature on group therapy with patients of different cultural backgrounds confirms the clinical impression that ease or lack of ease in verbal communication is consistently associated with good or poor outcome.

Man (1992) noted that clients with limited English skills should not be mixed with those who are fluent in English. Serrano and Holden (1989) reported several case studies in which language problems led to misunderstandings that disrupted effective pediatric care and relationships between family and staff. Tannenbaum (1990), who worked in English with groups of Vietnamese adolescents, stressed the importance of preference as well as proficiency in the use of language. Hardy-Fanta and Montant (1982) confirmed the experience of many authors about how personal feelings are more easily expressed in one's native tongue. They also advocated the use of culturally homogeneous groups and stressed that therapists need to be proficient in the members' language and culture. It can be hypothesized that the use of two languages would help bridge cultural gaps by providing increased familiarity and comfort and at same time enabling the new language to be learned within the context of the old one. Each dual-language group will find its appropriate voice.

Tomer (1993) pointed to the fact that the language barriers can contribute to psychopathology when youths who have average or above-average intelligence but who are doing poorly in school are excluded from socialization programs.

# ◆ Countertransference

Comas-Diaz and Jacobsen (1991), among others, emphasized that the therapist's attitudes, stereotypes, and prejudices should be openly examined even when he or she is part of the same ethnic group as the group members and is fluent in their language. The honest, open discussion of cultural and racial issues is essential to facilitate group formation; open communication is essential to foster a climate of mutual respect and to increase self-esteem. Culturally isolated group members often have a keen sense for recognizing biased feelings and insincerities in the therapist and group members. The powerful and personal issues of race and culture cannot be ignored in a population who are so sensitive to society's influences and who so desperately search for respect of their identity.

The group leaders must not only explore their own attitudes, but also examine their leadership role with group members to constructively receive the group members' perspectives and own distortions to achieve more congruent communication and foster needed change. Difference in status, social class, gender, and level of education can create additional problems and can often challenge the therapist's ability to be culturally effective and relevant.

Although knowledge of the language and of the culture is most useful, therapists with those skills are often not available. Sensitivity can be achieved in different ways. It is not essential for the therapist to be an expert on a particular ethnic group, provided that he or she is willing to be educated by group members, to collaborate with an experienced therapist, or to find suitable supervision and consultation. These are effective ways to deal with the most common countertransferential problems. They can help reduce an initial sense of insecurity and increase the cultural sensitivity of the less experienced therapist while helping him or her prevent possible cultural stereotyping. The culturally sensitive therapist avoids giving messages that may suggest that one culture is better than another.

In our review of the literature, we found no consensus concerning the significance of the therapist's own cultural and racial identity, although sensitivity was universally recognized as essential for effectively overcoming racial issues. Once again, the specific group goals and the availability of suitable therapists will dictate the matching of the therapist to the group. One of the reports documented how a group of African American youths was led effectively by white therapists (Lothstein 1985).

Both mixed and homogeneous groups were able to achieve success, although the challenges were obviously different. Intercultural conflicts were reported to play a greater role in mixed groups compared with homogeneous groups, where intracultural themes seemed to predominate and intercultural themes were secondary. In this limited sampling of the literature, the mixed groups took place within the setting of an educational system.

The reviewed articles have a generally optimistic tone; they report that cultural differences can be overcome.

We suggest exploring the use of culturally mixed groups after a successful experience with homogeneous groups. These culturally mixed groups can assist the movement toward increased bicultural participation of isolated minority individuals without a sacrifice of their basic cultural identity.

# ◆ Conclusion

The literature reporting cultural and ethnic issues in group psychotherapy with children and adolescents is relatively small. However, it demonstrates that there is solid evidence to support the effectiveness of group treatment modalities for minority populations in a variety of clinical and educational settings when these groups are conducted by culturally sensitive group psychotherapists.

# ◆ References

Bilides DG: Race, color, ethnicity and class: issues of bi-culturalism in school-based adolescent counseling groups. Social Work With Groups 13(4): 43–58, 1991

Bloombaum M, Yamamoto J, James G: Cultural stereotyping among psychotherapists. J Consult Clin Psychol 32:99, 1968

Comas-Diaz L, Jacobsen F: Ethnocultural transference and countertransference in the therapeutic dyad. Am J Orthopsychiatry 61:392–407, 1991

Dawkins M, Terry S, Dawkins M: Personality and lifestyle factors in utilization of mental health services. Psychol Rep 46:383–386, 1980

English R: The challenge for mental health: minorities and their world views. The second annual Robert L. Sutherland lecture, given at The University of Texas at Austin, School of Social Work, November 1983

Hardy-Fanta C, Montant P: The Hispanic female adolescent: a group therapy model. Int J Group Psychotherapy 32:351–366, 1982

Lopez J: Group work as a protective factor for immigrant youth. Social Work With Groups 14(1):29–40, 1991

Lothstein L: Group therapy for latency age black males: unplanned interventions, setting, and racial transferences as catalysts for change. Int J Group Psychother 35:603–623, 1985

Markward M: Group process and black adolescent identity crisis. School Social Work Journal 3(2):78–84, 1979

Man KH: Differential application of treatment modalities with Asian American youth, in Working With Culture: Psychotherapeutic Interventions With Ethnic Minority Children and Adolescents. Edited by Ross-Chioino J, Vargas L. San Francisco, CA, Jossey-Bass, 1992, pp 182–203

Scheidlinger S: Therapeutic group approaches in community mental health. Soc Work 13:87–95, 1968

Serrano AC, Holden P: Language barriers in pediatric care: clinical commentary. Clin Pediatr (Phila) 28:193–194, 1989

Serrano AC, Ruiz EJ: Transferential and cultural issues in group psychotherapy, in Psychoanalytic Group Theory and Therapy. Edited by Tuttman S. Madison, CT, International Universities Press, 1991, pp 323–333

Tannenbaum J: An English conversation group model for Vietnamese adolescent females. Social Work with Groups 13(2):41–55, 1990

Tomer A: Caring School Project–application of the group psychotherapy paradigm to the restructuring of public schools. Imperial County, CA, Office of Education, 1993

# CHAPTER 20

# Groups During the Gulf War Crisis: Intimacy and Transference Issues

*Stanley Schneider, Ph.D., and*
*Yechezkel Cohen, Ph.D.*

Emotionally disturbed children and adolescents need to learn how to negotiate the interface between their internal world and external reality as part of the therapeutic process. The complexities of intrapsychic feelings and emotions, family and peer relationships, school, and the social milieu have to be worked through and integrated for these children and adolescents to function more adequately. This chapter explores group therapy with emotionally disturbed children and adolescents in residential treatment in Israel during the Gulf War crisis. We examine how anxieties and stresses manifested themselves and were contained in the group psychotherapy sessions. Also, we note how intimacy was affected by the external threat of war and how these intimacy issues were enacted in the transference situation.

## ◆ Trauma and Anxiety: The Crisis of War

Freud (1926/1981) termed anxiety "an affective state" (p. 132) that "arose originally as a reaction to a state of danger and it is reproduced whenever a state of that kind recurs" (p. 134). In situations of danger, the ego anticipates a situation that it may not be able to master. Then, as Freud (1926/1981) states, "there are two reactions to real danger. One is an affective reaction, an outbreak of anxiety. The other is a protective action" (p. 165). The situation becomes traumatic when "the ego is reduced to a state of helplessness in the face of an excessive tension" (p. 141) that cannot be controlled. It seems, then, that there are degrees of severity regarding situations, as well as how the ego is able to respond.

In exposure to wartime situations, "no one exposed to war experiences comes away without some of the symptoms of the traumatic syndrome, however temporary these may be" (Kardiner 1959, p. 245). "The theoretical basis for psychological casualties during wartime has its roots in the concept of trauma" (Schneider 1989, p. 57). It would seem that war experiences, whether they are actual or only imminent or threatening, evoke symptoms of anxiety and trauma. One does not actually have to be in the traumatic situation. As Brenner (1955) suggests, the fear of danger can give rise to fantasies of the potential traumatic situation, which in turn cause signal anxiety, which may allow one to avoid a more traumatic condition. There seems to be a built-in loop (mechanism) that at one end perceives a real or imagined dangerous situation; then, this perception gives rise to a signal anxiety, which allows the ego to respond, thus forestalling a more serious situation (i.e., trauma).

We need to explore how this mechanism works in stressful circumstances. Freud (1920/1981) tried to relate external stimuli to the strength of the "protective shield barrier" *(reizschutz)*. If "external excitations" (p. 28) were strong enough to break through the barrier, they were called traumatic. Yet the way people respond to stressful or traumatic situations is very idiosyncratic. Does this mean that there are individual thresholds that are determined by the strength of the protective shield barrier? Or does everyone affected by very stressful or traumatic circumstances react to them in the same manner?

Several authors have theorized that parental attitudes to stress determine, in effect, how their children will respond (Freud 1956; Freud and Burlingham 1943). In reviewing children's responses to an air raid after Pearl Harbor, Solomon (1942) saw a direct relationship between children's behavior and the anxieties of their caretakers. Hartmann (1953/1964) and Anthony (1983) were interested in a "dynamic psychology of vulnerability" (Anthony 1983, p. 97) that evaluated the interplay between developmental and environmental aspects and the effect on the young child's vulnerability and resilience. "An insufficient constitutional protective barrier can generate vulnerability in two ways: by inducing unusual sensitivities, thereby increasing the barrage of stimulation from the outside, and also by developing a precocious ego with a high degree of secondary autonomy but lowered resistance to external impingements" (Anthony 1983, p. 97).

Kessler (1979) wrote that in children "the dynamic state of the child and the nature of his reaction should be emphasized rather than the kind and degree of stress" (p. 173). In her review of the literature on stress, Terr (1984) stated, "One important theme in the stress literature is that anyone may develop stress-related coping patterns, given unexpected, unsolvable, and intense enough conditions. This will occur regardless of the person's prior vulnerabilities, parenting and so forth" (p. 109). Rutter (1979) tried to look for protective factors that could reduce the risk for children living in disadvantaged environments. These factors included individual personality temperaments, a supportive family milieu, and the socializing influence of schools and administrators. Thus, although there are individual, idiosyncratic ways of dealing with stress and potential trauma and parental influences play a role, the socializing environment also can encourage and strengthen the child's ego system.

A crisis of war creates circumstances that evoke anxieties. If the person is actively involved in doing something, rather than being passive, the chances of a more severe trauma are diminished. As Fenichel (1945) states, "the blocking of external motor activity increases the possibility of a breakdown" (p. 117). Having discussions and sharing fears and anxieties (Schneider 1989) are active ways of reducing the anxieties by generalizing the circumstances (Schneider 1993). As Freud (1915/1981) stated, "The individual who is not himself a combatant, and so a cog in the gigantic machine of war, feels bewildered in his orientation and inhibited in his powers and activities. I believe that he will welcome any indications, however slight, which will make it easier for him to find his bearings within himself at least" (p. 275). The air raid sirens, running for shelter, and having to remain passively in the shelter contribute to feelings of extreme anxiety. Oftentimes, this anxiety leads to somatic symptoms and explosive reactions.

One needs to be aware of the aggression that is subsumed within the anxiety and trauma theories (Zetzel 1955, p. 379). The violence of the experience links up with the aggressive feelings of the child. A child's ability to talk about violence and aggression depends on his or her age (e.g., language, conceptual ability, concrete versus abstract thought): "The day after an air-raid the whole group of children would play air-raid" (Freud 1956, p. 155). Often a child who has seen or experienced actual violence will not talk about it: "The very violence of the experience seems, for the time being, to block the child's way to expression" (Freud 1956, p. 155).

The interplay between anxiety and aggression can best be viewed in the Kleinian tradition (Klein 1936/1988). The young child has aggressive feelings, impulses, and fantasies directed against his or her parents and projects these onto the parents. These unreal images then become internalized, and the child feels himself or herself to be controlled by dangerous and cruel parental figures. In effect, the superego turns on itself. The child facing intolerable threats because of the superego has a tremendous amount of anxiety, which is used to destroy objects, which causes the anxiety to increase in a vicious circle; more anxiety then again forces the child to turn against the objects. As the anxiety impulses diminish, the child finds better ways to adapt to social propriety and to master his or her anxiety. War anxieties intermix with normal/developmental) aggression, and this mix creates a complicated picture of anxiety, aggression, and a harsh superego.

Thus, Freud notes (1956) that children need to be helped to repress their aggressive instincts and sublimate them in spite of the external threat of destruction, death, and aggression. The danger to the child's psyche comes from the linkup of the real external threat of destruction (i.e., severe anxiety and trauma) with the internal aggressive and destructive feelings within the child.

The effect that wartime experience has on the child's psyche needs working through, because these traumas can affect the child as he or she grows into adolescence and adulthood.

An unconscious repetition compulsion is set in motion by the normal stresses of growing up. As Wangh noted (1968): "If, for instance, a whole generation of young men who suffered the traumatic stresses of war-time in their childhood, is faced on the threshold of manhood, a time of heightened anxiety under any circumstances, with economic crises and the threat of social displacement, they will be inclined, in defense against the resulting anxiety, to resort to the regressive patterns laid down in the war-time years of their childhood" (p. 319).

We now need to look at how the specific crisis of the Gulf War affected the children and adolescents who were in psychiatric residential treatment.

## ◆ The Gulf War: A Unique Crisis

Israelis are used to understanding the hardships children may go through in periods of war. Children may be affected by abandonments (e.g., father called up for army service, father and/or mother wounded or killed) or by emotional calamities felt by their primary caregivers (e.g., anxieties, loneliness, economic hardships). Thus, war may inflict a whole range of feelings and reactions directly on children, or it may affect the emotional makeup of the children indirectly, through the identification processes with their caregivers and the pressures the caregivers feel.

In addition, the impact of war also depends on the developmental phase the child is in, as well as on his or her personality structure (e.g., self-cohesiveness, ego strength).

The above brief description is sufficient to explain the difficulty in presenting a theory as to the impact of war in general on children. We believe that war, like any other potential traumatic event, has a full range of influences on the individual as a result of many factors, of which only a small portion may be known. Even reported cases of children who went through the Holocaust illustrate a variety of reactions to the most severe traumas (e.g., witnessing the killing of parents, being deserted in the woods, being hidden for a long period of time). However, there are such an extreme variety of reactions that we are unable to come to any general conclusions as to the influence of traumatic events like war on the child.

Therefore, we would like to try and explain our views on the impact of a particular war—the Gulf War—on a particular group of children—emotionally disturbed children and adolescents living in Israel and placed in residential treatment. Although this is a very specific group, it may shed some light on the larger topic of the effect of war on children.

The Gulf War for Israelis was a war totally different from any that had been experienced in the past. Prior wars in Israel were so different that one might expect unusual results from the Gulf War. In the past, the front lines were known and could be identified, which enabled each individual to define his or her nearness or distance from the front lines; thus, he or she could cope in more structured and controlled ways. In addition, soldiers who served in the army at the time of war or those who were recruited at that time were sent to the front line, meaning that they had to leave their families for different periods of time and for different, usually far-off, places. During the Gulf War, on the other hand, the front lines were unknown, unclear, and undefined. For the Israeli population, it was a kind of defenseless war in which every place could be the front line—a target for missile attacks—although the men were not enlisted and were not sent away.

One may compare the Gulf War to the blitz period in London during World War II, yet even the blitz was much more defined and much more localized. The Gulf War was also based on unknown potential weapons. During the entire war, people were warned that missiles might include biological, chemical, or atomic warheads and that the casualties could be much larger due to these weapons of mass destruction.

Schneider (1992) describes these civil defense procedures in Israel:

The civilian population of Israel were taught civil defense precautions several weeks in advance of the ultimatum that was given to Iraq. Israelis were issued gas masks. Adults had regular filter masks; children were given gas masks with a battery powered air filter; and infants were placed in special all-plastic enclosed cribs with air filter vents. Gas masks were to be carried on one's person, wherever one went. The gas mask kit also came equipped with an atropine self-injectable needle in case of a nerve gas attack and powder for removal of mustard gas, in the event of such an attack. (p. 25)

The uncertainty of the situation had people under the pressures of unknown potential traumas as to the location, the type of unexpected blows, and the extent of harm each missile hit might cause. This state of affairs provided the essential ingredients for creating all sorts of anxieties and fears, which in turn created feelings of insecurity, help-lessness, incompetence, and the like.

One additional factor potentiated the situation: the sealed room. Because there was a danger of biological, chemical, or atomic warfare, citizens were required to convert one room in each apartment or house into a sealed room. This sealed room had to be large enough to accommodate the entire family when they were required to stay there. Windows were sealed with plastic and thick plastic packaging tape. The doors were sealed along the sides with thick plastic tape, and the bottom jamb was covered with a wet towel, to prevent gas from leaking in. Whenever there was an alarm all over the country, the entire population was required to put on gas masks, enter the sealed rooms, and stay there as long was required. Each workplace followed the same routine.

The requirement for the sealed rooms forced the entire population to act simultaneously in the same manner. That may have resulted in a kind of unification that brought a feeling of togetherness. In this sense, it counteracted the alienation that characterized our day-to-day life. But more important, the fact that families stayed together in one room watching the television announcements, even during the night, had a dramatic effect on the joint experiences and feelings of together-ness that had been lacking in many families for long periods of time. We have here an excellent example of how it may be a mistake to discuss wars only in terms of their potential traumatic effects. Each case of this type should be judged according to the individual factors presented.

We now need to look at how this unique crisis manifested itself in the group psychotherapy sessions.

# ◆ The Group as a Facilitating Environment

What allows a therapeutic encounter to occur in the therapeutic situation has been referred to in the literature as an "atmosphere of safety" (Schafer 1983, p. 14). By maintaining a neutral attitude, without a moralizing stance and with a sympathetic and empathic understanding, we engender an atmosphere of safety. This "background of safety" (Sandler 1960, p. 352) allows patients a feeling of well-being in the regulation of their mental functioning. This "safety principle" (Sandler 1960, p. 352) is reinforced by the therapeutic factors of time, space, and abstinence. Patients regress in the therapeutic situation and need to enter into a dependent situation via an atmosphere of safety that can allow for "an unfreezing of an environmental failure situation" (Winnicott 1954/1982, p. 287). This is done by "the holding of the regressed patient in the clinical setting" (Winnicott 1954/1982, p. 289). Sufficient maturation of the ego to allow patients to hear and accept interpretations depends on an ability to be in a state of affective relatedness.

Winnicott wrote of the "holding environment . . . the facilitating environment" (1960/1985, p. 45). When group psychotherapy is carried out in an atmosphere of safety, this atmosphere will serve as a holding environment that can protect the patients "not only from . . . the dangers from without but also . . . from within . . . the holding environment provides an illusion that depends upon the bond of affective communication between the caretaker and the child" (Modell 1976, p. 290).

The analogy given by Winnicott and Modell—that the patient-therapist relationship re-creates the child-mother relationship—is echoed by Bowlby (1988) in his reworking of Mary Ainsworth's concept of "a secure base": "The therapist's role has been likened to that of a mother who provides her child with a secure base from which to explore" (Bowlby 1988, p. 152). Therefore, in anxious situations, such as war, children attach themselves to secure objects or persons, who serve as their secure base.

In effect, the atmosphere of safety of the holding environment functions as a transitional object (Winnicott 1953). "This transitional space allows the patient the possibility of regressing with clearly defined boundaries. The feeling of safety is engendered by the time, space and abstinence criteria of the therapeutic situation. The 'energy' for this is provided by the empathic stance of the therapist which consists of affect attunements as well as the empathic closure of the situation and the empathy conveyed by the therapist. . . ." (Schneider 1990, p. 82)

The therapeutic group functions as a therapeutic space that allows patients the ability to share in order to grow. It is a place where anxieties and fears can be contained and explored. The therapeutic group functions as a transitional object (Winnicott 1953), enabling the group members to bridge the gap between their dependent and independent struggles. The therapeutic group recreates the patient's anxieties (both external and internal) and allows a therapeutic space for experiencing them.

When therapeutic groups function within the therapeutic environment of a residential treatment center, there is a greater amount of containment, for "a child can let go of his false maturity, of his externalized independence that is based on fantasies of strength, greatness and omnipotence" (Cohen 1984, p. 36). The therapeutic space of the residential therapeutic community with emotionally disturbed children and adolescents serves as a holding environment. "It is the holding that constitutes therapy, when speaking of children who suffered ego defects in their development with resultant interference in the integration of their selves" (Cohen 1984, p. 39).

When individuals become severely anxious or traumatized, therapeutic groups can be useful in allowing for venting of feelings, especially feelings of anger and impotence. Therapeutic groups with children and adolescents can provide the structure that is needed "to create a consistent environment in which the children can feel safe and secure, knowing they will be taken care of by the group therapists" (Kernberg and Chazan 1991, p. 188). Groups that took place during the war crisis enabled the participants to reduce their anxiety levels and allowed them to channel their intense feelings and impulses in a manner that was not overwhelming to them or to the other group participants.

Yalom (1975) delineated the major curative factors of group psychotherapy: altruism, catharsis, cohesiveness, communality of problems, interpersonal learning, and recapitulation of the family experience. Although Yalom argued against the group leader's focusing exclusively on the group-level phenomena because this focus "is restrictive and severely limits the therapist's effectiveness" (p. 170), he did see an exception with "anxiety-laden issues" (p. 170).

In the Foulkesian model, therapists do focus on group-level phenomena, especially when dealing with anxiety-laden issues. This focus is the main thrust of a dynamic, analytic understanding of groups. As Foulkes and Anthony (1957/1984) described the resonance of the group: "Each member in the group will then show a distinctive tendency to reverberate to any group event according to the level at which he is 'set'" (p. 152). The unconscious connection that the children and adolescents in our groups made with one another allowed the group to move forward: "What is unknown and unknowable to each individual member is nevertheless activated by this common process and is in this way also fed back into the common matrix. It is as if all the events were specifically interrelated with each other in their vital meaning, and showed this interrelationship by resonating" (Foulkes 1990, p. 300).

Because the war crisis was ongoing and the therapists as well as the group participants were in a state of "anxiety limbo," not knowing what would happen or when, the fear of disruption, loss of family ties, and possible destruction of homes and possessions was very strong. This anxious situation resulted in very intense feelings, which were shared and acted out in the therapy groups. We need to explore this further in the light of transference and intimacy issues.

## ◆ Transference and Intimacy

The anxieties of the war crisis intensified the transferences that emerged in the group. Because an air raid alert could occur at any time, the fears and anxieties of the children and adolescents in residential treatment, as well as those of the staff, bounced off one another. The external anxiety about this potentially traumatic situation was brought into the group psychotherapy sessions. This made for multiple transferences within the group psychotherapeutic situation.

In the Foulkesian model of group analytic psychotherapy, the transference relationship is often more intense than the original relationship itself. With real anxiety impinging constantly from both outside and inside the group, the transference was intensified because the fantasies of the group members were flowing freely.

Often, this admixture of anxiety and transference made it difficult to tell the magnification of reality from fantasy.

### Case Example 1

Mike had professed over the past few months his unhappiness with the treatment center; he wanted to go home. However, when the war crisis began, Mike told the group how much he needed to stay because, as he said, "the country needed me." He put on an air of bravado and made a strong case for "supporting the allies and the only Western democracy in the Middle East." When the group conductor tried to clarify these statements in light of his previous attitude, Mike identified with "the Israeli soldiers, President Bush, and all the coalition partners."

In the residential treatment center that was treating emotionally disturbed adolescents, we found that the sealed room fostered intimacy and "quickened the fostering of a therapeutic relationship" (Schneider 1992, p. 30). Quite probably, the air raid alert, running to the sealed room (often in pajamas) where the entire unit (staff and patients) was together, putting on the gas masks, and turning on the radio and TV for instructions were the activities that were necessary to reduce the overwhelming anxiety. The forcing together of staff and patients in a sealed room, very often in intimate clothing, brought everyone together in a more familiar manner. Sometimes, therapists found themselves together with patients and counselor-support staff. There was a breakdown of therapeutic barriers.

The external, real crisis "created an intimacy that arose out of fear and anxiety. This was intensified in the sealed room when staff and patients were vulnerable together. Intimacy feelings were very strong for both patient and staff . . . strong countertransference feelings were engendered in the staff who, because of the joint vulnerability and reality of a frightening/anxious crisis, found themselves emotionally more available to patients" (Schneider 1993, p. 103).

### Case Example 2

Sandy expressed in the group her strong feelings for Sammy, the counselor. The group members accused Sandy of "running after anything in pants." The group conductor was able to direct the group members toward the issue of how warm feelings get brought up when "we're scared, away from home, and in close, cramped quarters." This interpretation enabled Sammy, nondefensively, to relate to how he had put his arm around Sandy when she became hysterical during an air raid alert.

We noticed that with the increase in intimacy, there was also an increase in the expression of aggressive feelings. We know that in group treatment with emotionally disturbed children there is often a mixture of love and hate, sometimes even in the same breath. As a result, the therapist may experience a wide range of emotions: "In doing group therapy with children . . . the therapist should expect to experience appreciable amounts of positive and negative feeling that may at times occasion guilt and shame or inadvertently discharge itself on to the children" (Foulkes and Anthony 1957/1984, p. 190).

### Case Example 3

Gideon was very restless in the group, running around the room and touching and throwing things. He found the counselor's keys and threw them out the window. The other children divided into two groups: one side cheered him on, and the other side moralized about how bad a boy he was. He ran out of the group with his therapist running after him. The therapist brought him back and was able to interpret to Gideon and the group how sometimes we feel lost and need to hold on to something like a key, to feel grounded and less anxious.

Because staff and patients experienced the same real external crisis, the feelings that emerged were legitimized within the group.

Group members became closer to one another; a stronger cohesive unit was formed; and the common enemy, Saddam Hussein, became the object of ridicule. The issue of intimacy struck at the core of dependence-independence and separation-individuation issues: "The pre-oedipal aspects of this 'encounter' in the group experience touched strongly upon feelings of shame (rather than oedipal feelings of guilt)" (Schneider 1993, p. 107).

### Case Example 4

Avi fetched toys from the shelves during his therapy session. He expressed a fear, which a lot of the other children had, that parts of the toys were broken, missing, and torn. He carried a nylon bag where he kept his gas mask and placed toys in the bag instead of the mask. He threw the broken toys in the garbage pail. The issue of separation from the residential treatment center and being home with his disturbed family reenacted for him the separation-individuation crisis. He needed the group as a "secure base" (Bowlby 1988).

## ◆ Summary

We have explored the topic of group psychotherapy with emotionally disturbed children and adolescents during the Gulf War crisis. While touching on how anxieties and stresses manifested themselves, we focused on group psychotherapy as a holding environment through the subthemes of transference and intimacy.

## ◆ References

Anthony EJ: Infancy in a crazy environment, in Frontiers of Infant Psychiatry. Edited by Call JD, Galenson E, Tyson RL. New York, Basic Books, 95–107, 1983

Bowlby J: A Secure Base. London, Tavistock/ Routledge, 1988

Brenner C: An Elementary Textbook of Psychoanalysis. New York, Doubleday, 1955

Cohen Y: Residential treatment as a holding environment. Residential Group Care and Treatment 2:33–43, 1984

Fenichel O: The Psychoanalytic Theory of Neurosis. New York, WW Norton, 1945

Foulkes SH: Selected Papers of S. H. Foulkes: Psychoanalysis and Group Analysis. London, Karnac, 1990

Foulkes SH, Anthony EJ (eds): Group Psychotherapy: The Psychoanalytical Approach (1957). London, Maresfield, 1984

Freud A: Special experiences of young children particularly in times of social disturbance, in Mental Health and Infant Development, Vol 1. Edited by Soddy K. New York, Basic Books, 1956, pp 141–160

Freud A, Burlingham DT: War and Children. New York, Medical War Books, 1943

Freud S: Thoughts for the times on war and death (1915), in The Standard Edition of the Complete Psychological Works of Sigmund Freud, Vol 14. Translated and edited by Strachy J. London, Hogarth Press, 1981, pp 273–302

Freud S: Beyond the pleasure principle (1920), in The Standard Edition of the Complete Psychological Works of Sigmund Freud, Vol 18. Translated and edited by Strachy J. London, Hogarth Press, 1981, pp 3–64

Freud S: Inhibitions, symptoms and anxiety (1926), in The Standard Edition of the Complete Psychological Works of Sigmund Freud, Vol 20. Translated and edited by Strachy J. London, Hogarth Press, 1981, pp 77–175

Hartmann H: Contribution to the metapsychology of schizophrenia (1953), in Essays on Ego Psychology. New York, International Universities Press, 1964, pp 186–206

Kardiner A: Traumatic neuroses of war, in American Handbook of Psychiatry, Vol 1. Edited by Arieti S. New York, Basic Books, 1959, pp 245–257

Kernberg PF, Chazan SE: Children with Conduct Disorders: A Psychotherapy Manual. New York, Basic Books, 1991

Kessler ES: Reactive disorders, in Basic Handbook of Child Psychiatry, Vol 2. Edited by Noshpitz J. New York, Basic Books, 1979, pp 173–184

Klein M: On criminality (1936), in Love, Guilt and Reparation. London, Virgo, 1988, pp 258–261

Modell AH: The holding environment and the therapeutic action of psychoanalysis. J Am Psychoanal Assoc 24:285–308, 1976

Rutter M: Protective factors in children's responses to stress and disadvantage, in Social Competence in Children. Edited by Kent M, Rolf JE. Hanover, NH, University of New England Press, 1979, pp 212–242

Sandler J: The background of safety. Int J Psychoanal 41:352–365, 1960

Schafer R: The Analytic Attitude. New York, Basic Books, 1983

Schneider S: The chaplain/rabbi as a reducer of stress. Journal of Psychology and Judaism 13:57–68, 1989

Schneider S: Transitional objects, the holding environment and empathy, in Boundaries in Adolescence: Family, School, Individual and Group Therapy (in Hebrew). Edited by Schneider S, Deutsch C. Jerusalem, Israel, Summit Institute, 1990, pp 77–82

Schneider S: Intimacy and the eroticized transference: psychotherapy under the threat of war, in Clinical Social Work in the 90s. Edited by Cummings RE. Silver Spring, MD, American Board of Examiners in Clinical Social Work, 1992, pp 25–35

Schneider S: Group analytic psychotherapy under the threat of war: the Gulf Crisis. Group Analysis 26:99–108, 1993

Solomon J: Reactions of children to black-outs. Am J Orthopsychiatry 12:361–362, 1942

Terr LC: Children at acute risk: psychic trauma, in Psychiatry Update, Vol 3. Edited by Grinspoon L. Washington, DC, American Psychiatric Press, 1984, pp 104–120

Wangh M: Psychogenic factor in the recurrence of war. Int J Psychoanal 49:319–323, 1968

Winnicott DW: Transitional objects and transitional phenomena. Int J Psychoanal 34:89–97, 1953

Winnicott DW: Metapsychological and clinical aspects of regression within the psycho-analytical set-up (1954), in Through Paediatrics to Psycho-Analysis. London, Hogarth, 1982, pp 278–294

Winnicott DW: The theory of the parent-infant relationship (1960), in The Maturational Processes and the Facilitating Environment. London, Hogarth, 1985, pp 37–55

Yalom I: The Theory and Practice of Group Psychotherapy. New York, Basic Books, 1975

Zetzel ER: The concept of anxiety in relation to the development of psychoanalysis. J Am Psychoanal Assoc 3:369–388, 1955

# CHAPTER 21

# Cults and Children: A Group Dynamic Perspective on Child Abuse Within Cults

*David A. Halperin, M.D.*

The catastrophe at Waco, Texas, presents a grim reminder of the potential within cults for the abuse and death of children. Throughout the 51-day siege, the fate of the children sequestered within the Branch Davidian compound hung as a fearful backdrop to the negotiations ostensibly being conducted between David Koresh (a.k.a. Vernon Howell) and the federal government. The failure of these negotiations and the Branch Davidian's amalgam of theological obscurantism, distortions of biblical prophecy, and paranoia led to a tragedy of proportions surpassed only by the hecatomb of Jonestown, Guyana. During recent legal actions undertaken by governments in Australia, Spain, and Argentina material produced during proceedings illustrated the potential for abuse within a marginal group: The Children of God (a.k.a. The Family). This chapter examines the group

I would like to express my appreciation to the members of the Community Services of Victoria (Melbourne, Victoria, Australia) for giving me the opportunity to participate in their protective action and to review their extensive survey of the literature produced by the Children of God, as well as for the personal communications in which they shared their concerns.

processes active within cults and cultlike groups that have led and may lead to the abuse and death of children at the hands of their ostensibly loving caretakers.

## ◆ Child Abuse Within Cults: A Historical Perspective

In 1984, Markowitz and Halperin noted the potential for child abuse within cultic contexts: "While child abuse need not be a necessary consequence of familial affiliation with a cult the very characteristic of the cult organization and life-style provides significant predisposing factors" (p. 145).

West and Singer described how

> the preeminent characteristic of a cult is the totalitarian control of the members' life by a leader claiming a special relationship with God or some suprahistorical force. Within the cult, there is the development of a deep emotional dependence, a prohibition of critical analysis and independent thinking, the creation of exploitative working conditions that often leave members with little time for family-centered activities, and the development of communities characterized by exclusivity and isolation. Within such a context, there is little to restrain the cult leader from instituting his most whimsical ideas on childbearing. (Halperin 1983b, p. 226)

These criteria accurately characterize a cultlike group active on a worldwide basis: The Children of God. A group dynamic perspective is particularly applicable to this group in understanding the potential for child abuse within cults.

## ◆ Historical Background on The Children of God

The group named The Children of God is the creation of David Berg. Berg was born in 1919 in Huntington Beach, California. His mother was a fundamentalist Christian missionary. After his marriage, Berg, his wife, Jane, and their four children, Aaron, Hosea, Deborah, and Faithy, joined Berg's mother in her ministry. On his mother's death in March 1968, Berg assumed control of this marginal, minute organization. Initially, Berg's group was simply another one of the "Jesus freak" groups active in California. But in April 1969, he left Huntington Beach and changed the group's name to Teens for Christ, proclaiming: "We are the one and only absolute and total genuine revolution in the whole world! We are it! We are God's children!" (D. Berg, Mo Letters, [unpublished documents], 1983) [1]

By denominating his followers as revolutionaries, Berg defined them as an isolated and elite group—initiating a process of increasing cultic withdrawal from the outside world. In addition, Berg started the relationship with Karen Zerby (a.k.a. Maria, now the primary leader of The Children of God). By 1970, Berg claimed to "talk in tongues" and to have acquired a "spirit guide," Abrahim, a thirteenth-century Gypsy King from Bulgaria. In 1973, Berg prophesied that the United States would be destroyed by the comet Kohoutek. His preachings increasingly began to focus on *end time,* and he began to style himself Moses David, The End-Time Prophet (as well as Grandpa, Dad, Father David, and The King).

It was also around this time that he began to issue his Mo Letters—communicating with his followers from a concealed place because of his being pursued by Satan/Antichrist. The Mo Letters appealed to his followers through a combination of the exhortative ("We are the one and only absolute and total genuine revolution in the whole world"), the revelatory ("In each case, the one I was making love to would suddenly turn into one of these strange and beautiful goddesses, and I would immediately explode in an orgasm of tremendous spiritual power while at the same time prophesying violently in some foreign tongue"), the confessional ("Sometimes I almost go crazy in the night, I get so terrified and so paranoid!"), and the grandiose ("I have the wisdom of all ages"). The organizational and group dynamics of The Children of God are depicted in succinct terms:

---

[1] The Mo Letters are documents by Berg that were distributed occasionally to his followers.

We have often compared ourselves with. . . a guerilla [sic] army. . . .

You are supposed to love, honor, respect and obey your leadership . . . let's learn to follow leadership, follow suggestions and learn to respect authority. . . .

And if you can't take an order, you're not going to be *obedient,* let me tell you, you're not going to be in the *Family* very long! Because this is an *Army* run on basic army principles, and one of the main ones is that you've got to be able to follow *orders* and take commands! (D. Berg, Mo Letters, 1979)

The implications of this totalitarian governance are directly reflected in the authorized approach to child discipline: "I had one little method that was very effective, the kids didn't like it either. The skull is a pretty safe place to crack 'em once they're a little older, and I used to take my knuckles and go bang bang bang right on the head, and boy, they didn't like that!" (D. Berg, Mo Letters, 1983)

Despite the garrulous, avuncular paternal persona presented in the Mo Letters, there is a consistent emphasis on a totalitarian discipline, a preoccupation with establishing a rigid hierarchy, and a paranoid fear of persecution.

The Children of God expanded into a worldwide organization during the 1970s. During the early 1970s, Berg promulgated his most distinctive practice: *flirty fishing.* Flirty fishing encourages female members to become prostitutes as a means of recruiting new members (hookers for Jesus) and of raising money. Women who refused to participate and husbands who opposed their wives' participation were labeled backsliders or considered *systemites* (a term of opprobrium indicating adherence to the mainstream system). A corollary to this exploitation of female members is the practice of *family sharing,* in which all male members could demand to have their sexual needs met by female members; refusal by a female member to participate was also labeled backsliding.

Not surprisingly, the response of the broader society to these practices has been very negative. The response by The Children of God to this criticism has been twofold: 1) to deny that flirty fishing or family sharing are current practices and 2) to adopt a nomadic pattern of existence in which members rarely remain in the same place for more than 3 months. This nomadic existence as "pilgrims" encourages the members to huddle together in a fight-flight group, fearful of the noncult world and increasingly dependent on their "divinely or-dained" leader. [2]

Other consequences of this life-style include 1) that members are unable to maintain regular employment and resort primarily to beg-ging or hustling as a means of support, 2) that educational opportuni-ties for children are severely limited, and 3) that children have no opportunity to form relationships outside of the cult group, leaving them particularly subject to group processes designed to inculcate this very particularistic worldview.

The primary residences of The Children of God remain outside the United States, but a recent article notes:

> Some 200–250 members of the Children of God, now calling them-selves The Family, have moved from various international locations back to the United States and set up communal living situations in ten major American cities, with headquarters in Anaheim, CA. . . . ("Children of God Returning to U.S." 1993, p. 2)

## ◆ The Abuse of Children Within The Children of God

Child protective services agencies have been concerned about poten-tial and actual child abuse within The Children of God since 1974. Since the 1974 study by the attorney general of New York State, authorities have been concerned about the destructive impact of The Children of God on the children of members. The group's practices that have elicited concern include the following:

**Continuing lies, deception, and propaganda.** Children are ex-posed only to group-approved literature. Television is censored by

---

[2]
Such a group is termed a *basic-assumptions* group—a non-task-oriented group organized around a controlling leader. Basic-assumptions groups are discussed below in the section "Group Dynamic Processes in the Evolution of Cults: A Brief Overview."

elders within the group before being viewed by children. Thus, the group presents to children a harshly polarized view of the world in which everything outside the group's boundaries is portrayed as "satanic"—the product of systemites. Family members who are not group members are also portrayed as evil or only intent on stealing children from "God's army." However, for its own survival, the group justifies as "witnessing" actions of deception, including lying to child-care authorities and presenting a mainstream facade.

**Rigorous control.** Actions or activities not specifically sanctioned by the group or its leader are automatically viewed as suspect. Separation from the group for any purpose or at any level is viewed as treacherous—thus, children taken into child protective services agencies for evaluation would vigorously deny any interest in mainstream activities, even though they would rapidly begin to watch mainstream, uncensored television.

**Nomadism.** Members of The Children of God accept being dispatched on missionary activity without question. In addition, children are ordered to prepare "flee bags" containing their few personal belongings to enable them to decamp at a moment's notice. This nomadism exacerbates the sense of transience and heightens group members' dependence on the group.

**Obsession with persecution and security.** The life of children within The Children of God is dominated by constant warning that the Antichrist is relentlessly attempting to destroy the group. Thus, children, even during contact with the noncult world, are warned against forming any relationship with nongroup members except if it appears that the contact will afford an opportunity for fund-raising or recruitment. Moreover, during contact with the nongroup world, children are encouraged to present a pathetic appearance to raise funds.

**Sexual practices.** David Berg detailed in the Mo Letters his approval of sexual activity between children, irrespective of age. Limitation on the contact between children and adults appears to primarily reflect public relations concerns. Psychotherapy with a former group member clearly revealed that he joined the group at age 16 because the promiscuous atmosphere presented opportunities for sexual activity. In addition, the intensity of the sexual activity within the group heightened the sense of group polarization vis-à-vis the noncult world.

**Child-rearing practices.** Child-rearing practices within cult groups often reflect the cult's demands rather than the child's needs. Thus, child rearing is viewed primarily as an opportunity for indoctrination rather than as preparation for an autonomous adulthood. Contact with the noncult world is minimized, demonized, or virtually destroyed (unless relatives may be sympathetic or offer an opportunity for fundraising). Contact between children and a parent if the parent has left the group has been almost impossible to arrange with any consistency. Even if both parents are group members, contact with biological parents is often very limited. Parents may be absent for long periods of time, leaving children to be raised primarily in a communal setting with little individualized contact with caretakers. Children raised in such a group context often appear to develop a protective facade marked by affective flattening and blunting of affect. In addition, their primary identification appears to be with the group. What individualized caretaking occurs is often between siblings. In this context, older siblings are saddled with the responsibility for their younger siblings—a responsibility they discharge with rigidity, harshness, and a concern that these younger siblings might disclose group secrets to nongroup members.

Within The Children of God, group concerns are primary. Children are routinely denied any privacy (they may sleep 10–12 to a small room), are exposed to adult sexuality at a very early age, are denied personal objects (toilet paper may be reused), and are disciplined with unusual harshness. Of particular barbarism is the practice of isolating a nonconforming child from any contact with other individuals for extended periods of time.

**Educational practices.** The Mo Letters explicitly deny the importance of children being exposed to a higher education or to any outside educational experience that might encourage dissent. Education is limited to the basics within a home schooling context, which prevents children from being exposed to outside ideas. Children who were evaluated in child protective services agencies would lecture their caretakers about the evils of public education.

Naturally, in this context, low value is placed on the education of females, who in any event are portrayed in stereotypical terms with their activities limited to childbearing. Adolescents are also limited in their educational opportunities by being placed in special teen camps focusing on indoctrination for work within the group. The removal of adolescents deprives younger children of potential role models and heightens their identification with the group.

**Bigotry and anti-Semitism.**   When groups organize themselves in opposition to the outside world, it is hardly surprising that they will seize on some group as a particular foe. David Berg is said to have lived with the Libyan dictator Muammar al-Qaddafi for 3 years, so it is unexceptional that The Children of God are virulently anti-Semitic. For example, a former member's fear that Jews controlled medicine, psychiatry, and the world of affairs was a primary issue that had to be addressed in treatment.

**Health practices.**   Totalistic groups such as The Children of God are very skeptical that any non-cult-oriented knowledge may play a positive role in child care. They do not deny that mainstream medicine may be helpful, but their doctrine states that illness is a "spiritual malaise." Thus, when an individual is symptomatic, the group's primary focus is curing the spiritual illness. In this context, children deny symptoms because being sick is equated with the loss of spiritual value and the loss of status within the group. Moreover, the group's nomadic life-style prevents children from establishing a trusting relationship with caretakers or receiving any continuity in their medical care.

## ◆ The Branch Davidians: A Historical Perspective

However, The Children of God are not unique. A comparison with the Branch Davidian movement is instructive. The Branch Davidian movement was a mutation of an earlier Adventist splinter group. The Davidians trace their roots to Victor Houteff, a Bulgarian immigrant, who was expelled from a Los Angeles Adventist church in 1929. Houteff had become obsessed with passages in the Book of Ezekiel in which an angel of God divides the faithful from the sinful before Jerusalem's fall to Babylon. Believing that passage to be a warning to Adventists, Houteff established a splinter organization in 1935 on the outskirts of Waco, in the deeply religious prairie land of Texas.

When he died 20 years later, his widow Florence assumed leadership of the sect. She dissolved it after the failure of her prediction that the last days of creation would commence on April 22, 1959. . . . ("Cult of Death" 1993, p. 36)

David Koresh joined the remnants of the Branch Davidian movement in 1984. After a power struggle with the leader of the remnant of the Branch Davidians, Koresh assumed leadership in 1989. Even at that time, it was a well-armed group, and the final dispute between Koresh and his rival, George Roden, involved violence. It was at that time that Koresh began to promulgate an "apocalyptic theology converged with secular survivalism, with its programs for hunkering down amid stockpiles of food and ammo to endure a nuclear holocaust or social collapse" ("Cult of Death" 1993, p. 36).

This convergence of apocalypse and survivalism has been noted in many contexts. With messianic zeal,

Koresh began to preach that his followers should ready themselves for a final battle with unbelievers. The Waco settlement, once a collection of old cottages scattered around 78 acres of scrub pasture and woods, was consolidated into a compact fort the size of a city block" ("Cult of Death" 1993, p. 36).

David Koresh's apocalyptic theology reflected a strain within the Great Awakening that transformed religious life within the United States in the 1840s. However, his fusion of apocalyptic theology, survivalism, and sexual control reflects other more individual and group dynamic issues. A comparison with The Children of God in terms of its evolution is intriguing.

## ◆ Group Dynamic Processes in the Evolution of Cults: A Brief Overview

The apocalyptic scenario that created the backdrop for the tragedy at Waco and the underpinning of both The Children of God and the Branch Davidians reflect group dynamic patterns common to these and other cult groups. Kernberg has noted, as quoted in Halperin (1983a),

> The Messianic temptations of small groups such as the search for "instant intimacy," or the breaking of ordinary sexual boundaries, illustrate the appeal of the various contemporary group movements that have exploited these processes in more or less sensationalistic ways. (p. 260)

When an appeal to instant intimacy and family formation is imbued with a perspective that views the nongroup world in terms of total polarization (i.e., absolute good resides only within the group, and absolute evil [Satan/Antichrist] pervades the nongroup world), the bond within the group becomes extraordinarily intense. The cult leader is then in a position to intensify further the individual's bond with the group by constant reiteration that he or she alone possesses the knowledge and magic to enable the group to survive the persecution of an inimical outside world and to enable the individual to survive imminent apocalypse.

Bion's work on basic-assumptions groups (defined above) is particularly relevant in enhancing an appreciation of the linkage between end time and cultic commitment. I have noted that

> averting or surviving the apocalypse is a task of such a nature that any task orientation becomes ill-defined and both individual and group feel ill-equipped to cope with their "responsibility." Thus, the group members are encouraged to huddle around the group leader in defense of the impending end. (Halperin 1983b)

The position of the cult leader is further enhanced by his or her unique possession of a gnosis that will putatively enable the group to survive. The leader's uniqueness is granted a magical quality that will armor the group against all threats and enable it to survive all dangers. The cult leader enhances his or her position by declaring that the followers are not a fringe minority but rather an elite who will have a unique role in the governance of the new age that will follow the apocalypse.

However, magic is not enough. David Koresh assembled a significant armory. The Children of God have adopted an alternative strategy that calls for dispersal into small groups that are constantly prepared to flee persecution or nuclear attack. A similar strategy was adopted by the Sullivanian Institute/Fourth Wall Theater Company, which maintained a fleet of buses in constant readiness for flight and controlled members by insisting that they wear beepers enabling them to be summoned in the event of nuclear attack. Like The Children of God, the Sullivanian Institute raised children communally and would ostracize parents who showed too personal an interest in their children.

Basic-assumptions groups may evolve from the fight-flight position to the pairing position. It is an evolution from a position of "being forcefully controlled by him [the group leader] to experiencing closeness in a shared denial of intergroup hostility, and to project[ing] aggression onto an outgroup" (Halperin 1983b, p. 26) to a position in which the group or cult directs its energies in a more ostensibly creative fashion and deals with its fear of termination by pairing to produce a new successor group. Because children produced within the cult constitute this successor group, their behavior and status are charged from birth with an ideological importance.

## ◆ Child Abuse Within Cults: Group Issues

Children present the cult with both a challenge and the potential for affirmation and validation of the cult's theology. In view of the Soviet Union's current state of disorganization, it is difficult for nonresidents to appreciate how seriously ideologists in the former Soviet Union took their propaganda about creating the new Soviet man: homo sovieticus. Cults, like larger totalitarian societies, envisage themselves as creating a new superior race to justify the deprivation and isolation that they impose on their members and to rationalize the privileges that their leadership cadre enjoys. If a child acts in a nonconforming manner, the group experiences it as a challenge to the group theology and considers it to be the manifestation of some malign outside force at work. The child may then become subject to correctional "treatment" to expel the "demonic forces" felt to be at work.

Thus, David Berg subjected children in The Children of God to decidedly unpaternal behavior because he considered any unusual behavior, including learning disability, to be a manifestation of spiritual impurity and advocated an approach of triage for the nonconforming. In this army there is no place for the sick or those unable to accept the cult's discipline (irrespective of age). Among punishments imposed is silencing. As has already been noted, this may consist of solitary confinement of an offending child for periods as long as 3 months, during which all other group members, including the child's family, are expected to treat the child as a pariah. In the cultic context, ordinary reprimands may be capricious or confusing:

> No one knows exactly what the children's lives had been like inside the compound [Branch Davidian], which had no indoor plumbing. But there have been reports of Mr. Koresh's reproaching them for hours about their sins, and showing them his arsenal of weapons. While there is considerable evidence that the children were well cared for, discipline was rigidly enforced. Children were spanked with a paddle, relatives said. ("Growing Up Under Koresh: Cult Children Tell of Abuses" 1993, p. B11)

Dr. Bruce Perry, who has worked with the surviving children, described the confusion experienced by these children:

> Even after their release and as they described their treatment by Mr. Koresh, nearly all the children have talked about their love for him . . . their feelings were something else. "Fear is what it was. . . ." They learned to substitute the word 'love' for fear. . . . The cult leader controlled everything—sex, school, play and even diet. ("Growing Up Under Koresh: Cult Children Tell of Abuses" 1993, p. B11)

In this totalitarian environment, any individuality expressed by a child was seen as a challenge to the claim that the cult alone possessed the knowledge and the ability to "perfect" individuals—a challenge met with harsh treatment.

A factor of prime importance in how children are treated within cult groups is the cult's total focus of all sexual cathexis on the cult leader. David Koresh enforced celibacy on all males within the group but allowed himself to form relationships with any female member irrespective of age. Female children were exposed to sexuality, and Koresh himself married and/or was sexually intimate with women who were in early adolescence. Previously married male group members were told to "donate" their wives to Koresh. Koresh's insistence on the destruction of the marriages of other group members reflected his accurate perception that the persistence of the family and family ties, no matter how diluted in form, constituted a barrier to total immersion within the cult group. His actions and the dilution of the biological family within the Branch Davidians conform to Freud's appreciation that the mob resents any individuality and perceives any other bonds as a challenge to the group mentality (Roth 1994). In these cult groups, parental ties with children—even if the parents and children are group members—were perceived by the cult and cult leader as a threat to their dominion.

The refusal of cult groups to use mainstream medical practices is another example of the cult leader's considering any alternate form of expertise as a challenge to his or her omniscience. Infants in The Children of God (and in groups such as the Island Kingdom Church of Vermont) died because of marginal sanitary facilities or lack of inoculations. Mainstream medical care is suspect within cult groups because of their primary focus on seeing illness only in "spiritual" terms. The cult leader regards the medical doctor with his or her objective medical knowledge as the possessor of a noncult source of knowledge and therefore as inherently suspect. Comparably, The Children of God and the Branch Davidians disparaged education because education—particularly of female members—might undermine the cult group's pretensions to being the sole repository of wisdom. Like totalitarian societies in Germany and Russia, objectivity was stigmatized as "bourgeois," "non-Aryan," or "unChristian."

# ◆ Summary

This chapter describes and places within a group dynamic perspective the widespread and fearful abuse of children with cult groups. The extent to which children have been and continue to be brutalized by quasi-totalitarian organizations under an ostensibly religious aegis has not been recognized by mainstream society. As mental health professionals, we should appreciate the extent of the abuse and the reality that it is an inevitable aspect of the group processes active within a wide variety of cult groups.

# ◆ References

Children of God returning to U.S. Cult Observer, October 5, 1993

Cult of death. Time, March 15, 1993, pp 36–39

Growing up under Koresh: cult children tell of abuses. The New York Times, May 4, 1993, p B11

Halperin DA: Gnosticism in high tech: science fiction and cult formation, in Psychodynamic Perspectives on Religion, Sect and Cult. Edited by Halperin DA. Littleton, MA, John Wright-PSG, 1983a

Halperin DA: Group processes in cult recruitment and affiliation, in Psychodynamic Perspectives on Religion, Sect and Cult. Edited by Halperin DA. Littleton, MA, John Wright-PSG, 1983b

Markowitz A, Halperin DA: Cults and children: the abuse of the young. Cultic Studies Journal 11:143–156, 1984

Roth BE: Revised model of internalization derived from group psychology, editorial introduction. Group 18(1):3–5, 1994

# SECTION V

# Research

# CHAPTER 22

# Status of Adolescent Research

*Fern J. Cramer Azima, Ph.D.*

This review of the present status of adolescent group psychother-apy research is a follow-up of earlier reviews by Tramonata (1980) and Azima and Dies (1989). Studies were selected from a computerized Medline search (1986–1992) of group journals and books that demonstrated adequate methodology and were concerned with current issues relevant to the practice of group psychotherapy with adolescents. The goal was to evaluate a selected group of studies, rather than to perform an exhaustive review, which is beyond the scope of this chapter. Investigations that used more recent evaluation instruments and research methodology were included. Implications for future research in this area is the final focus of this chapter.

## ◆ General Overview

In general, child and adolescent individual and group psychotherapy research has lagged behind investigations of adult group psychother-apy (Azima and Dies 1989; Barrnett et al. 1991; Kazdin 1991; Shaffer 1984). On a practical level, it is not clear whether equal funding is provided for researchers investigating child and adolescent groups, nor is it clear whether research teams centered in university and large hospitals are investigating child and adolescent groups. Doing re-search on children and adolescents sometimes involves questions of motivation, developmental factors, compliance, concerns about confidentiality, ambivalence about family interference, and ethical issues.

As with other areas of mental health delivery, group psychotherapists have adopted time-limited, briefer therapy modules to produce cost-effective treatment. This selective overview assesses short-term treatment, to the neglect of long-term follow-up studies. Outcome studies of efficacy are much more prevalent than investigations of process variables, leadership, and composition. Outpatient studies are much more prevalent than inpatient group treatment.

In a recent review, Piper (1993) detailed not only the economic pressures but also the methodological and conceptual pressures involved in research on group psychotherapy. The effort has been to apply the research rigor involved in the areas of individual therapy and pharmacotherapy. The comparison of group therapy with other types of therapy or with control conditions has become fashionable, as the present survey notes. Although "patient allocation involving matching and random allocation have become the expected standard" (Piper 1993, p. 674), I cogently point to the difficulty in applying these same criteria to assembling a group of patients who may decide not to attend or to drop out. The need for a large pool of suitable patients is likely met only in large psychiatric services. The consequence is that little significant research can be undertaken by private-practice therapists or small clinics, who carry out a large proportion of adolescent group therapy.

From the conceptual-research point of view, the stress on multidimensional models has increased (Azima and Dies 1989; Dies and Dies 1993; Piper 1993). A minimum list of variables includes patient-patient, patient-therapist, patient-group, and therapist-group plus the combined interaction matrix effects. The task of computing ongoing group interaction has remained largely unsolved other than by brief time-sampling methods.

## ◆ Efficacy Studies

A pioneer study by Smith et al. (1980) used a metanalysis approach in the evaluation of 500 outcome studies done on a wide range of clinical studies. Metanalysis is a method of calculating the effect size for each study. The effect size is obtained by dividing the mean difference of the outcome scores between the treatment and control groups by the standard deviation of the control group. Studies are then compared as to their efficacy, with the standard quantitative effect indexes. The general conclusions were that psychotherapy was effective (as compared with the control condition) and that no one therapy modality was superior to another. Put otherwise, group psychotherapy was just as effective as individual psychotherapy, and both were significantly more effective than the control condition. Approximately 20 of these 500 studies were of children and adolescents; but because these data were not analyzed separately, no effect size of these studies was given. However, one can assume that the overall trend was for better outcome of psychotherapy compared with the control condition. It is of some interest that a correlational analysis in the Smith et al. study showed that the patient's age had little effect on treatment outcome.

Many investigators confirmed the lack of appreciable difference between group psychotherapy and individual psychotherapy (Budman et al. 1988; Kaul and Bednar 1986; Orlinsky and Howard 1986; Pilkonis et al. 1984; Tillitski 1990).

# ◆ Adolescent Group Psychotherapy Research Reviews 1969–1989

The early review by Tramonata (1980) identified a total of 6 clinical and 13 experimental adolescent group psychotherapy investigations between 1967 and 1970. Of these, only five studies showed adequate methodology and research design. The author criticized the deficits in data collection and the lack of sufficient information related to patient, therapist, process, and outcome variables. Nonetheless, Tramonata thought that the five studies demonstrated the efficacy of group psychotherapy compared with no therapy.

In the Toseland and Siporin review (1986) scanning a total of 74 investigations, there were 6 child and adolescent studies, 4 college studies, and 2 family studies, all of which showed no significant differences between individual and group treatments. Schoolchildren ages 12 and 13 with self-control problems did better in group therapy; children with home problems such as noncompliance, tantrums, and fighting did better in family group therapy; and adolescents with psychoses showed a trend for greater improvement in group therapy. The overall findings revealed no superiority for individual therapy, and there was an edge for group therapies.

Azima and Dies (1989) reported on 10 selected studies between 1977 and 1986 in the areas of outcome, process, and leadership. Some of these studies used standardized research instruments, observer ratings, and structured interviews. It was noted that no study used control or contrast groups and, further, that difficulties inherent in adult group research were magnified for adolescent group research. On the whole, statistical design was weak, and follow-up of results was limited or absent. The authors outlined guidelines and directions for future research in the area of adolescent group therapy.

## ◆ Selective Survey of Adolescent Group Psychotherapy Research 1986–1993

The following investigations were chosen, in the main, on the basis of good research design and because they represent the current application of group therapy with adolescents in different settings.

The studies are categorized into outcome research with special populations and process research. Descriptions and evaluations of the studies and surveys are included to provide guidelines for future research.

### Outcome Research With Special Populations

**Eating disorders.** The application of time-limited group psychotherapy to the treatment of bulimia has proved very rewarding in terms of short-term gains. The group formats have in general been eclectic, combining cognitive-behavioral, psychoeducational, and psychodynamic theories, alone or in combination with pharmacotherapies (Azima 1992). Mitchell and his colleagues (1990), in a well-designed study, compared antidepressant therapy with structured, manual-guided group therapy for a total period of 12 weeks (2 weeks for baseline evaluation, followed by 10 treatment sessions). One hundred and seventy-one women aged 18–40 years were randomly assigned to one of four treatment cells: 1) antidepressant treatment with the tricyclic imipramine hydrochloride, 2) placebo treatment, 3) imipramine combined with intensive group psychotherapy focused on the treatment of bulimia nervosa, and 4) placebo treatment combined with participation in the outpatient group psychotherapy program.

The overall finding of the study was that the addition of the antidepressant treatment to the intensive group psychotherapy component did not significantly improve outcome over that obtained with intensive group psychotherapy combined with placebo treatment in terms of the eating disorder, but it did result in more improvement in the symptoms of depression and anxiety. At 6-month follow-up (Pyle et al. 1990), 30% of the 68 subjects who had participated in the initial study had relapsed. Initial treatment with group psychotherapy plus placebo or imipramine was associated with a lower relapse rate than was initial treatment with the medication alone. The investigations also noted that neither attendance at the maintenance group sessions nor imipramine maintenance was associated with better outcome.

These studies were well designed and used a large sample that could be randomly allocated to contrasting treatment or control groups. The baseline assessments included DSM-III diagnosis (American Psychiatric Press 1980), global functioning of severity, eating disorders questionnaires, nutritional counseling, a data sheet for routine information, and the Hamilton scales for depression and anxiety (Hamilton 1969a, 1969b). These instruments were used periodically at outcome and at 6-month follow-up.

Statistical analysis indicated that the treatment responders' substantial reduction in binge eating at the end of initial treatment was maintained at 6-month follow-up. The authors concluded that the most important factor in preventing relapse was the initial treatment with group psychotherapy, regardless of maintenance treatment. An interesting finding was that the support-group attendance during the 6-month maintenance period was less than 50%. The relapsers attended the majority of group sessions, whereas the majority of those who never relapsed attended fewer than 50% of the group sessions. The authors interpreted this fact to mean that the subjects who were in better control of their eating behavior did not want to continue in treatment. The confounding problem is that longer treatment is necessary to deal more thoroughly with symptom reduction. However, the longer the treatment, the less compliant were the subjects. An 18-month follow-up study is now in progress. The general questions are the degree of subject compliance in follow-up studies and the difficulty in assuming that nonattenders are in the improved group. An additional step in future studies would be the identification of personality correlates of those subjects who improved with the group therapy.

**Depression.** Although depression and suicide rates in adolescents are very high, there are few research studies either of individual or group treatment modalities. Reynolds and Coats (1986) compared 30 moderately depressed high school students (11 males and 19 females) who were randomly assigned to cognitive-behavior treatment, relaxation training, or a control waiting list. The two treatment groups met for 50-minute sessions over 5 weeks for a total of 10 sessions in a high school setting. The subjects were initially screened with the Reynolds Adolescent Depression scale (1986) from a total of 800 adolescents. A battery of tests were administered, including measures for depression, self-esteem, and anxiety. The cognitive-behavior and relaxation training groups were superior to the waiting list groups in the reduction of depressive symptomology, improvement in self-esteem, and academic self-concept. The findings indicated that both treatment groups were equally effective in decreasing depression in adolescents identified in a nonclinical population.

Fine et al. (1991) reported on the comparison of two forms of short-term group therapy for a sample of 66 outpatient adolescents clinically diagnosed as depressed. Subjects were randomly assigned either to a social skills training group or a therapeutic support group. Posttreatment, adolescents in the therapeutic support groups showed a greater decrease in depressive symptomatology and significant increases in self-concept (Offer et al. 1982) compared with subjects in the social skills training group. At 9-month follow-up, the adolescents in the therapeutic support groups maintained their improvements, but the adolescents in the social skills group had caught up in their improvement between posttreatment and follow-up. The findings suggest that depressed adolescents be treated in psychotherapy groups before being referred to social skills groups—that is, that they will be able to problem solve when they are less depressed.

The group climate questionnaire (MacKenzie 1981) was used as a process measure, and the adolescents in the therapy support group tended to be more engaged and less avoidant than those adolescents in the social skills group. It is to be noted that many of the adolescents in the study were in other concurrent therapies. On the latter issue, the authors agree with Teri and Lewinsohn (1986) that concurrent therapy was contraindicated for positive outcome in group treatment for depressed adults.

The Fine et al. investigation (1991) is a well-designed study, identifying a diagnosed population, the use of a contrast group, the inclusion of a process instrument in the outcome study, and good statistical analysis. Fine et al. themselves comment on the need to follow up the sample to judge the duration of improvement and remission rates. They point to the need to identify the specific therapeutic factors in group treatments for adolescents. They postulate that a sequential approach may be more effective, commencing with therapeutic support in early sessions followed by social skill strategies in later sessions. Additionally, they suggest that it is important to identify the demographic, characterological, environmental, and symptomatic predictors of successful outcome.

**HIV-seropositive patients.** Levine et al. (1991) reported a pilot study of a single group of six patients (five men and one woman) between the ages of 18 and 55 years identified as seropositive for the human immunodeficiency virus (HIV) who were being treated for major depression with fluoxetine. The group consisted of 20 sessions combining psychoeducational, supportive, and cognitive orientations. The members had been psychiatrically diagnosed and were administered the Hamilton Rating Scale for Depression (Hamilton 1969a), the Hamilton Anxiety Scale (Hamilton 1969b), the Global Assessment Scale (Spitzer et al. 1975), a diagnostic evaluation form for anxiety disorders, a modified Structured Clinical Interview for the DSM

(SCID) (Bystritsky 1987; Spitzer et al. 1988), and the Symptom Checklist—90 (Derogatis 1975). Outcome results were given for the four patients who participated.

As could be anticipated, the sample was too small and the number of variables was too large. The reported trends were that the group therapy was an effective, cost-efficient treatment method and that there was a decrease in depression, anxiety, and symptoms. The battery of tests is well identified, but the generalizations from this pilot study need to be further replicated with a larger sample and a control or contrast group. At the same time, if the pilot study promotes future research, its goal will have been met.

**Sexual abuse.** The use of group approaches with children, adolescents, and their families has been widely advocated, but there are few adequate research investigations to demonstrate their efficacy. The study of Furniss et al. (1988) with sexually abused adolescent girls is a description of 10 girls aged 12–15 years who attended group therapy for 2 years, as well as a follow-up of the progress of 9 girls. Seven of the nine girls had improved levels of self-esteem and victim behavior, relationship with peers, ability to discuss the traumatic events with parents, and overall social adjustment. The therapy groups with both adolescents and parents were part of a multipronged treatment program, including family therapy and individual therapy. Groups were held weekly and run in parallel with family sessions in which various family members were seen at three to four weekly sessions. Basic descriptive data about the subjects and the nature of sexual abuse were given. The overall goals of the group were to provide direct help to the adolescents themselves in the areas of the self, relation to parents and family, and peers. A psychoanalytic (Bion) interpretative model was used, but the therapist often had to intervene directly and restrain the girls from dangerous acting out. Information about sexual development and child care was provided, as well as drawing materials for nonverbal members, role playing, and video feedback.

The Furniss et al. study falls short of adequate research methodology, but it is an illustration of how clinicians have tried to assess case-by-case changes in behavior and relationships with others without benefit of controls or test-retest. In summary, the authors concluded that at outcome the girls were less anxious, showed less sexualized behavior and more ability to trust (and express anger toward) therapists, and had improved self-esteem and a decline in suicidal, self-mutilating behavior. The authors pointed out that the goal-oriented treatment proved a "viable and valuable" treatment for girls sexually abused within their families and "group work facilitated changes not easily achieved in direct work with the family . . . in particular, the girls developed both their self-esteem and their capacity for assertiveness" (p. 104). At follow-up, improvements were maintained for the majority of the patients.

A more systematic pilot study of sexually abused preadolescents effectively treated in time-limited group therapy was reported by Corder et al. (1990). The design could be applied to the adolescent group as well.

**Substance abuse programs.** Programs for the treatment of eating disorders, substance abuse, and delinquency often use a variety of group treatment modalities. Although it is very difficult to disentangle the therapeutic components of group therapy from the remainder of the program, it seems appropriate to include them in this survey because of the current evaluation of these inpatient, or residential, programs for a large population of adolescents.

Friedman and Glickman (1986) reviewed 30 drug-free outpatient treatment programs involving 5,789 adolescents. A partial cross-validation study was conducted on the analysis of two annual client subsamples. The program, not the individual subjects, was the unit of analysis. With multiple regression analysis of the differences between programs, among the characteristics statistically predictive of outcome were the employment of therapists with at least 2 years of experience working with adolescent drug users; the provision of psychoeducational services, including vocational counseling and birth control services; the use of crisis intervention, gestalt therapy, music or art therapy, and group confrontation; and freedom of expression and spontaneous action, which were important features of the programs (compared with authority-dominated programs).

Several collection instruments were used to gather the program data: forms for administrators and therapists, and the Community

Oriented Environment Scale developed by Moos (1974). The results indicated that the most significant variable for positive treatment outcome was the number of hours of counseling services. The provision of special services (vocational, school, recreational) in large, well-funded programs with more experienced therapists bore a more positive relationship to outcome than any of the therapies used (gestalt, art or music therapy, or confrontation).

Although the analysis of the Community Oriented Environment Scale showed equivocal findings, there were positive trends for positive ratings of liberal, well-organized, factual programs, where clients felt helped with their personal problems. The authors commented on an unexpected finding: that the confrontation technique used in the outpatient program showed a positive outcome trend. Apparently, adolescents appreciated this type of "hot-seat" technique of direct challenging and disciplining of uncooperative or negative behavior. Azima (1989) also discussed the differential use of confrontation, empathy, and interpretation. It may be that many of the drug-addicted teenagers preferred direct confrontation to a more passive, empathic, less verbal clarification of problem issues. The overall findings suggest that problem-oriented, psychoeducational groups have more practical use with this population than interpretative, unstructured groups.

In a review by Hoffman et al. (1987) evaluating chemical dependency treatment programs for adolescents, the suggestions were for more sophisticated methodology and statistical understanding to conduct such program research and for more systematic outcome variables besides simple abstinence from drug abuse (e.g., reentry into school, home, decline in symptoms and antisocial behavior). Additionally, these investigators advocated the use of measuring the response to treatment process—for example, the ability of the teenager to participate in confrontational sessions and self-reflect on past behavior.

These authors reviewed an interesting, but less common long-term family program that works with both adolescents and their parents. Parents must agree to be active coparticipants in the treatment program. An adolescent entering the treatment program is removed from the parental family and lives with a family whose adolescent has progressed to a certain program criterion. The senior adolescent assumes responsibility for the junior participant (an arrangement bene-fiting both). Parents must attend informational and therapy sessions until they also reach a level of change, at which time they serve as the host family to a newly admitted adolescent. Follow-up is up to 1 year. No evaluation of the program is presented.

**Residential treatment.** In his survey of residential treatment of children and adolescents, Curry (1991) evaluated the deficits in out-come research in these multimodal programs, especially the limita-tions of single-sample designs without control groups. Curry's suggestions for future research included more powerful designs, such as 1) between programs and between treatments, 2) between treat-ments and within programs, and 3) across programs. He proposed, in agreement with others, that treatment components be identified at baseline and outcome be measured at different levels and followed up sequentially at several time periods.

## Process Research

Curry's evaluation (1991) points to the paucity of process research, as noted above. Investigators have been trapped into using preoutcome-postoutcome models without identifying ongoing changes that affect a wider range of improvement and without determining the effective-ness of various therapeutic factors in these group-oriented programs (Fuhriman and Packard 1986).

Chase (1991) investigated a group of 33 adolescents and 11 chil-dren in two psychiatric inpatient units to assess their perceptions of the curative factors in group therapy. All subjects were diagnosed accord-ing to DSM-III criteria. Three measures were completed by the child-care technician at intake: a demographics list, the Level of Functioning Scale (adapted from the Global Assessment of Functioning Scale [GAF], American Psychiatric Association 1987, p. 12) and the Revised Behavior Problem Checklist (Quay and Peterson 1983); the latter two measures were repeated after 23 sessions. The Yalom 60-item Q sort (1970) was revised for children and was administered after the 7th and the 23rd group sessions. Most of the subjects met daily in groups

(28-day inpatient stay), with the exception of one unit that met once weekly. Each subject was asked to rate the curative factors clustered in five categories on a 4-point scale of helpfulness. The findings pointed to modest differences: children valued "hope" more than adolescents, whereas a "sense of not being unique" was more important for the adolescents. Least valued curative factors included "identification" and "family reenactment," irrespective of age, type of group, level of functioning, or time in treatment.

Chase commented that adolescents would find it difficult to endorse the identification items as written, because adolescents are in search of their own personal identities. Low valuing of family enactment, rated an important curative factor for psychoanalytic theory, corroborated the earlier adult study by Butler and Fuhriman (1980). Rather, child and adolescent patients respond "best to experiences that are a-historical and focus on the here-and-now aspects of their interpersonal style. Functional problem-solving aspects should be emphasized. Attempts at genetic insight and characterological change will likely meet with resistance and failure" (Chase 1991, p. 106). Adolescents consistently rate curative factors less highly compared with children, which is a confirmation of the earlier findings of Corder et al. (1981).

Reviews of adult groups indicated that cohesiveness, learning from feedback, and insight are highly valued, whereas family enactment and guidance are devalued. Outpatient psychotherapy groups valued learning and understanding, and inpatients valued morale building and support (Bloch and Crouch 1985; Butler and Fuhriman 1980; MacKenzie 1987; Piper 1993).

An important finding in the study by Chase (1991) was that both children and adolescents rank group cohesion as extremely important. This may reflect their need to deal with their sense of isolation and homesickness. On the basis of the present data, I found that there was no need to separate the adolescents into specifier groups according to their level of functioning, with the exception of the exclusion of psychotic patients. Publication of the Yalom curative factors for children and adolescents, reworded by Chase, and an indication of the groupings of the 12 curative items would have been helpful additions to this important article.

# ◆ Implications and Trends

Careful scanning of the literature reveals that there are relatively few substantive research studies of adolescent group psychotherapy, compared with adult investigations. However, on the positive side, the quality of the research has improved, especially when adolescents are included in the adult sample, as in the treatment of eating disorders, drug abuse, and depression. If the adolescent sample size is large enough, a separate analysis of outcome results would be useful in future research. Control and contrast groups, as well as comparisons with alternate therapy and drug treatments, have greatly enhanced the efficacy results. Comparison with previous surveys suggests that the present status of adolescent group research is improving, especially with the availability of better evaluative instruments, and that future developments are promising.

In general, how to control for the large number of variables and what constitutes the ideal linkage of process, outcome, and follow-up measures are questions that still haunt researchers in the field. Studies with adolescents are constrained by developmental, motivation, compliance, family, confidentiality, and ethical issues. At the same time, there is the positive advantage that adolescents often prefer peer groups over individual treatment. From a pragmatic viewpoint, there may be fewer well-funded large university centers committed to ongoing research on group treatments of adolescents. Minimum sample sizes are necessary for subject allocation and for studies of control and contrasting approaches.

The present review indicated more outcome studies than process studies. In fact, only two process studies were identified (Chase 1991; Corder et al. 1981), both of which studied curative factors. At this point, it seems important to identify priority lists of curative factors for children and adolescents compared with adults. Follow-up studies still continue to be difficult in view of the diminution of the returning sample.

Large-program and residential research with outpatient research suggests that highly structured psychoeducational, manual-guided formats addressing here-and-now issues are highly effective. It is not clear whether this effectiveness is based on patient and therapist character-istics (e.g., intelligence, severity of disorder, psychological minded-ness, differences in therapists' training). It seems that the theoretical position of the therapists often falls by the wayside in actual practice with teenagers, and therapists are forced to become more active. Additionally, short-term modalities pressure therapists to complete the specified tasks and strategies. Problems of working through often cannot be resolved. It is still to be determined whether early recovery rates in time-limited treatments will be maintained at longer-term follow-up. Long-term studies are needed, but these require a large investment of time and money. Future research will, it is hoped, address the issue of which subjects should receive short-term as op-posed to long-term therapy.

Missing from the survey is research linked to composition, leader-ship, group interaction variables, and subject characteristics. The fact that only one well-designed inpatient adolescent group investigation (Chase 1991) was found for inclusion in this overview points to the pressing need for research in this area. At present, budget cuts and minimal short-term hospitalization do not forecast much improve-ment. One strategy would be to supplement the inpatient demograph-ics and diagnostic evaluation at intake with a minimum of evaluation procedures that could be repeated sequentially or at a midpoint and again at discharge from the group program. The addition of specified process measures—such as group climate, therapeutic alliance, cura-tive factors, and consumer satisfaction—may provide a minimal re-search strategy linking outcome with process data.

Questions that still face us include the therapeutic efficacy of multiple-person feedback, characteristics of a good therapeutic group member, and how peers influence each other in the ongoing group interactive process. Although recording group interaction measures remains complex and difficult, sequential observer ratings and ad-ministration of relevant tests to the subjects, therapists, and observers may be effective ways to clarify process measures, indexes of caring, support, learning, insight, group cohesion, and climate. Adolescents value and profit from a confrontational approach in the group modality.

Large-scale, well-designed studies are needed to produce efficacy results that are statistically significant. However, one must encourage clinicians to conceptualize, describe their observations, and let the nature of the group interaction guide meaningful research. Group psychotherapy remains a challenging, important area for both clinicians and researchers to pool their resources to advance the understanding and treatment of adolescents.

# ◆ References

American Psychiatric Association: Diagnostic and Statistical Manual of Mental Disorders, 3rd Edition. Washington, DC, American Psychiatric Association, 1980

American Psychiatric Association: Diagnostic and Statistical Manual of Mental Disorders, 3rd Edition, Revised. Washington, DC, American Psychiatric Association, 1987

Azima FJ Cramer: Confrontation, empathy, and interpretation issues in adolescent group psychotherapy, in Adolescent Group Psychotherapy. Edited by Azima FJ Cramer, Richmond LH. Madison, CT, International Universities Press, 1989, pp 3–19

Azima FJ Cramer: Adolescent group treatment, in Group Psychotherapy for Eating Disorders. Edited by Harper-Giuffre H, MacKenzie KR. Washington, DC, American Psychiatric Press, 1992, pp 233–247

Azima FJ Cramer, Dies K: Clinical research in adolescent group psychotherapy: status, guidelines and directions, in Adolescent Group Psychotherapy. Edited by Azima FJ Cramer, Richmond LH. Madison, CT, International Universities Press, 1989, pp 193–225

Barrnett RJ, Docherty JP, Frommelt GM: A review of child psychotherapy research since 1963. J Am Acad Child Adolesc Psychiatry 30:1–14, 1991

Bloch S, Crouch C: Therapeutic Factors in Group Psychotherapy. Oxford, Oxford University Press, 1985

Budman SH, Demby A, Redondo JP, et al: Comparative outcome in time-limited individual and group psychotherapy. Int J Group Psychother 38:63–86, 1988

Butler T, Fuhriman A: Patient perspective on the curative process: a comparison of day treatment and outpatient psychotherapy groups. Small Group Behavior 11:371–388, 1980

Bystritsky A: UCLA Anxiety Disorders Program Initial Evaluation Form, Modified SCID. Los Angeles, CA, University of California, Los Angeles Press, 1987

Chase JL: Inpatient adolescent and latency age children's perspectives on the curative factors in group psychotherapy. Group 15:95–108, 1991

Corder B, Whiteside L, Haizlip T: A study of curative factors in group psychotherapy with adolescents. Int J Group Psychother 30:345–354, 1981

Corder BF, Haizlip T, DeBaer P: A pilot study for a structured, time-limited therapy group for sexually abused pre-adolescent children. Child Abuse Negl 14:243–257, 1990

Curry JF: Outcome research in residential treatment: Implications and suggested directions. Am J Orthopsychiatry 61:348–357, 1991

Derogatis LR: The SCL-90-R. Baltimore, MD, Clinical Psychometric Research, 1975

Dies R, Dies K: The role of evaluation in clinical practice: overview and group treatment illustration. Int J Group Psychother 43:77–105, 1993

Fine S, Forth A, Gilbert M, et al: Group therapy for adolescent depressive disorder: a comparison of social skills and therapeutic support. J Am Acad Child Adolesc Psychiatry 30:79–85, 1991

Friedman AS, Glickman NW: Program characteristics for successful treatment of adolescent drug abuse. J Nerv Ment Dis 174:669–679, 1986

Fuhriman A, Packard T: Group process instruments: therapeutic themes and issues. Int J Group Psychother 36:399–425, 1986

Furniss T, Bingley-Miller L, Van Elburg A: Goal oriented group treatment for sexually abused adolescent girls. Br J Psychiatry 152:97–106, 1988

Hamilton M: Diagnosis and rating of depression. Br J Psychiatry 3:76–79, 1969a

Hamilton M: Diagnosis and rating of anxiety. Br J Psychiatry 3:80–83, 1969b

Hoffman NG, Sonis WA, Halikas JA: Issues in the evaluation of chemical dependency treatment programs for adolescents. Pediatr Clin North Am 34:449–459, 1991

Kaul T, Bednar RL: Experiential group research: Results, questions and suggestions, in Handbook of Psychotherapy and Behavior Change, 3rd Edition. Edited by Garfield S, Bergin A. New York, Wiley, 1986, pp 671–690

Kazdin AE: Effectiveness of psychotherapy with children and adolescents. J Consult Clin Psychol 59:785–798, 1991

Levine SH, Bystritsky A, Baron D, et al: Group psychotherapy for HIV seropositive patients with major depression. Am J Psychother 45:413–424, 1991

MacKenzie KR: Measurement of group climate. Int J Group Psychother 31:287–296, 1981

MacKenzie KR: Therapeutic factors in group psychotherapy: a contemporary view. Group 11:26–34, 1987

Mitchell JE, Pyle RL, Eckert ED, et al: Antidepressants vs group therapy in the treatment of bulimia. Arch Gen Psychiatry 47:149–157, 1990

Moos R: Community Oriented Environment Scale (COPES). Palo Alto, CA, Psychologists Press, 1974

Offer D, Ostrov E, Howard KI: The Offer Self-Image Questionnaire for Adolescents, 3rd Edition. Chicago, IL, Michael Reese Hospital and Medical Center, 1982

Orlinsky DE, Howard KT: Process and outcome in psychotherapy, in Handbook of Psychotherapy and Behavior Change, 3rd Edition. Edited by Garfield SL, Bergin AE. New York, Wiley, 1986, pp 311–381

Pilkonis AA, Imber SD, Lewis P, et al: A comparative outcome study of individual, group and conjoint psychotherapy. Arch Gen Psychiatry 41:431–439, 1984

Piper WE: Group psychotherapy research, in Comprehensive Group Psychotherapy, 3rd Edition. Edited by Kaplan HI, Sadock BJ. Baltimore, MD, Williams & Wilkins, 1993, pp 673–682

Pyle RL, Mitchell JE, Eckert ED, et al: Maintenance treatment and 6 month outcome for bulimia patients who respond to initial treatment. Am J Psychiatry 147:871–875, 1990

Quay H, Peterson D: Revised Behavior Problem Checklist. Coral Gables, FL, University of Miami, 1983

Reynolds WH, Coats KA: A comparison of cognitive-behavioral and relaxation training for the treatment of depressed adolescents. J Consult Clin Psychol 54:653–660, 1986

Reynolds WM: Assessment of Depression in Adolescents: Manual for the Reynolds Adolescent Depression Scale. Adessa, FL, Psychological Assessment Resources, 1986

Shaffer D: Notes on Psychotherapy research among children and adolescents. Journal of the American Academy of Child Psychiatry 23: 552–561, 1984

Smith MH, Glass GV, Miller TI: The Benefits of Psychotherapy. Baltimore, MD, John Hopkins University Press, 1980

Spitzer RL, Gibson M, Endicott J: The Global Assessment Scale (GAS). New York, Biometrics Research Department, New York State Psychiatric Institute, 1975

Spitzer RL, Williams JB, Gibbon M, et al: Structured Clinical Interviews for DSM-III-R, Patient Version (SCID-P). New York, Biometrics Research Department, New York State Psychiatric Institute, 1988

Teri L, Lewinsohn PM: Individual and group treatment of unipolar depression. Behav Ther 17:215–228, 1986

Tillitski CJ: A meta-analysis of estimated effect sizes for group versus individual versus control treatments. Int J Group Psychother 40:215–224, 1990

Toseland RW, Siporin M: When to recommend group treatment: a review of the clinical and the research literature. Int J Group Psychother 36:171–201, 1986

Tramonata MG: Critical review of research on psychotherapy outcome with adolescents: 1967–1977. Psychol Bull 88:429–450, 1980

Yalom I: The Theory and Practice of Group Psychotherapy. New York, Basic Books, 1970

# Index

*Page numbers printed in **boldface** type refer to tables or figures.*